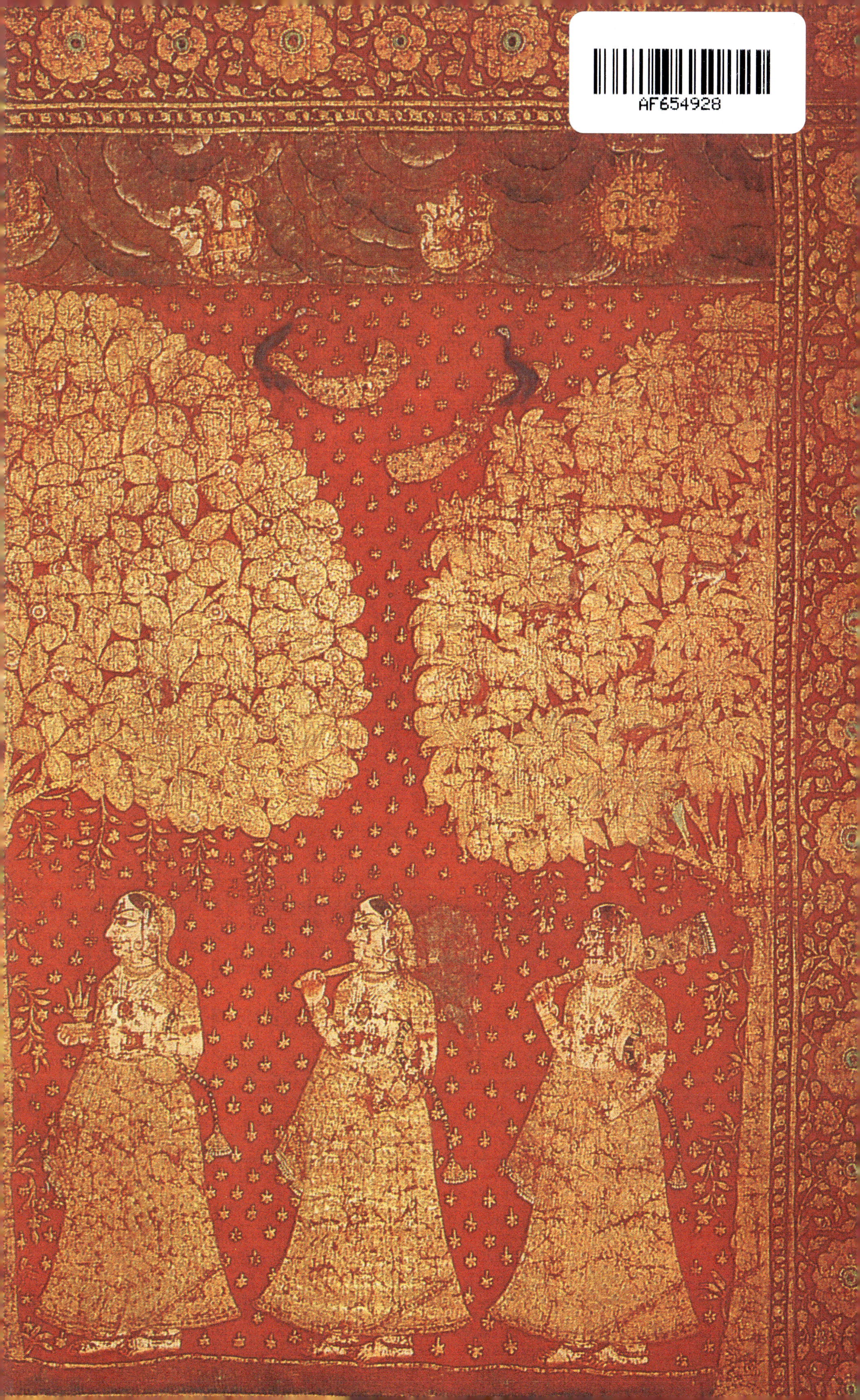

THE NEW AGE KAMA SUTRA FOR WOMEN

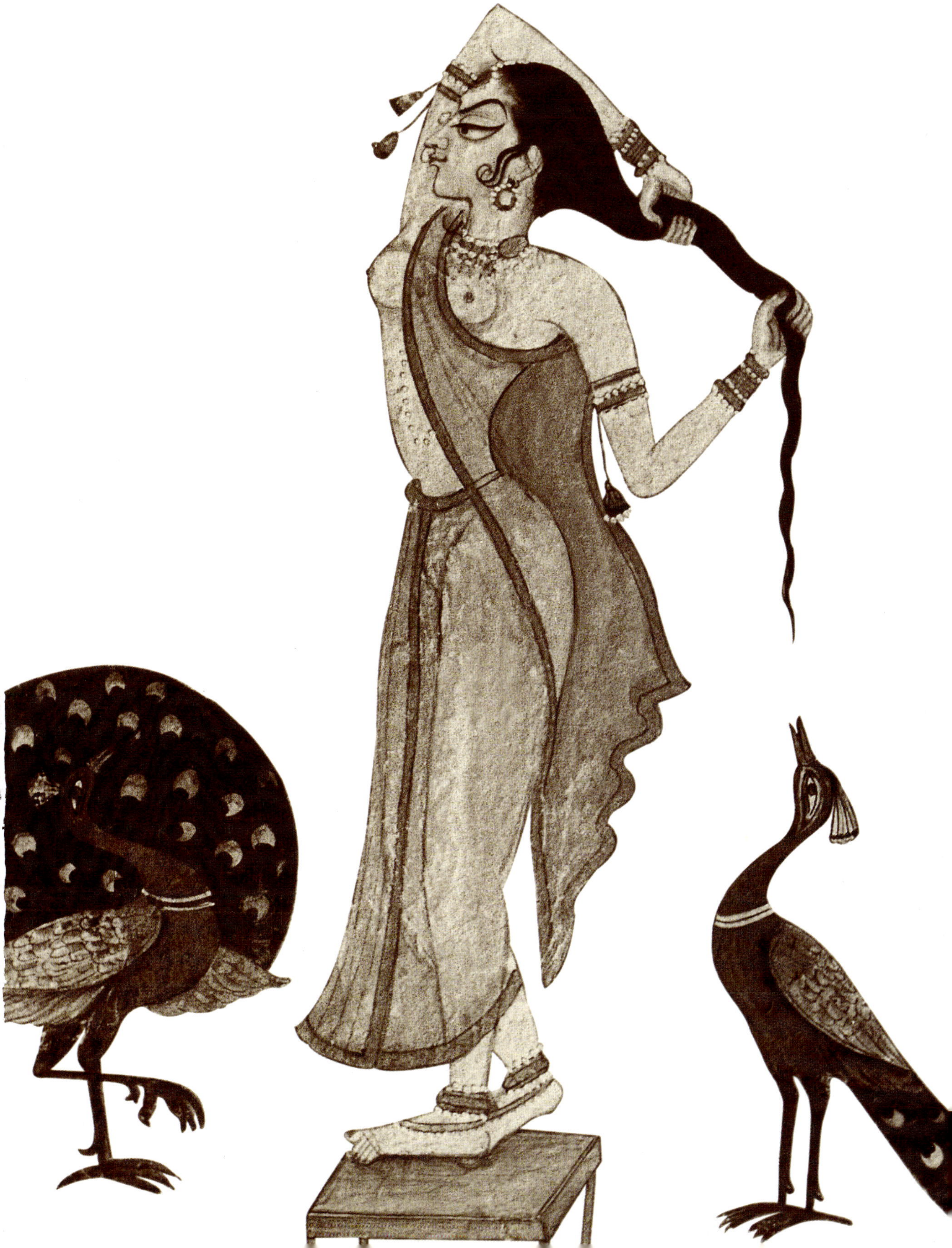

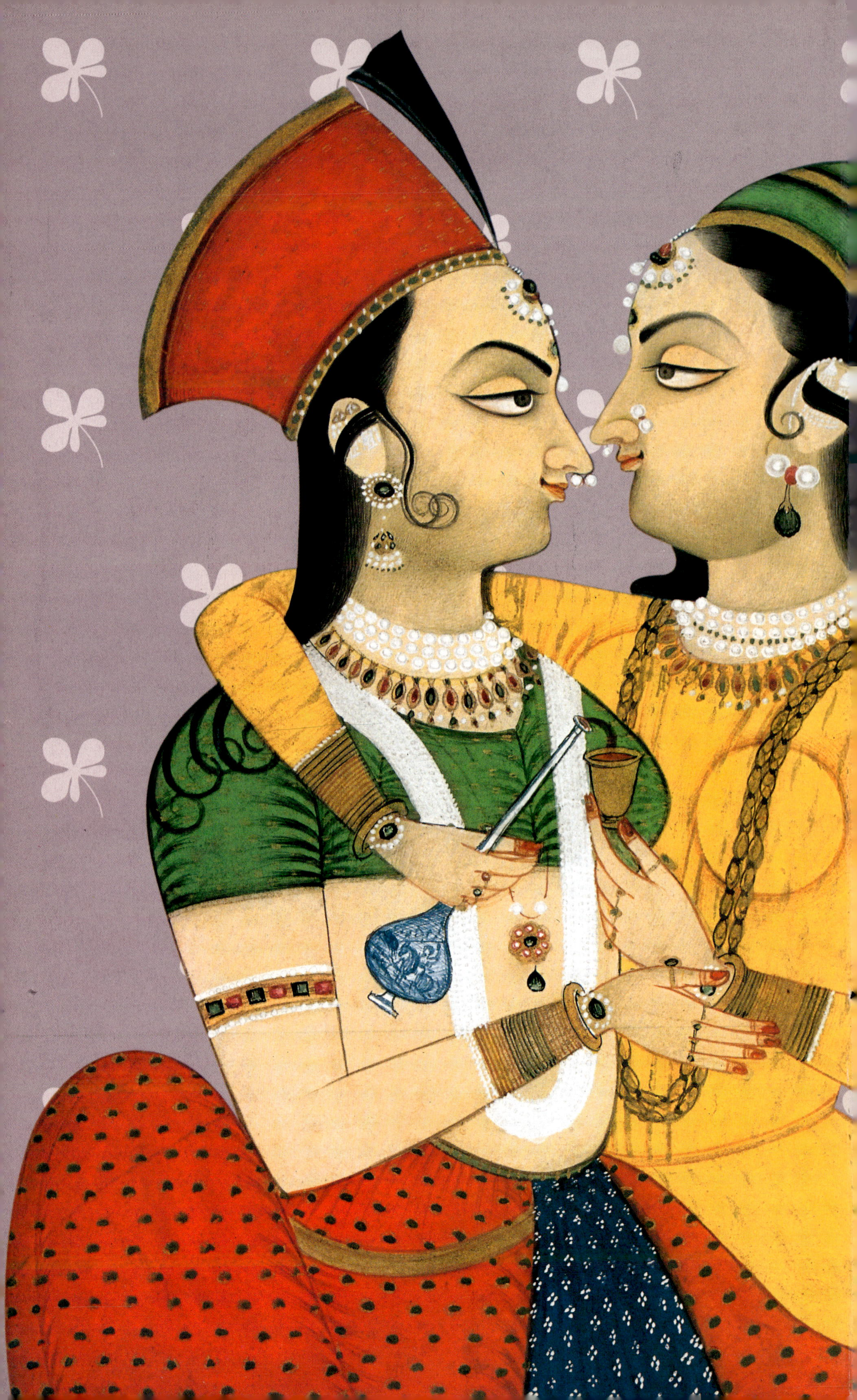

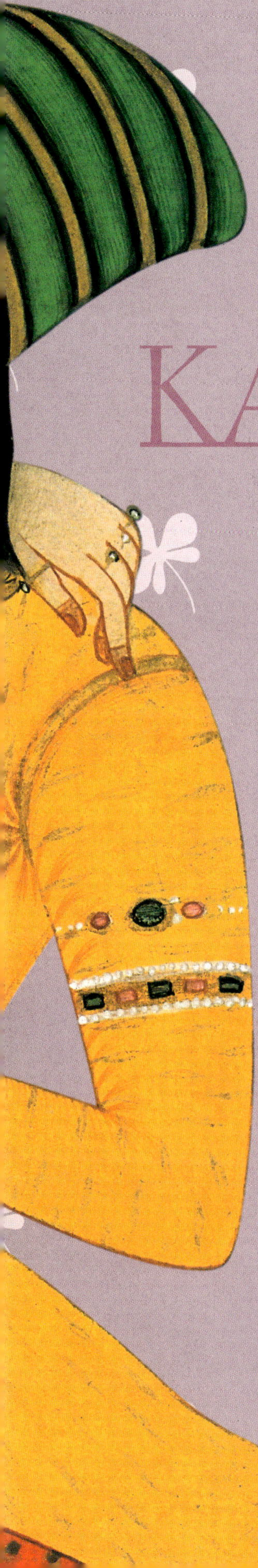

THE NEW AGE KAMA SUTRA FOR WOMEN

Dr. Alka Pande • Lance Dane

BRIJBASI

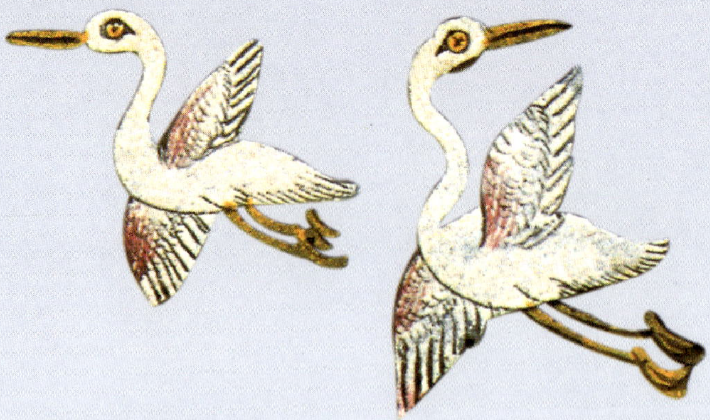

Published by Brijbasi Art Press Ltd.
E 46/11 Okhla Industrial Area, Phase II
New Delhi 110020
E-mail: brijbasi@touchtelindia.net
www.brijbasiartpress.com

Text by Dr. Alka Pande
Editor: Veena Baswani

Designed by: Yogesh Suraksha Design Studio
www.ysdesignstudio.com

ISBN 81-8385-098-7

Processed, printed and bound at Brijbasi Art Press Ltd.

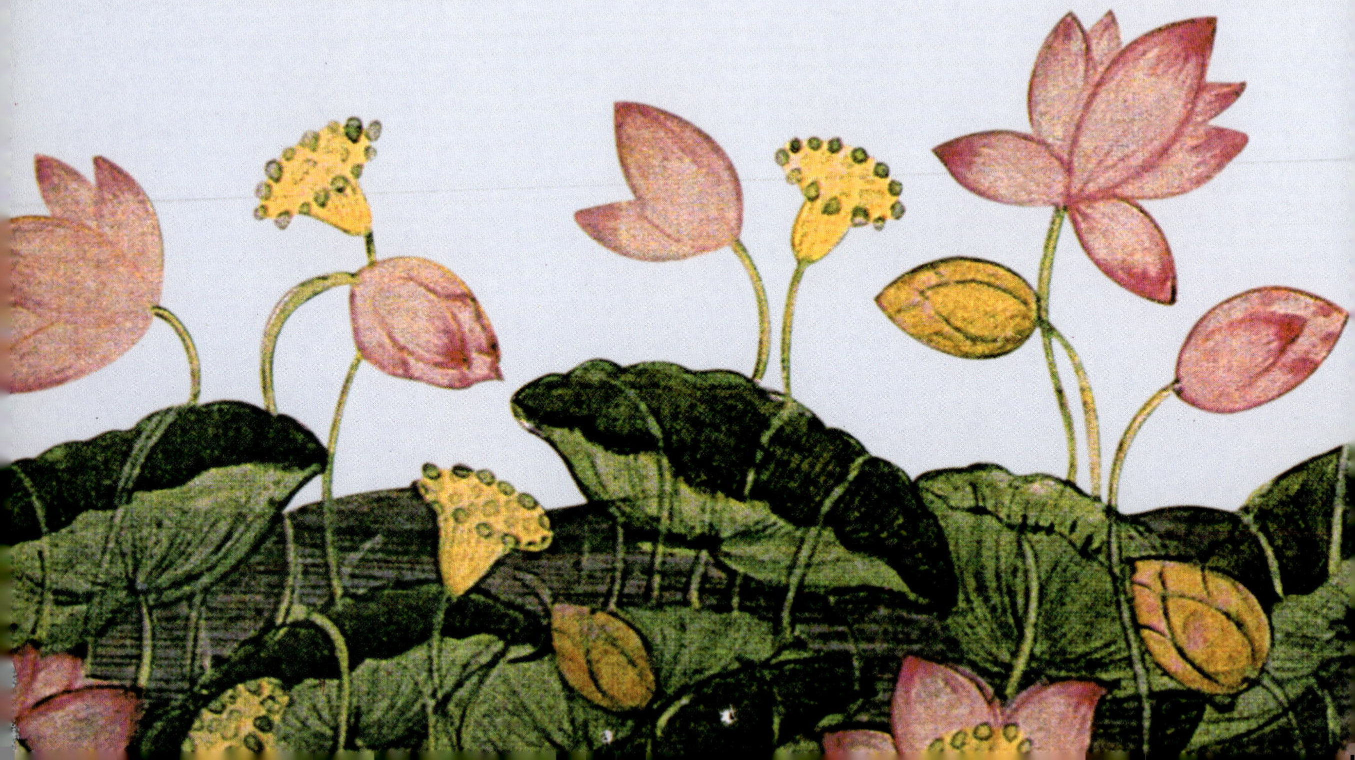

CONTENTS

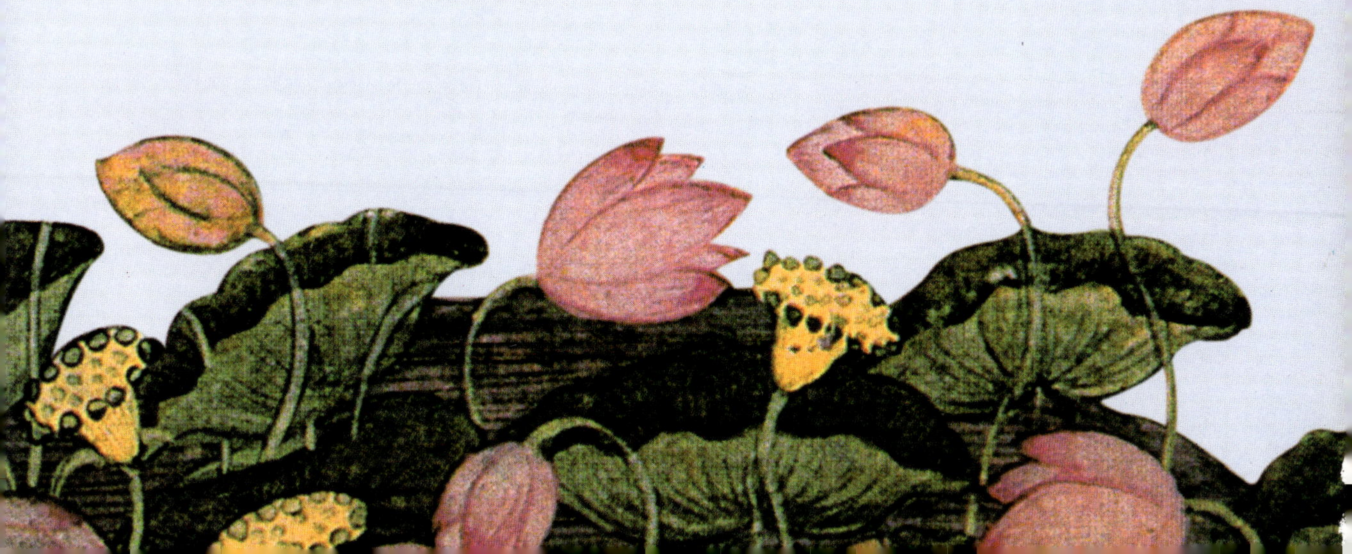

Preface

It is wonderful to be alive.
But heavenly to be young...

As I slip smoothly into the autumn of my life and leave behind many seasons of joyousness, of celebration, of deep sorrow, and deep love, all I know is that at this point of my life I aspire only to celebrate life with the *navrasas* of life, where the horrific and the sublime walk hand in hand.

The New Age Kama Sutra for Women is a continuation of the thought process of my previous book *Indian Erotica.* In fact it is a natural corollary to *Indian Erotica* and the *Kama Sutra.* With the coming of age of the Indian woman, very much an inherent part of my personal history - *The New Age Kama Sutra. for Women* is a text written from the gaze of a woman. Most of the translations and interpretations of the *Kama Sutra* have been written by men and, therefore, the gaze has been patriarchal. In this book I attempt to celebrate and articulate the sensitivities of being a woman, of what it means to be a complete woman and to live the life of a woman. This book is an equal must-read for men, for how can any man truly enjoy his *grihastya ashrama* if he does not understand the complex nature of women.

The New Age sensitive, yet self-assured metrosexual man also keeps his woman happy and content, and he cannot be successful in this complex operation till he truly gets into the skin of the woman. The New Age brings with it a complex and new sensibility, often leading to a shift between the relationship and the role of the male and the female. It is an age when gender roles are changing: men have moved from being gruff, rugged, strong men to becoming metrosexual. A metrosexual man is silent, more evolved than his predecessors, and often takes over roles that have been stereotypically dominated by women. The woman of *now* is the power woman, exploring new facets of her sexuality. She has the privilege of walking out of a marriage and choosing her own partner. Releasing herself from the feminine mystique of domesticity, her true liberation is achieved with economic empowerment. Gender, thus, becomes an important tool in crafting a new identity.

The days of the female eunuch are over, where Germaine

Greer sought to revolutionise the repression that women underwent within societal norms. 'Women have somehow been separated from their libido, from their faculty of desire, from their sexuality. They've become suspicious about it. Like beasts, for example, who are castrated in farming in order to serve their master's ulterior motives - to be fattened or made docile - women have been cut off from their capacity for action. It's a process that sacrifices vigour for delicacy and succulence, and one that's got to be changed.'

With all transactions there are paradoxes. Often the power woman forgets the *woman* in herself, and thus, an imbalance arises in her. Whether she is a CEO of a company or a shy bride in a traditional male society, the woman's natural urges and attributes, if celebrated, make a society more sumptuous, beautiful and credible. She should not misread and miscast her femininity; instead she should celebrate the nuances of being a woman.

This book is not about judgements or opinions but evolves and emerges from observed behaviour. It is as much for the male as for the female; it is about sharing and caring, and bringing them together in fruitful union. While each couple plays its own roles, evolves its own balances, some basic formulas are common to all, and often the mundane and the forgotten ones can weave in a magic and an excitement in a relationship - thus the *Kama Sutra.*

The *Kama Sutra* is a celebration of the relationship between men and women in different civilisations across the globe. Erotica is an inherent part of social relations. *Kama* or sexual copulation is an important aspect of physical life. In the Hindu way of life and thought it also becomes an important aim on the path to deliverance.

The *Kama Sutra* is the first ever literary document on sexual enjoyment. It has been the brightest star in the firmament of Indian Exotica and Erotica. It is not a pornographic text providing ingenious and acrobatic sexual positions, as frivolously explained away by some, but a timeless classic. It is a 'human document'. The axiom of the *Kama Sutra's* eroticism is the discovery of the woman as a full recipient of a man's lust. It reflects and fosters a woman's enjoyment of her own sexuality. The *Kama Sutra* is more a manual, an erotic text that asserts the importance of sexual enjoyment, which is complementary to the moral, material and spiritual well-being of a person. It was regarded as natural as sight and scent, not something to be hidden in shame and then brooded upon with guilt. The raison d'etre of the *Kama Sutra* and the erotic sculptures on the façade of the medieval temples in India was to foreground the importance of sex in everyday life. Images on the temple facades served to educate. Nowhere in the world has the feminine form been so celebrated as in the temples of Khajuraho. From the seductive *Alasya kanyas* to women performing their toilette, women are represented in their complete glory.

The *Kama Sutra* takes its place along with *The Perfumed Garden* and *The Arabian Nights*. It comprises the 'Aphorisms of Love' sourced by *Vatsyayana*, containing about one thousand, two hundred and fifty *shlokas*, verses, which are divided into seven books and thirty-six parts. This treatise was composed according to the precepts of the Holy Writ, for the benefit of the world. In ancient India, the study of the erotic science, *Kama Sutra*, was on par with the study of the *dharma shastras* and *artha shastras*, and it was said that 'man should study the *Kama Sutra* and the related arts and sciences, in addition to the study of the arts and sciences contained in *Dharma and Artha*. Young maids should study the *Kama Sutra* along with its sixty-four arts before marriage'.

The *Kama Sutra* sought to provide to its readers, both men and women, a 'guidebook' encyclopedic in its scope, and replete with detailed advice. It also set the framework in which erotic experiences were to be viewed: in other words, the social and moral underpinnings were elucidated. The *Kama Sutra* became a canon and laid the grid for subsequent texts on *kama*. Texts in this genre became the muse for a number of fine artists and performers through the passage of time. There have been at least a hundred translations of the *Kama Sutra* in different shapes and sizes, from luscious coffee-table books to small pillow books, but *The New Age Kama Sutra for Women* is a singular feminine voice. It is the celebration of the feminine, of female sexuality, of complete equality between man and woman, where the sixty-four arts lead to refinement of tastes.

The first translation of the *Kama Sutra* is that by Sir Richard Burton. He brought alive to the world an important text that would otherwise have remained within the sanctum sanctorum of a specialised Sanskrit *gurukul*. However, being a translation in English, the first 'loss in translation' lay in the change of the language itself. Secondly, it emerged from the consciousness of a Victorian man, and so had its own drawbacks, particularly in topics relating to female sexuality.

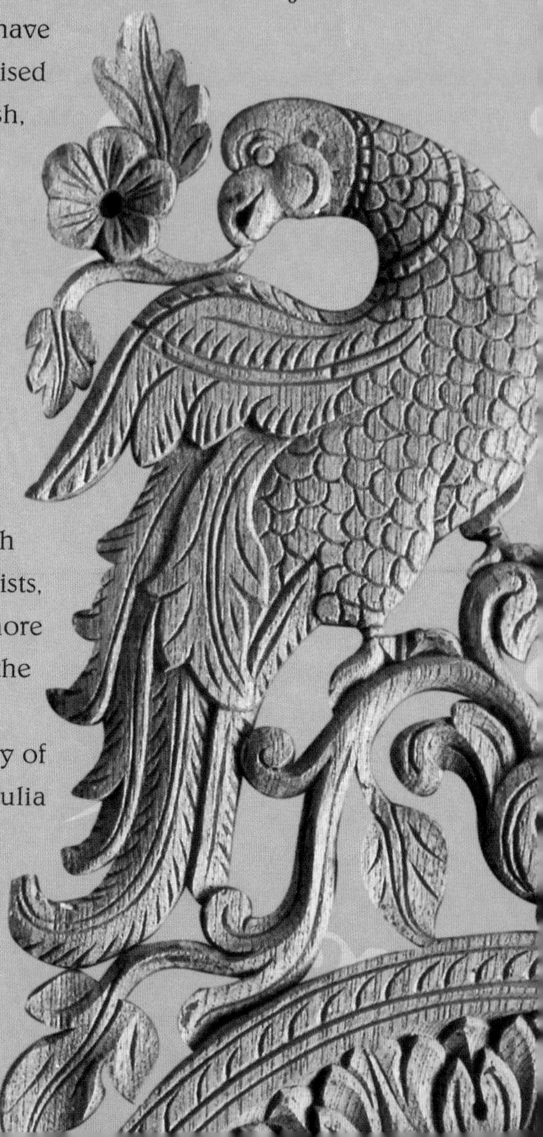

The Sanskrit commentary by Yashodhara and the Hindi commentary by Devadutta Shastri influenced the translation of the *Kama Sutra* by yet another brilliant scholar, Allen Danielou.

I have, in the course of this book, referred to Wendy Doniger's interpretation of the *Kama Sutra*, which though it could go against the grain of many scholars and theorists, I wanted to include it as a diverse voice - even a more feminine stringent voice, which would also signify the scholarship of the 'other'.

In the same genre I have also included the trajectory of psychoanalysts and key feminist thinkers like Julia Christeva, Luce Irigaray, Helen Cixous, Judith Butler, Simone de Beauvoir, Virginia Woolf, and our own Indian poets and writers like Kamala Das, who have written on the subject. With these multiple voices I have looked at the thought processes of the *bhakti* poets and the *riti* poets of medieval India like Jayadeva and Keshavadas. Whether it is the *Bihari Satsai* or the *Rasikapriya* of Keshavadas, it is the beauty of women that has been extolled. Jayadeva's *Gita Govinda* belongs completely to the genre of *bhakti*, where exultation of love is pitched high to the tuning of the *bhakt*, where both the subject and the object are feminine in the respective form of the *nayika* and the *devi*. In his *Amaru Shataka*, Amaru's poetry centres around women who have been described variously as a haunting melody; a glorious sunset; a lovely rustic belle flaunting her robust charms, wearing a necklace of strikingly colourful beads, her dark eyes smeared with lampblack. Women have been celebrated in the mythic pasts as divine and semi-divine beings; they were considered sacred and pure, nurturers, mother goddesses, earth mothers, protectors . . .

It is only as Eve, the temptress, that women entered into another domain. As a seductress, any woman enjoying sex is either a mistress or a courtesan. Amrapali, the courtesan of Pataliputra, became the protagonist in Buddhist tales; she became Buddha's disciple, as was Mary Magdelene a disciple of Jesus. The representation of women has been of two extremes - that of the mother or the temptress.

Women should be nurtured with every tenderness and attention by their fathers, their brothers, their husbands and their brothers-in-law, if they desire great prosperity. Where women live in affliction, the family soon becomes extinct, but when they are loved and respected, and cherished with tenderness, the family grows and prospers in all circumstances.

(Extracts from Manu's Shloka 55)

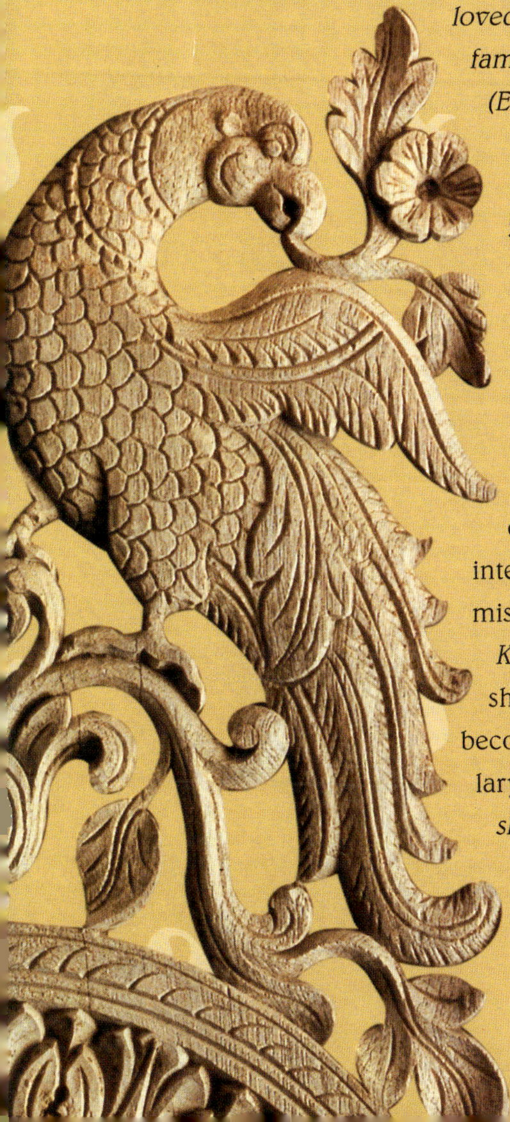

Literary evidence suggests that kings and towns were destroyed because a single woman was wronged by the State. For example, Valmiki's *Ramayana* teaches us that Ravana and his entire clan were wiped out because he abducted Sita. Ved Vyasa's *Mahabharata* informs us that all the Kauravas were killed because they disgraced Draupadi in public.

The idea behind *The New Age Kama Sutra for Women* was to include disparate voices, leaving it open for readers to draw their own interpretations. Perusing numerous interpretations of the *Kama Sutra*, which have often been misunderstood, misread, and misinterpreted, *The New Age Kama Sutra for Women* is also my own journey of scholarship, heavily laced with my personal history, which becomes the most potent ingredient of any written vocabulary. It veers between the Kanatian sublime and the Indian *shringara*, and this becomes the voice of the book. I felt the need to recontextualise and re-read the canon that is the *Kama Sutra*.

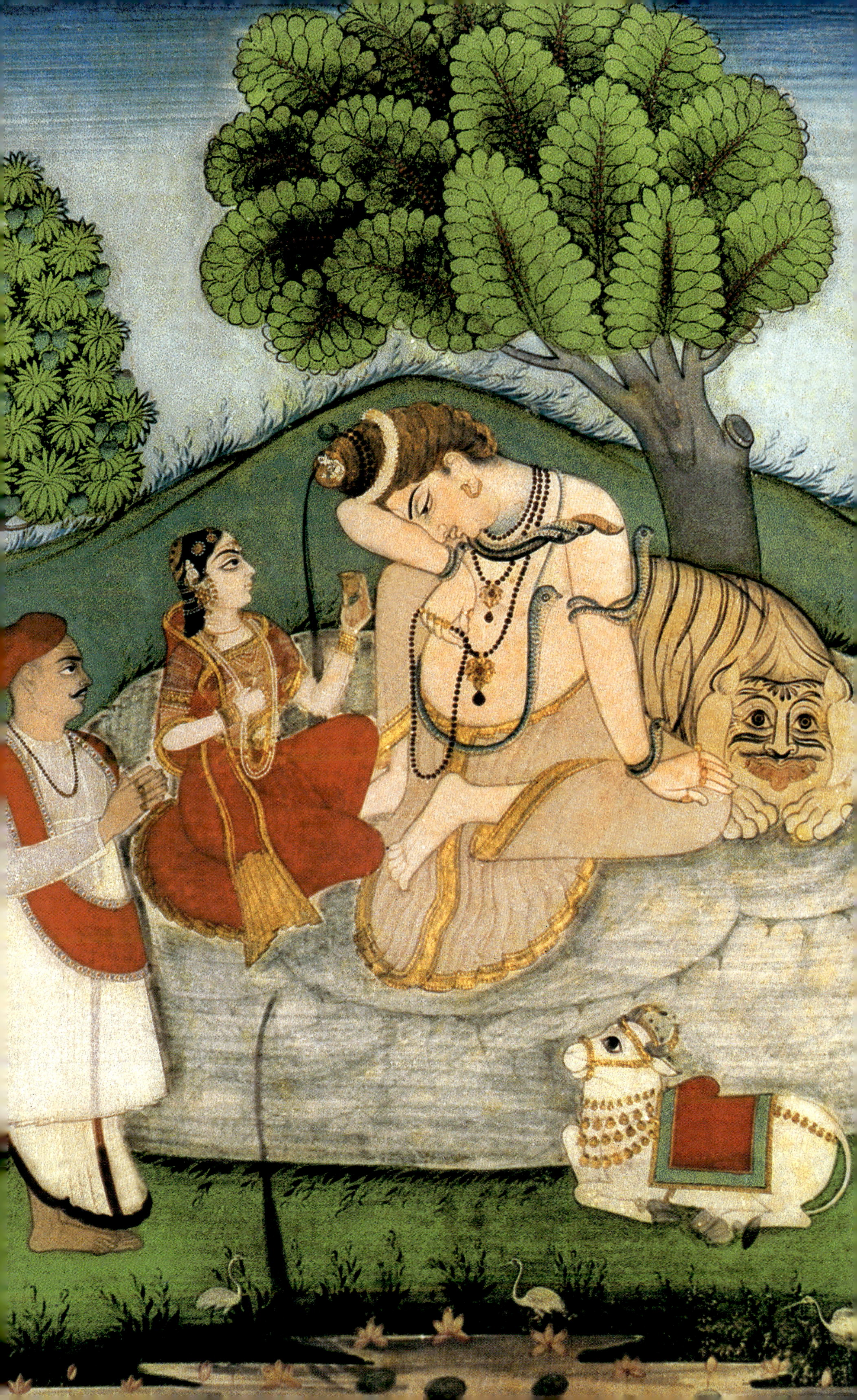

the female PERSPECTIVE

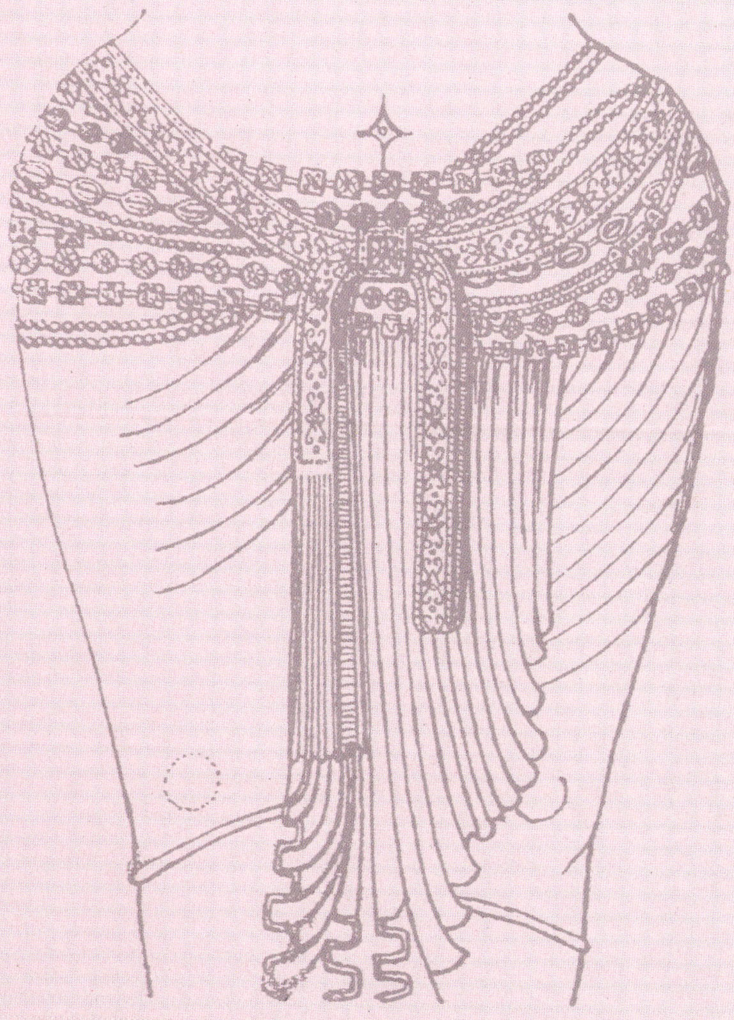

To live in the glory of your love, have I been born!
My beloved; I seek fulfillment in the light of your beauty.
Say what you will, love is great,
The art that joins this world with the other;
If that anger has vanished, Come fill my body and mind

Cover: **Bani Thani** - The eternal Radha. The 'nom de plume' given by Raja Sawant Singh, fitted the role of Radha - Bani Thani, 'All dressesd up and ready to go.' Their captivated and unwavering devotion as *bhakti* and *bhakta* - they were noted for their complete attachment and fervent devotion. The Raja absolved his birthright and together they became *gopa* and *gopi*, cowboy and cowgirl. They adopted the attitude of deeply beloved as Radha and Krishna. *Miniature painting, Kishengarh, Rajasthan, mid 19th century. Private collection*

Endpaper: Pichhavai, *a decorative backdrop cloth, Deccan, late 18th century. Gold painted on cloth. Museum of Fine Arts, Boston.*

Page 1: **The *nayika*, heroine at leisure:** Artists are the most conscious and have filled every book with artistic reproductions of the beautiful pastimes of their heroines. Here, the artist has provided hidden spots in the setting, to expose the body to the warm sunrays as one flushes oneself with gushing cold water in the company of no one else but peacocks who are shown quenching their thirst from the maiden's hair. *Miniature painting, Kishengarh, Rajasthan, early 20th century. Private collection.*

Page 2-3: **Flirting beauties:** Two women of the royal family sharing wine from the same goblet and having fun by flirting homosexually. *Nagaur, Rajasthan, late 18th century.*

In *Sanskrit, kama* means sensuous love or an emotional feeling of attachment. For lack of a better word in English, it is better to use the term 'erotica' to represent *kama*, although erotica may essentially connote arousal. Two thousand years ago, the sage Vatsayana wrote his landmark manuscript, the *Kama Sutra* (erotic codes). Though written from a male perspective, it emphasises gender equality in terms of sexual gratification, which is complementary to the moral, material and spiritual well-being of an individual. Sex is as natural as sunshine and rain, as food and drink, as sight and scent. Pleasure is as essential as food for our existence, yet it must be pursued with moderation and caution.

Sexuality permeates all of human life. It is a kind of all-pervasive life force or energy that emanates from a certain space in the body and causes specific physiological reactions. Total satisfaction and salvation are the two goals of human life according to ancient Indian wisdom. The former is achieved through various material pursuits in a lifetime and the latter through the intangible spiritual path. One of the main components of material satisfaction is sexuality. In fact, in the Upanishads, the sexual act becomes the sacred means of salvation itself - the fusion of man and woman where each becomes both and together they are freed of all bonds and merge with the cosmos.

THE CULT OF THE FEMININE

Through the ages and all over the world, the feminine has been adored, loved and worshipped. A woman dons numerous faces - a young girl, a submissive wife, a giving mother, a fiery enchantress, a lover possessed . . . She is the ageless woman who is portrayed in Indian literature as the pious Sita, the sensuous and seductive Mohini, the fierce Kali, the goddess of plenitude - Lakshmi, the stupendous

Previous page left: **Uma-Maheshwara-Uma, Sakti:** An artistic miniature painting representing Shiva, who has just arisen from a state of deep meditation, his body embraced in close physical bond, which his limbs hold, finds his tender and devoted consort-Parvati in close proximity. The artist has brought a gentle smile, in recognition and pleasure, alighting on his visage. *Miniature painting, Pahari Hills, Kangra style, early 19th century, Private collection.*

Facing page: **Durga, *Mahisasuramardini* - she who destroys the demon:** The goddess Durga was anointed by the gods to subdue Mahisasura, who was over confident of his powers and disrespected the gods. Armed with weapons given to her by the gods, Durga is represented as the supreme victor. Ably assisted by her *vahana* (vehicle), the tiger, she overpowered the demon. This image of Durga is a magnificent representation of the glorious triumph of womanhood by virtue of her *Shakti*, feminine energy. *Wood, Thanjavur, Tamil Nadu, 20th century. Private collection.*

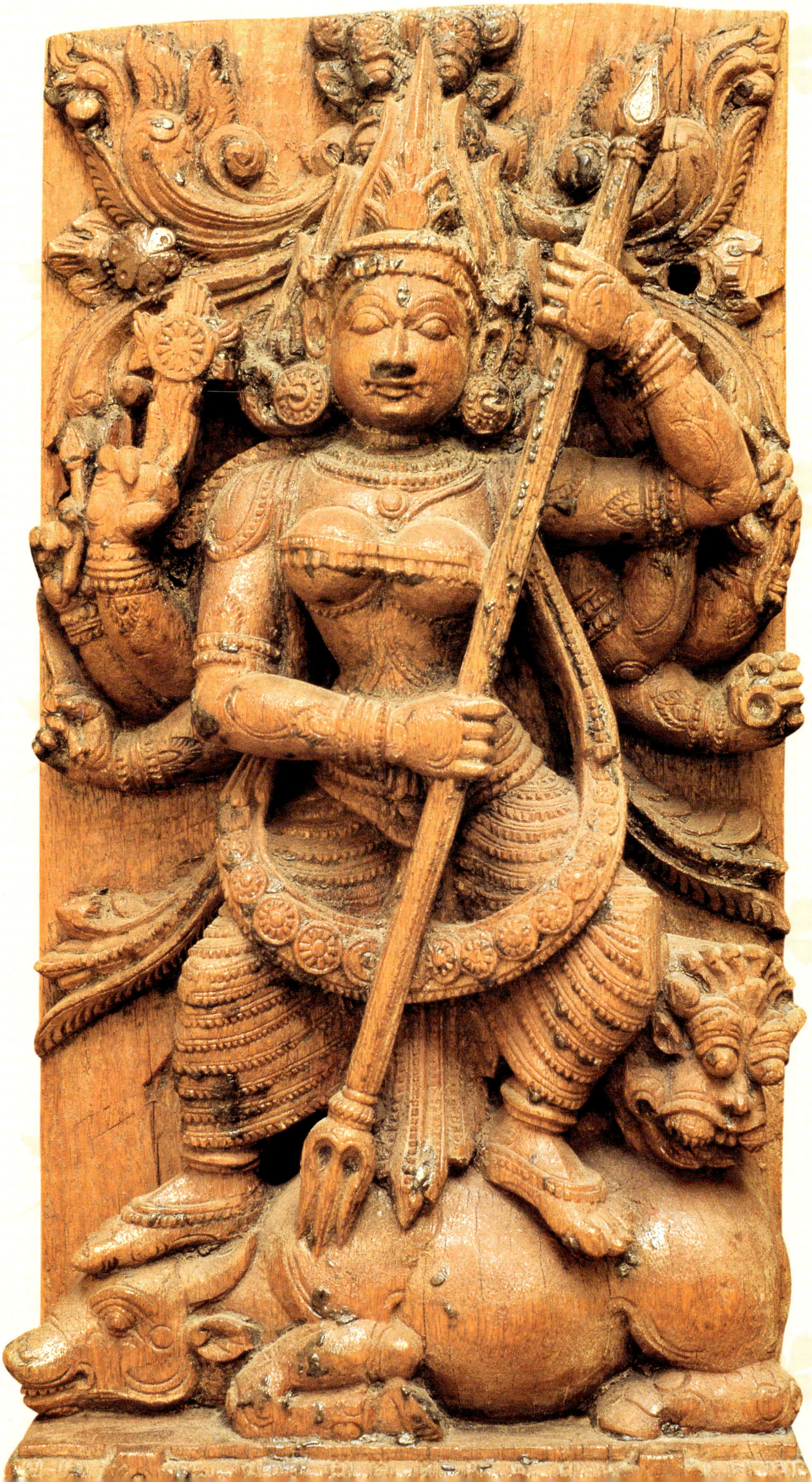

Durga and the lovelorn Radha.

Myths and legends in different cultures across continents celebrate and validate the varied and diverse aspects of women. Beauty, grace and charm, the classical attributes that make the quintessential feminine woman, have led to them being celebrated in the mythic pasts as divine or semi-divine beings. In Greek mythology, springing from the primordial chaos, the woman is Gaia, the Earth, the supporter. In Chinese mythology, she is familiar as Hu-tu; in Mesopotamian culture, she is acknowledged as Ninhursag. The Romans celebrated her as the Goddess Minerva, the Goddess of arts and crafts.

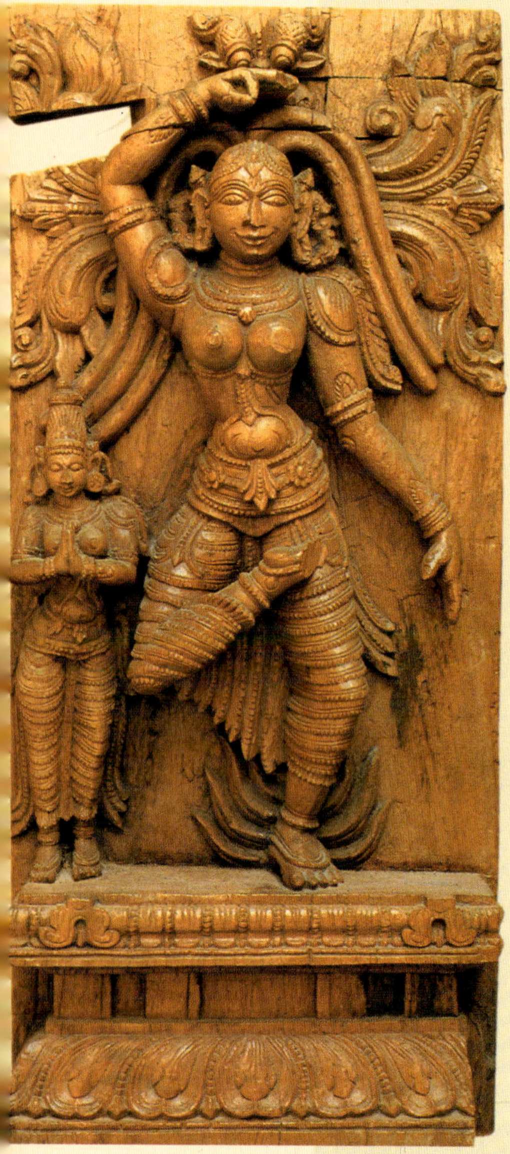

The abundance of examples in cross-cultural manifestation abound. One of her many forms in India is that of Durga. Worshipped as the fertile womb of the world, giving birth to all life, every woman is considered to be her personification. As the cosmic womb, her icon in a shrine or temple is called the *yoni*, vulva. She is *shakti*, the cosmic energy, the divine force that cannot be destroyed. She supports, sustains and nurtures life. While the man, the masculine principle, implants the seeds of creation, contained in the seminal fluid, it is the female anatomy that is the location where the seed of life unites and bursts forth as an entity unto itself.

The *Kama Sutra* is not solely a text about the art of love making that lists the famous sixty-four positions to satisfy one's desire. It emphasises the specificity of men and women to the experience of pleasure, within the larger, holistic context of creation.

Sita, heroine of the *Ramayana*: She was so named by Janaka, her father, when she materialised in a 'furrow' during a sacrificial rite to plough for progeny. After the long exile and their return to Ayodhya, Sita, to prove her innocence and purity had to undergo the legendary trial by fire. Her beauty and grace is glorified in this wood sculpture and her innocence is laudably commemorated in this artistic rendition of such charm and simplicity. *Wood sculpture from temple ratha, chariot, Thanjavur, Tamil Nadu, 20th century. Private collection.*

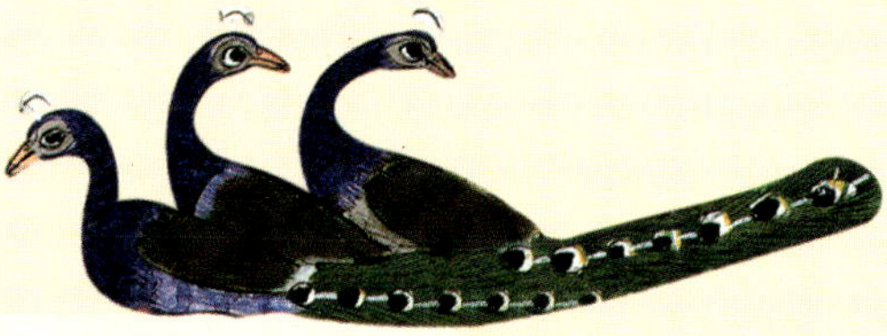

'SHAKTI' IN THE TWENTY-FIRST CENTURY

The New Age woman has, in the 21st century, absorbed tradition and is fast infusing modernity into her being. By the day, she labours through office, and by dusk, she attends to her family and friends as the epitome of love and hospitality. She is the seductress who embraces and shields her man in a combination of aggressive passion and tender care. While quenching the desires of her partner, she reaches out for hers as well. Sometimes, there is a head-on collision between the old and the new. Often confronted with pragmatic issues such as female infanticide, lack of equal opportunity, pandering to

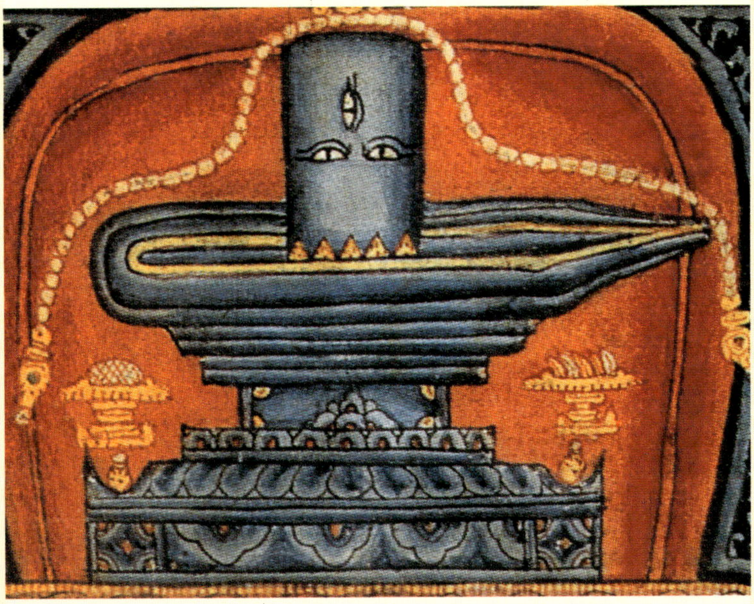

her husband's whims, denial of inheritance of property, she is under constant pressure. But she is now reaching for the stars. She is becoming smart and savvy, and increasingly confident of what she wants, and who she is or wants to be. Her persona is changing dramatically.

The stress on gender equality is more than ever before. With the increase in access to education, social structures are altering vastly and women are emerging as co-players.

The composite symbolic aspect of Shiva and Parvati: This is consolidated in the form of the *linga*, the creative phallaic aspect of Shiva, resting upon the *yoni*, the symbolic aspect of Parvati. The aspect of this tremendous iconographic form, is widely depicted in stone and metals, artistic paintings and symbolic forms, which represent this artistic manifestation of the icon including the face of Shiva, which is described as *Mukha Linga. Manuscript painting, Nepal, 17th century. Private collection.*

Ritual oil lamp: This terracotta object of tribal origin is hand moulded from clay. The lamp bowl is the *yoni*, the feminine aspect. The male aspect is a graceful handle shaped as the *linga*. *Terracotta, Maria Gonds tribal art, Narainpur, Bastar, Madhya Pradesh. 20th century. The National Museum of Arts and Crafts, New Delhi.*

Facing page: **Yakshi and her parrot:** Many such columnar pillars circumambulate the stupas. An excavation at Bhuteshwar revealed many richly decorated pillars with numerous *yakshis*, symbolic of good fortune. They were chosen to serve Kubera, lord of all the treasures of the Earth. They are elemental beings *Punya-jana*, 'propitious'. Physically fulsome, they were voluptuous and playful. They could rap with parrots and other birds, availing their guidance on the whereabouts of precious jewels, who directed them to these concealed places. *Red sandstone, Kushana period, Bhuteshwar, Mathura, Uttar Pradesh, 2nd century. Indian Museum, Kolkata.*

Sensitivity to the innate differences between men and women, however, needs to be enhanced.

In Indian mythology, Parvati was the consort of Shiva, the Destroyer. She was the provider or *shakti*, signifying the concept of male and female energies working together as equal partners in the universe. This concept is carried further to its logical climax in the form of *Ardhanarisvara*, formed by the fusion of Shiva and *Shakti* in one body, each occupying one half of the body, denoting that one is incomplete without the other. This equality of the male and female balance of power is again embodied in world cultures. Every god has an accompanying goddess as his consort, as for example, Isis and Osiris in Egyptian mythology, and Rhea and Cronus in Greek mythology.

The concept of *Shakti* has empowered Indian women and has been the flag bearer of Indian feminism. In fact, feminism is not a Western import; it has its roots in the *Shakti* cult of old and is now on the road to rediscovery.

The sacred literature of the Hindus is filled with myths and legends of feminine dreams and themes, either grating with female fury or submission. There has always been a duality, a paradox, and black and white existing in the interpretation and representation of the woman.

KAMA SUTRA: THE FEMALE PERSPECTIVE TODAY

There is a paradox in the status of women in India, where as a daughter, wife and mother, she is adored, and as a single woman she could perhaps be looked upon as a modern-day temptress and seductress. In the ancient past there were tales of goddesses who struck children with fever nymphs who seduced sages: one such story is about Menaka, the celestial maiden, who destroyed the ascetic discipline of the sage Valmiki.

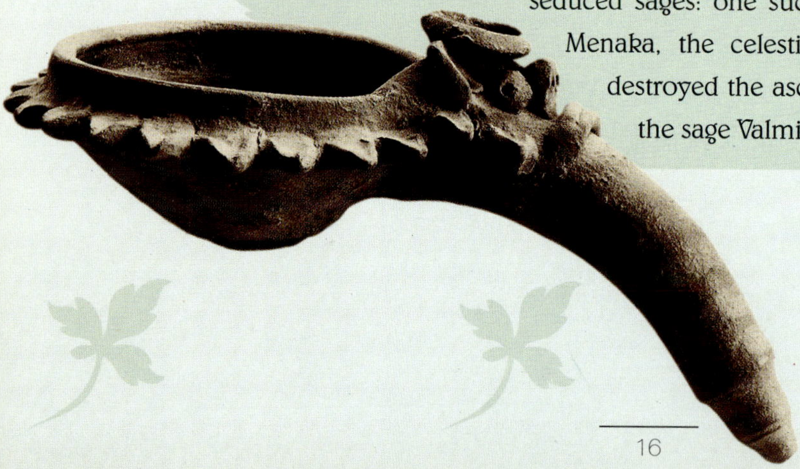

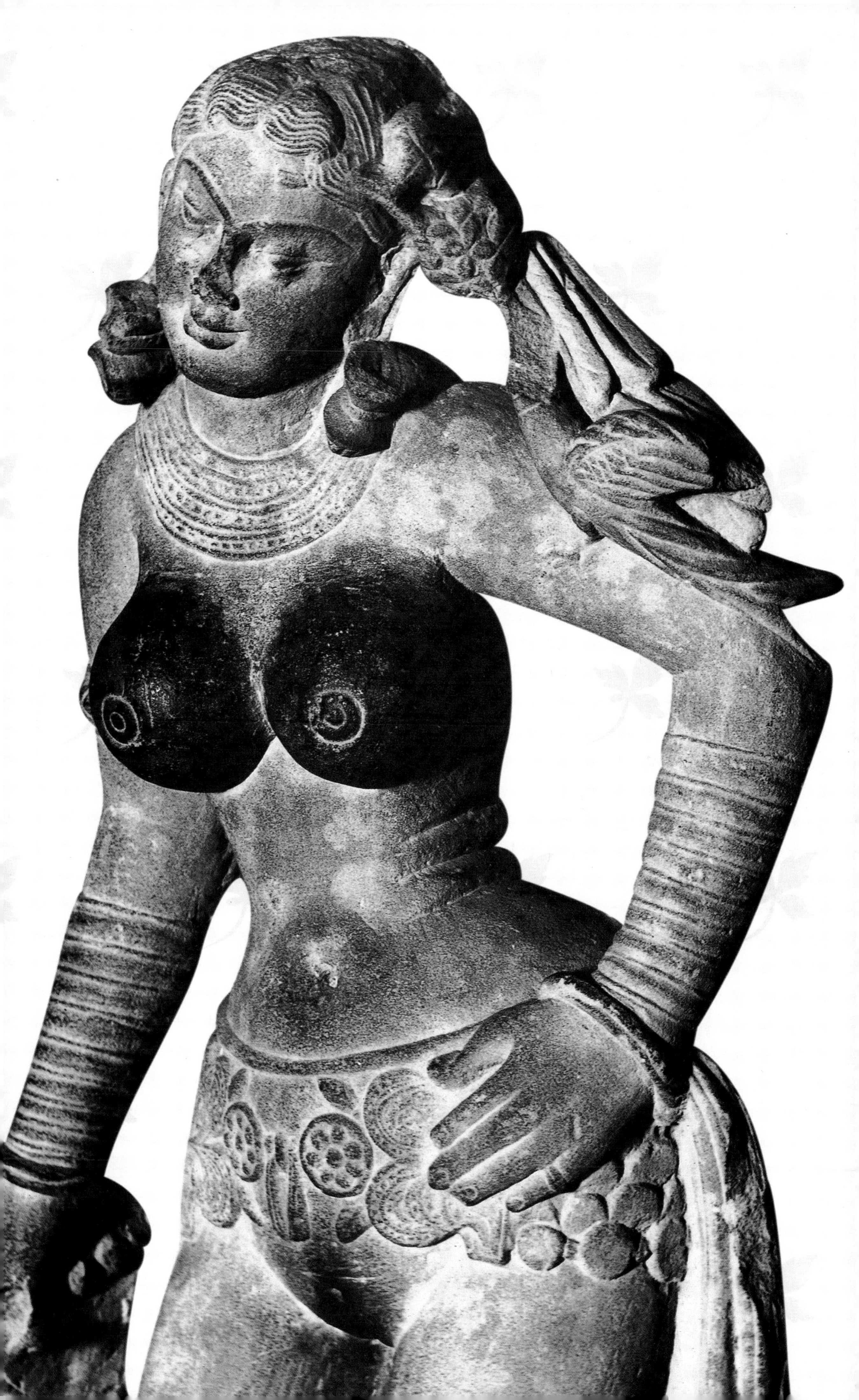

Somewhere from the past lore has emerged the beating heart of the ageless woman: the pious Sita, the sensuous Radha, the seductive Mohini, the fierce and demonic Kali, and the bountiful Lakshmi. In the West, issues relating to gender have often been misunderstood or increasingly thought of as being part of a stereotyped feminist discourse, that started with bra-burning, making that gesture symbolic of demanding equality with men. That aspect of the feminist discourse is, however, a limiting one, and following the feminine trajectory, femininity gets marginalised. The *power* of being a woman becomes labeled and packaged as a commodity, and the celebration of the feminine self gets lost. But the feminist discourse of the West does not find a similar resonance in India. The Indian woman of today is proud of her femininity and aware of her power. She revels in it, arouses and obtains pleasure from it, and most of all - asks her male companion to acknowledge *her* special needs as being *equally* as important as his.

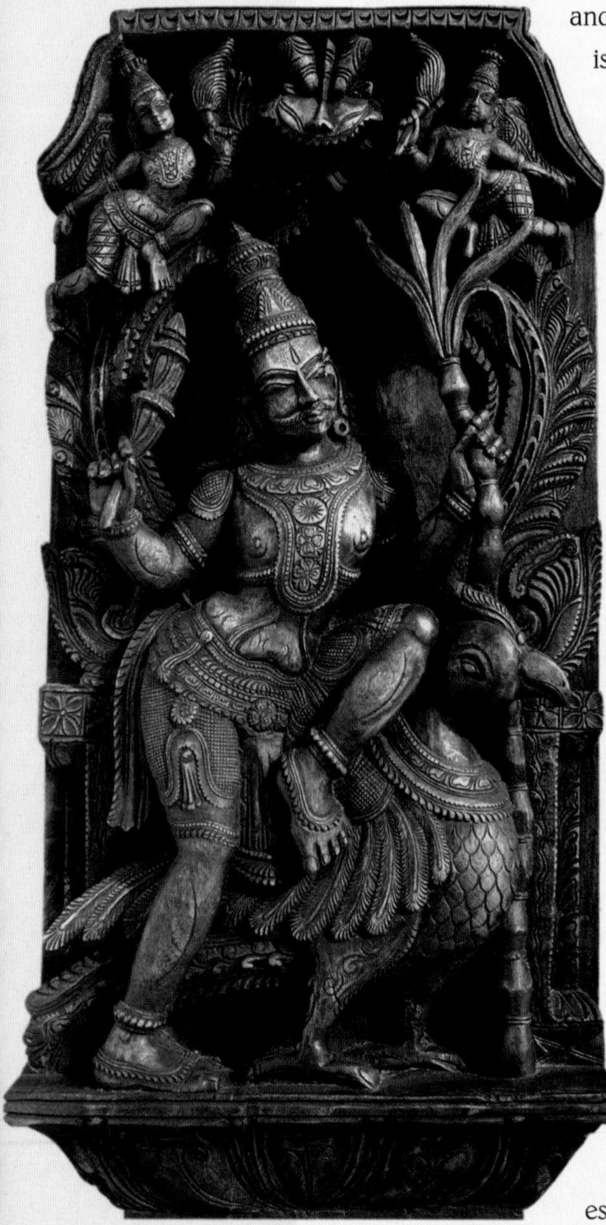

The *Kama Sutra* reflects the Hindu tradition where sex is essential to life and therefore worthy of serious study. It not only respects a woman's sexual needs but also empowers her. It reflects and fosters a woman's enjoyment of her sexuality. It is said in the *Kama Sutra* that

Kama Deva, Manmatha, and his consort Rati Devi: *Kama* (desire), first stirred at the dawn of creation, is a handsome youth and the god of abounding love. In the *Atharva Veda*, he is exalted as a creator. Rati Devi is *Kama-Priya*, 'beloved of Kama'. *Kama* is a valiant lover, handsome and dashing. His *vahana*, vehicle is the parrot. He is armed with his weapon of mass-connection, a sugar-cane bow, which is strung with woven threads of longing made up of buzzing bees and is a lively repository for his arrows, which are tipped with lotus flowers. Highly decorative sculptured carvings from a wooden *ratha*, temple chariot. As a part of the rituals in South Indian temples, these very heavy carts are hand pulled from one destination to another during the festivals. Hundreds of youths voluntarily perform this task. *Wood, Tamil Nadu, 20th century. Madame Florence M de Surmont collection, Switzerland.*

women derive more pleasure from sex than men. The story of King Bhagashwana in the *Mahabharata* affirms this belief. Bhagashwana was cursed to become a woman and as a woman, he produced many sons, who fought and killed each other. He asked for mercy to revive his sons. When Indra asked which set of his sons he wished to revive, Bhagashwana replied the ones who called him Mother. When asked whether he wanted a male or female body, he replied: 'A female one so that I can get more pleasure'.

The *Kama Sutra's* heritage is worthy of care and protection, be it portrayed within the configurations of modern life. *Sat-chit-ananda*, truth-consciousness-bliss: this is the founding principle of Indian thought and a universal that cannot be challenged by any definitions of time or space.

The shifting and contested boundaries of female sexuality reflect the coming of age of empowerment in women. A new map of power, proliferation of ideas, desires and identities, have seen the emergence of a revolution wherein the woman of today is exploring new facets of her sexuality and coming to terms with it.

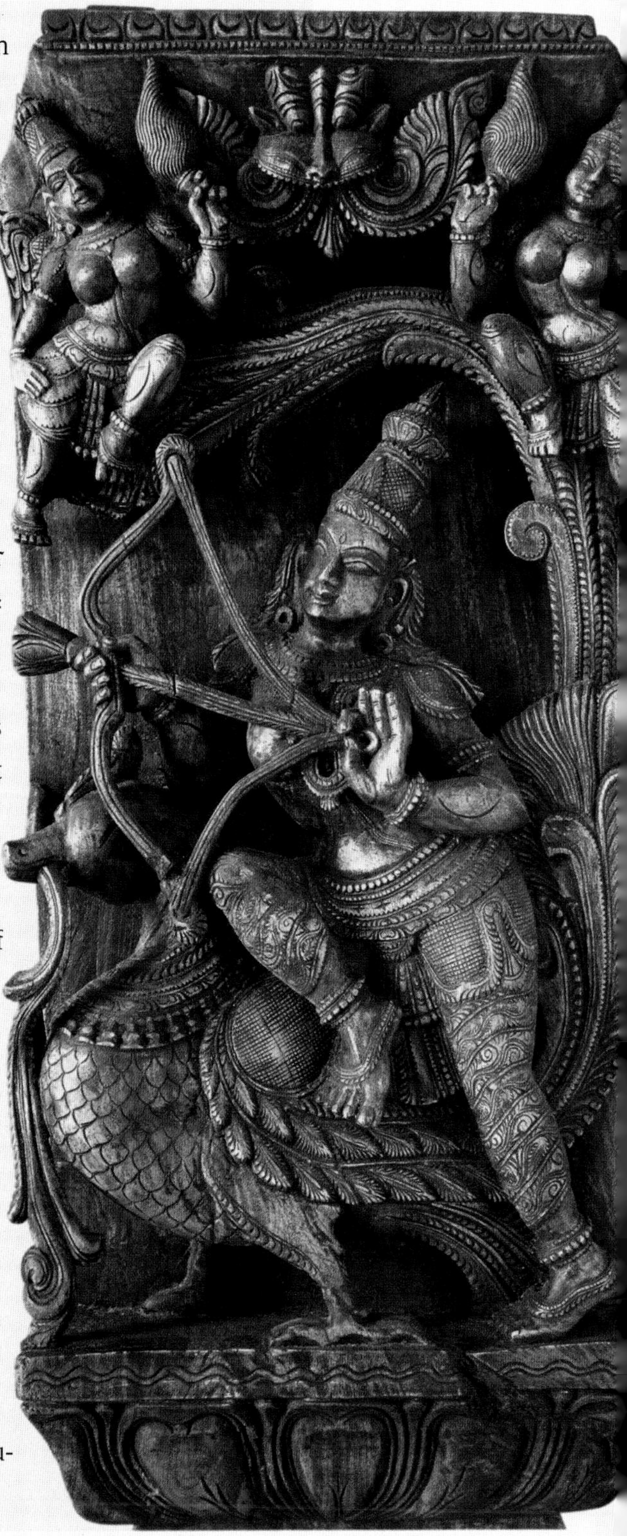

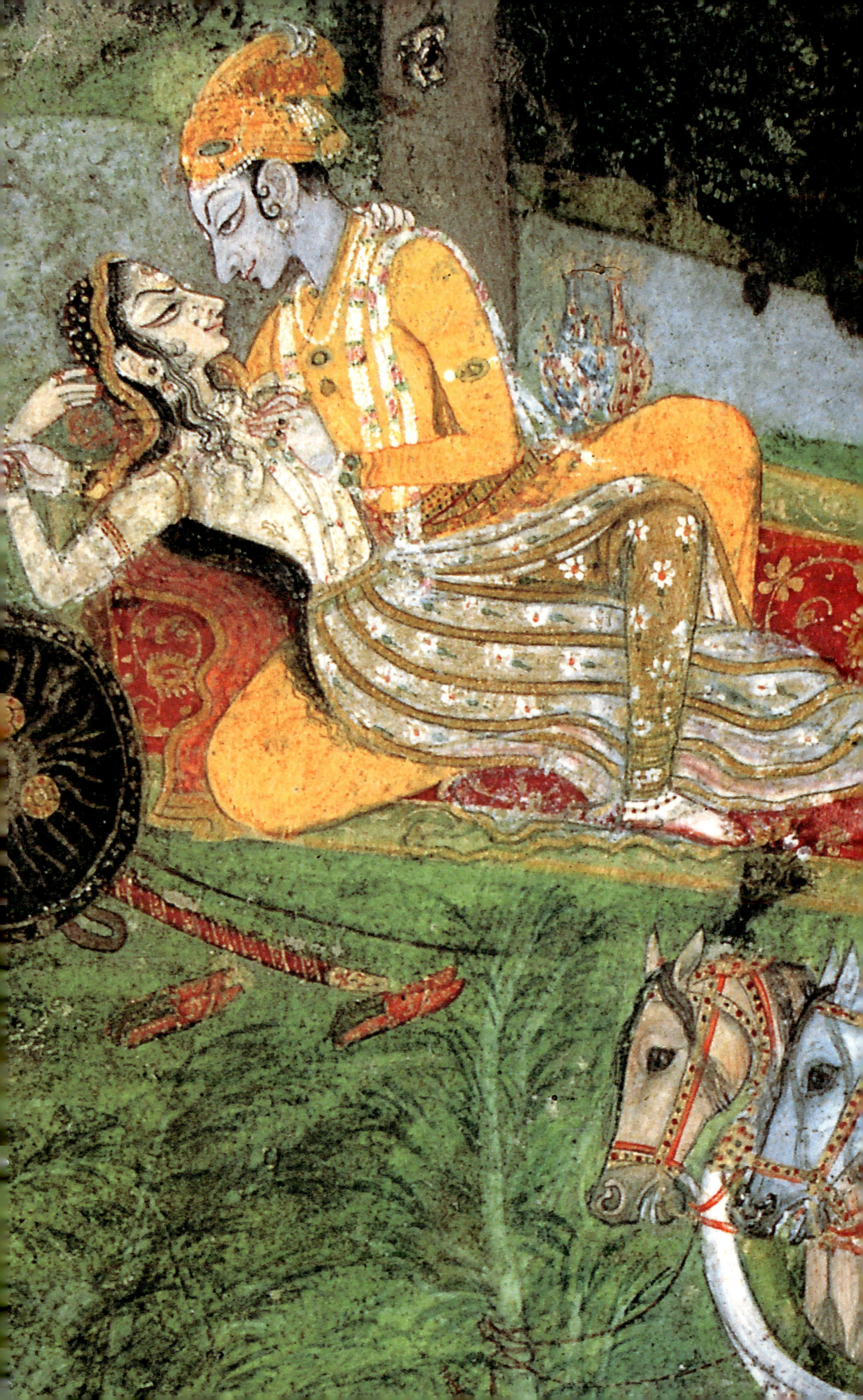

*By the union with men the lust, desire, or passion of women is satisfied,
and the pleasure derived from the consciousness of it is called their satisfaction*

Kama Sutra

the art of COURTSHIP

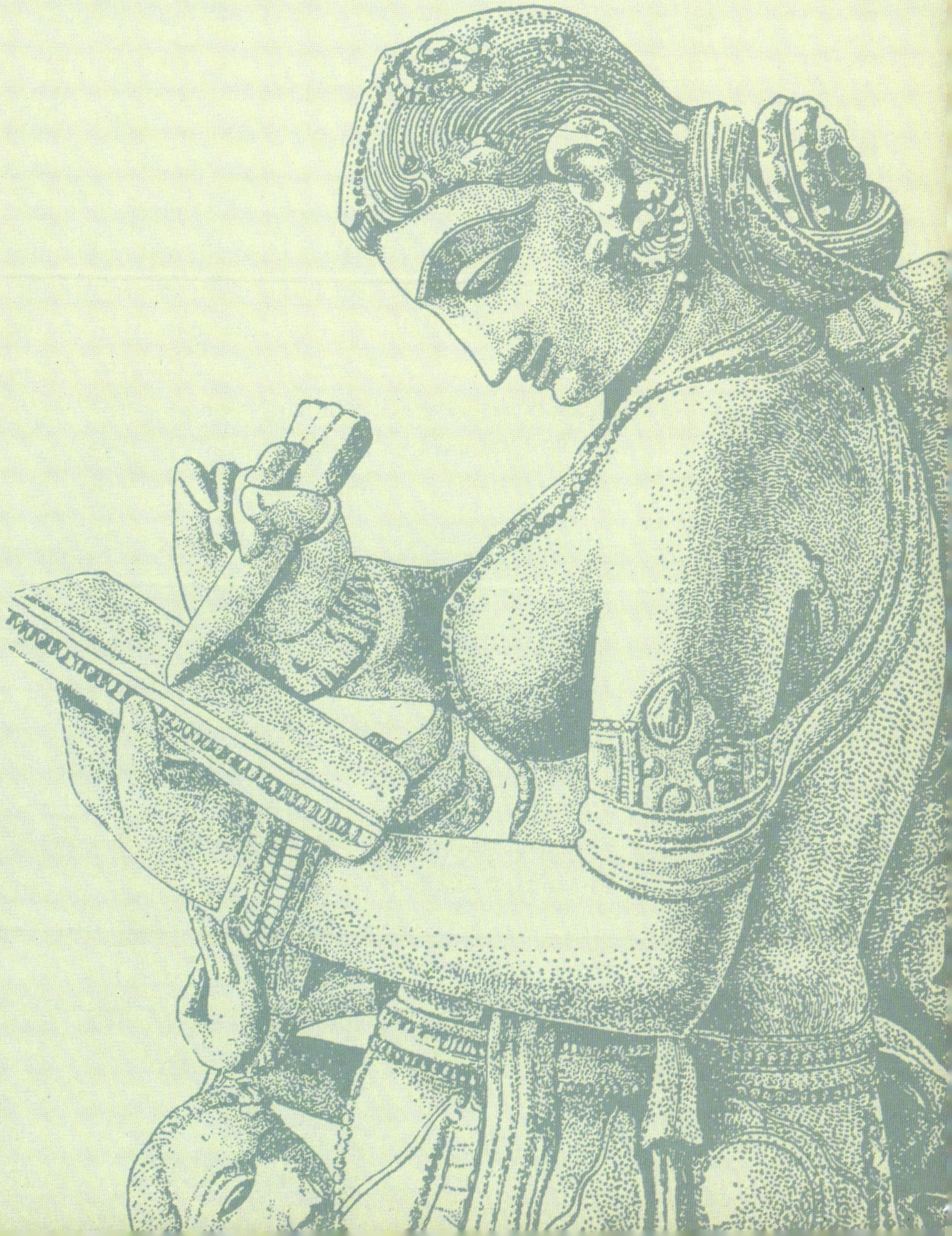

Previous page left:
Krishna and Radha, hero & heroine courting:
The most active protagonist and favourite subject of artists is Krishna, the handsome young boy. His adventures with Radha involve a great deal of love making. He portrays all the characteristics of a hero - tall, dark, and handsome with a well built physic and airs of a village youth. He was also very strong and feared nothing and no one. He loved to venture here and there, and knew many secret places in the forest. Radha, the darling of his heart and all the *gopis*, cow-girls were in constant attendance. His devotions in the service of the fair sex, knew no limits. The *gopis*, who dallied with him in the forests around Gokula, are a favourite subject of romantic literature and art. Among his *bhaktas*, devotees were Sawant Singh, artist, poet and the prince of Kishengarh and his beloved Bani Thani. They were totally attuned in their daily life and they lived together as if they were Radha and Krishna. Here they are portrayed in a style of painting identified by their distinct facial features, raised eye brows, fish eyes, and small mouth. They gaze at each other with constant love and longing and their long and tender fingers flutter and fondle each other. *Miniature painting, Kishengarh, Rajasthan, 19th century. Private collection.*

Courtship, as a word, has old-world connotations but remains a crucial and determining moment in a relationship, which plants the seeds of a more long-term companionship. It is a time when a couple considers the prospects of their relationship, gauges its potential and addresses each other's needs while together. It is a time for testing.

A man acting in accordance with the inclinations of a girl should try and gain her over so that she may love him and place her confidence in him. A man does not succeed either by implicitly following the inclinations of a girl, or by wholly opposing her, and he should, therefore, adopt a middle course. He, who knows how to make himself beloved by women, as well as to increase their honour and create confidence in them, becomes an object of their love. But he, who neglects a girl, thinking she is too bashful, is despised by her as a beast, ignorant of the working of the female mind. Moreover, a girl forcibly enjoyed by one who does not understand the hearts of girls becomes nervous, uneasy and dejected, and suddenly begins to fear the man who has taken advantage of her; and then, when her love is not understood or returned, she sinks into despondency, and becomes either a hater of mankind, or, hating her own man, she has recourse to other men.

A meeting in the lush green park, or on the stunning remains of an old monument, by the quiet river or lake, still awaken dreams of romantic interludes, but even if the environment has changed, the delicate sanctity of a man-woman relationship

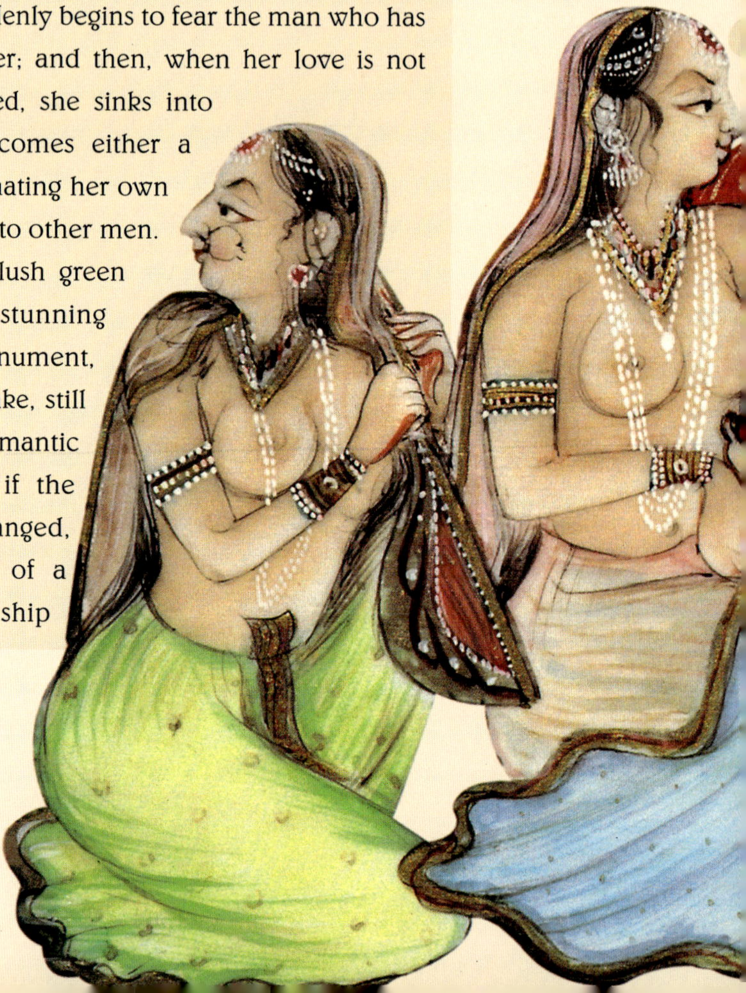

remains the same. Building a woman's confidence is as crucial today as before. The *Kama Sutra* advises that when a boy has started to woo the girl he loves, '*he should spend his time with her and amuse her with various diversions fit for their age and acquaintanceship*'.

This is the time to soak and immerse themselves in each other's company. There is no better way than by going smooth and easy, and taking one's own time to open up.

TENDER BEGINNINGS

Ancient texts have rightly said that women being of a tender nature, desire tender beginnings. Innovation, humour, quietude, silence - all these are *bhavas*, emotions, that help to nurture the *rasa*, essence, of togetherness. A man should start by doing whatever a woman enjoys and get for her what she likes.Vatsyayana iterates:

Such things should be given at different times whenever he gets an opportunity of meeting her, and some of them should be given in private, and some in public, according to circum-

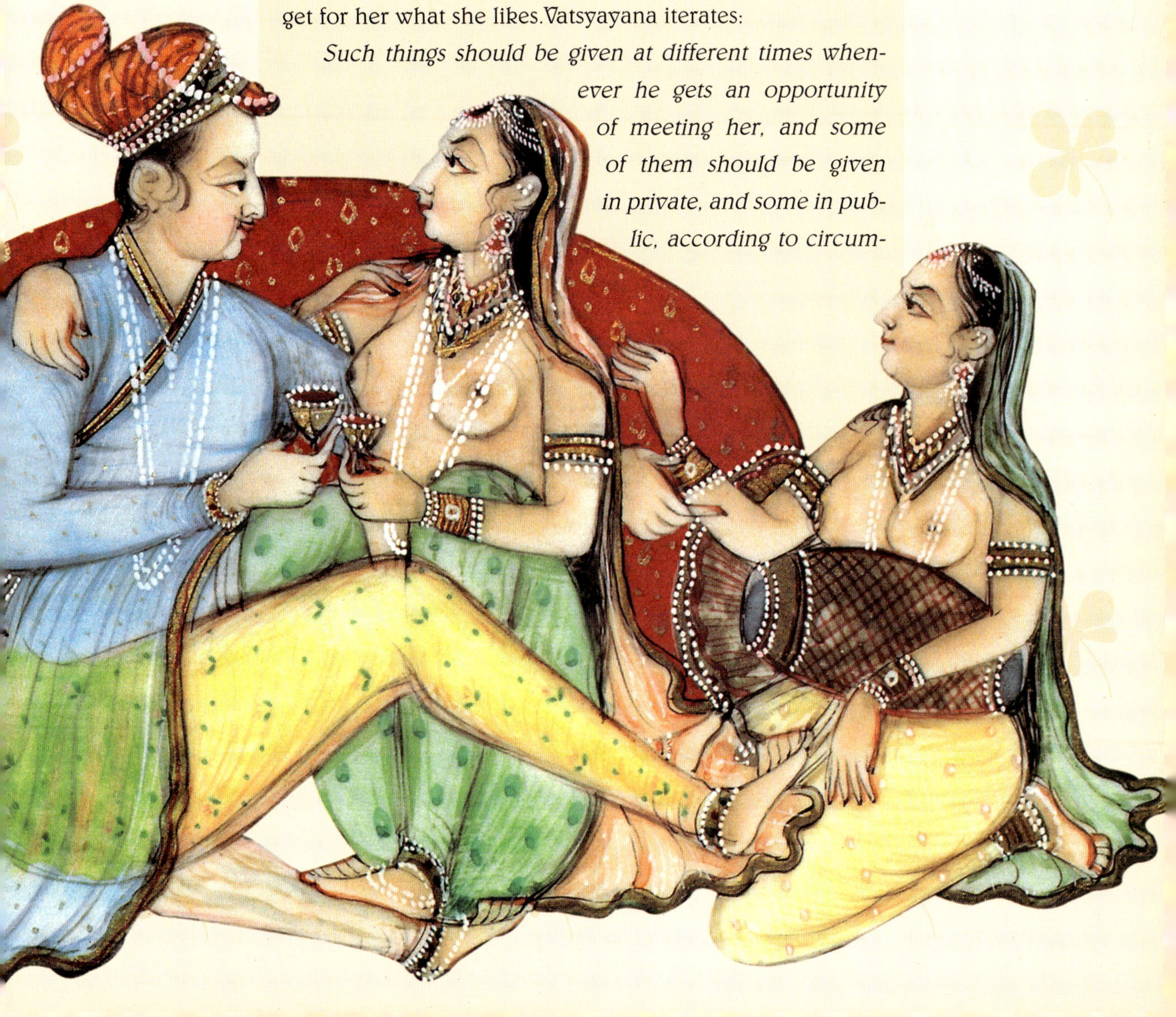

Revelry: A beautiful woman, educated, socially accustomed and with grace represents the most joyous companion for an evening out. No experience can match the resulting companionship. They make a perfect subject for painting commissioned from an artistic memorabilia. When such a gathering of party goers get together, and all concerned participate, the air is luminous and vibrant with expectation. *Painting on ivory, Rajasthan, 20th century. Private collection.*

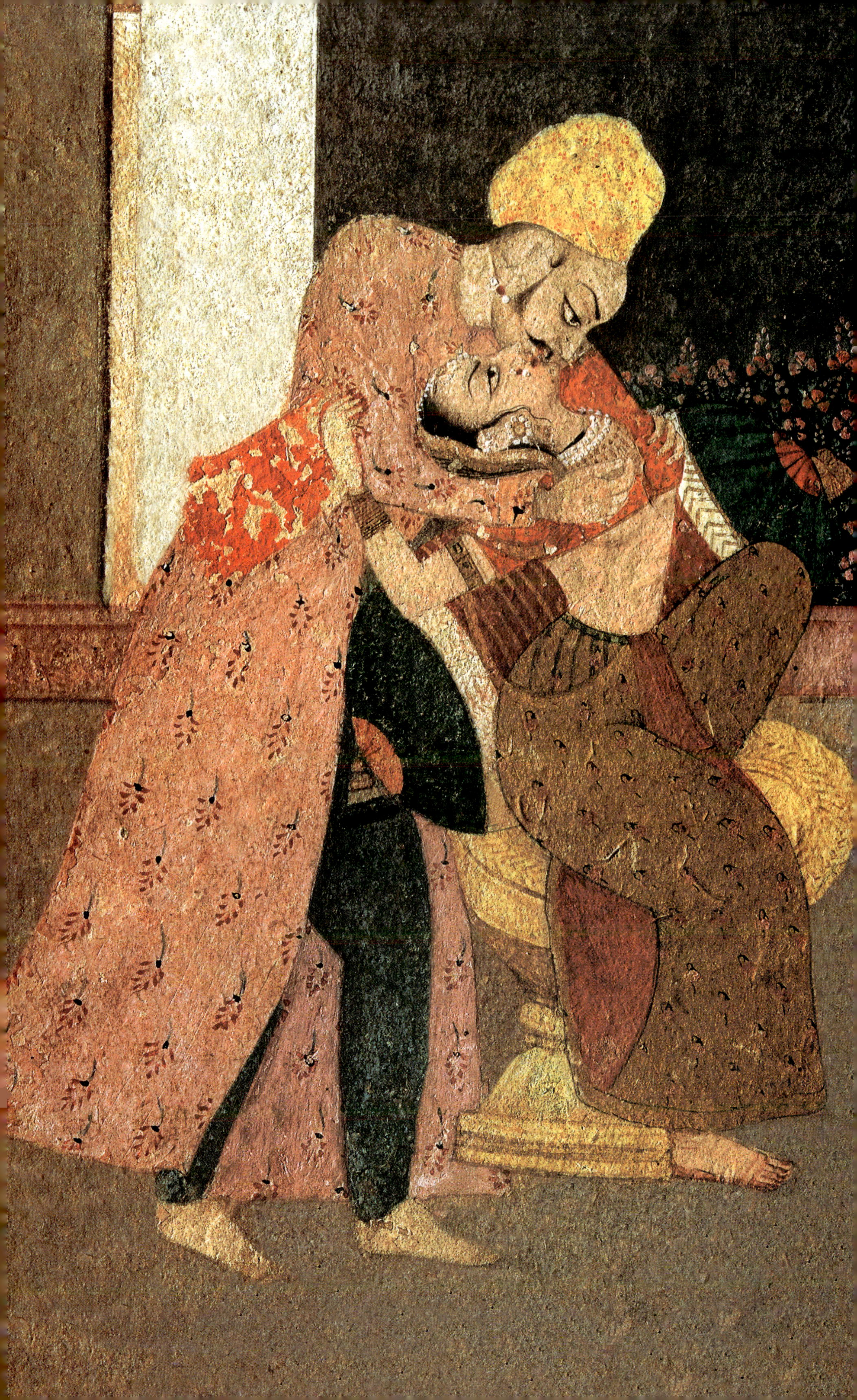

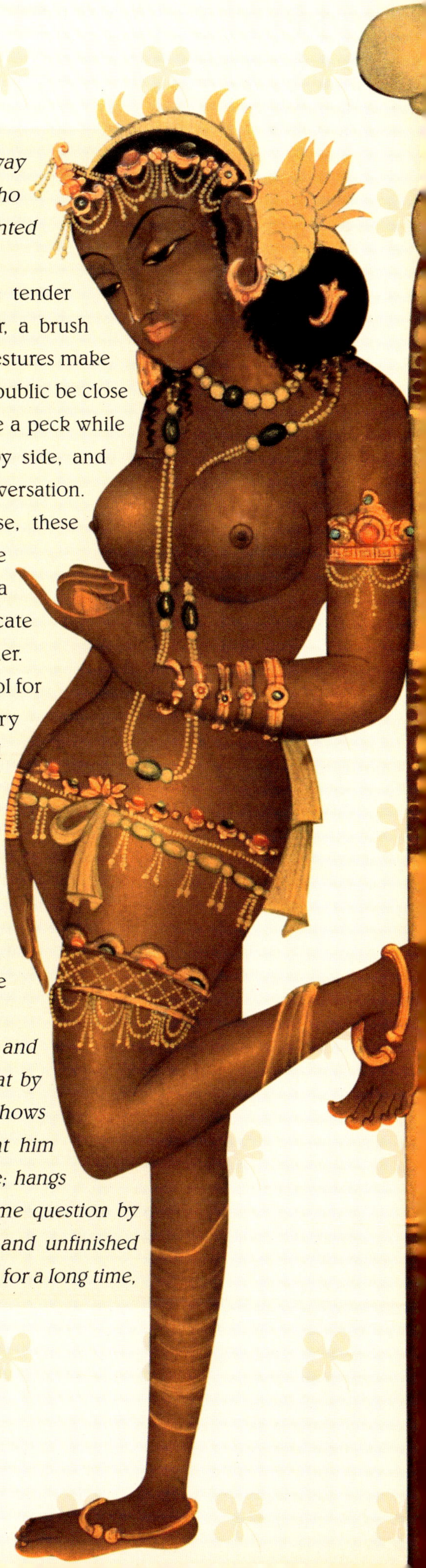

A lacquer painting: It is modelled on a mural from Ajanta. The Ajanta cave frescoes were painted between A.D. 200-650. *Contemporary painting, Nirmal, Andhra Pradesh. Private collection.*
Facing page: **The art of kiss:** Sanskrit and Pali legends outline the tale of Chitraleka, who drew portraits identifiable as Aniruddha, whom she had seen in a dream, and had fallen head over heals in love with. Similarly, literature has provided countless interpretations of the kiss. The hero takes the heroine by surprise from behind. She turns, and pleased, she tilts her head to receive his passionate kisses, petting and caresses. The throbbing deep passion provides the lovers with a wonderful flow in their body language. The artistic semblance is full of the fire of delight and fiery ardour, suggesting artistic ability of some merit. The costumes are also an important clue, typically regional Deccan in style. *Miniature painting, Deccan, Andhra Pradesh, early 17th century.*

stances. In short he should try in every way to make her look upon him as one who would do for her everything that she wanted to be done.

A soft kiss, a light embrace, some tender moves, gentle strokes through her hair, a brush against her skin now and then - these gestures make you aware of each other's presence. In public be close and share gentle physical exchanges like a peck while greeting, a brush while walking side by side, and holding hands when together in conversation. When performed with grace and poise, these gestures not only give the right message to the people around, they also build a woman's respect for the man and indicate to her his intentions in a dignified manner.

Language too, can be more than a tool for communication. A delicate vocabulary succeeds in conveying one's desires and skills; and also reduces the inhibitions of the girl. During the initial courtship, there is a mild shyness in the air and feelings merely formulate into actions or signs. A whole new language evolves with its own distinct vocabulary and communicates what words cannot. The *Kama Sutra* says of girls:

She never looks the man in the face, and becomes abashed when she is looked at by him; under some pretext or other she shows her limbs to him; she looks secretly at him though he has gone away from her side; hangs down her head when she is asked some question by him, and answers in indistinct words and unfinished sentences, delights to be in his company for a long time, speaks to her attendants in a peculiar tone with the hope of attracting his attention towards her . . .

On her part too, a girl should express her keenness in a relationship and adopt means to endear herself to the young man she is interested in.

Try meeting your loved one in lonely places and on the odd occasion shower him with flowers. Show him your skills in the fine arts. Discuss with him things he likes to talk about as well as the numerous ways in which one can win the love of a girl.

There is a flow that evolves when togetherness is punctuated with simple recreational gestures: picking flowers together, watching the sun set, an evening of music or dance, appreciating works of art . . . None of this, however, should be performed at the cost of a woman's dignity. As favourable as a woman may be, when a man expresses his desires towards her, she should show no change in her demeanour, receive his manifestations of love as if ignorant of his state of mind, oppose him a bit when he tries to embrace or kiss. These are no prescriptions, but mechanisms to gauge the intensity of his desires.

THE *KAMA SUTRA* STATES:

A man who has seen and perceived the feelings of the girl towards him, and who has noticed the outward signs and movements by which those feelings are expressed, should

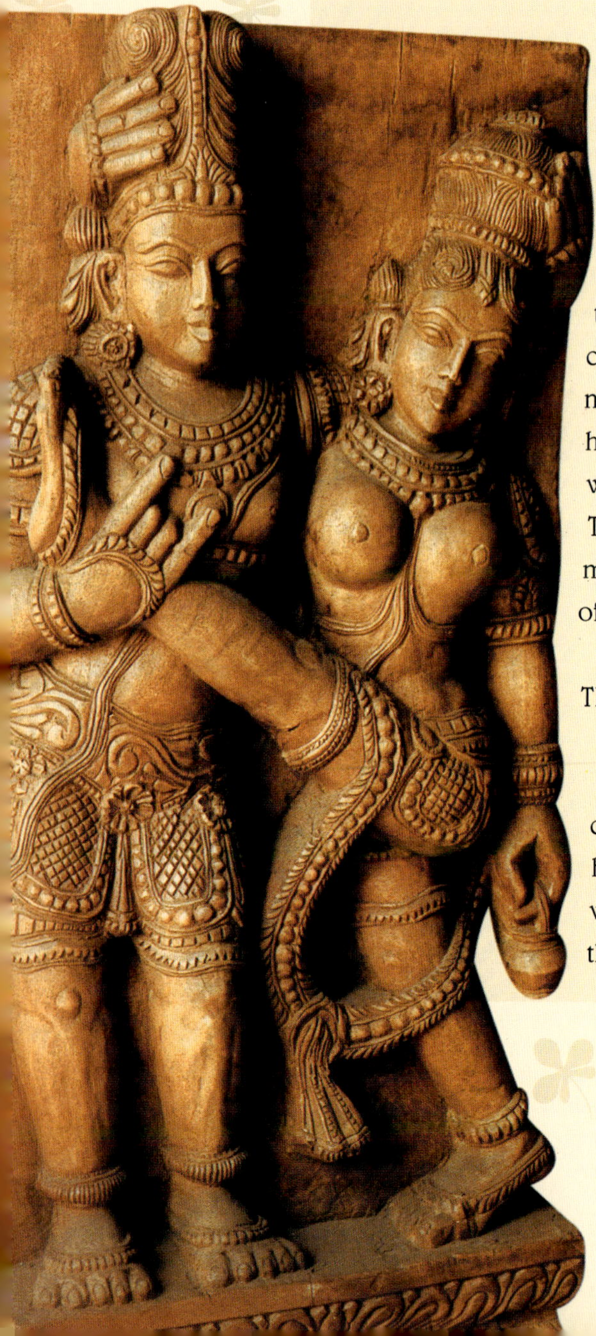

Krishna at play: Two wood carvings from a Vaishnavite temple show Krishna's exploits with the village belles. Theatrical in composition, they are figments of the vivid imagination and skill of the sculptors, who enriched the decor of temples with such works based on Hindu myths and legends. Lord Vishnu appeared on earth in many *avatars*, reincarnations, Krishna being one of them. The two examples are regionally identifiable - the lower left Mithuna loving couple from *Chitambaram* and on the right from *Thanjavur, Tamil Nadu, 20th century. Private collection.*

do everything in his power to effect a union with her.

GETTING CLOSER

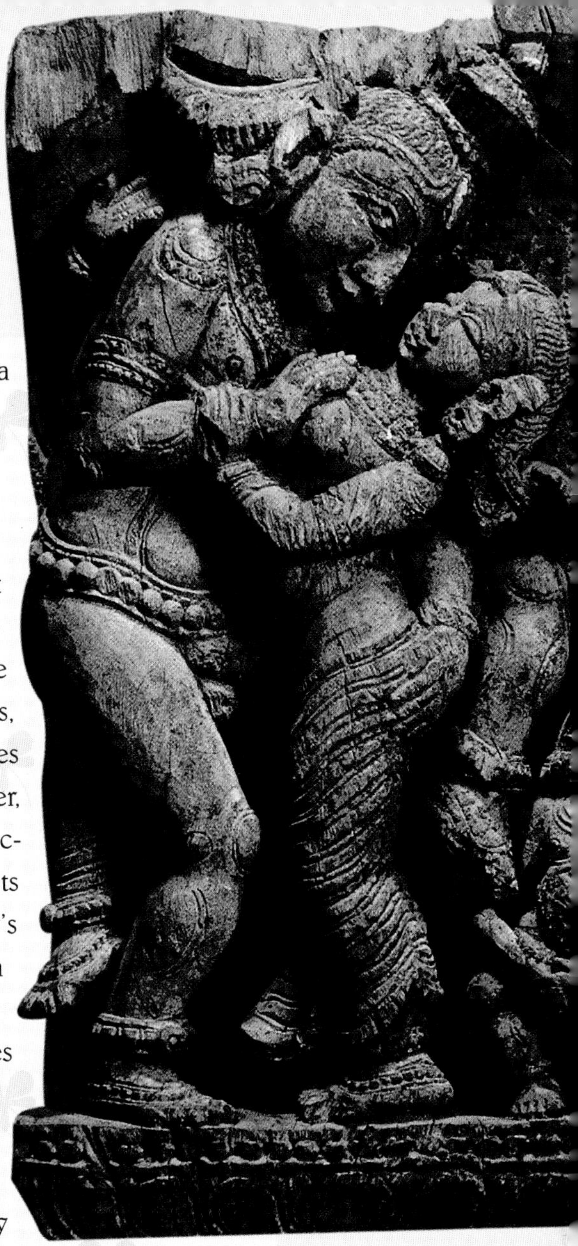

The *Rasikapriya*, a medieval text written by Keshavadas, in which the nine sentiments or emotions are expressed at length, says: 'When eyes, speech and minds are united, bodies also wish to unite.' Taking this further, the *Kama Sutra* maintains that embracing removes distances and acquaints one with the comfort of the partner's body. The first embrace advised is a tender one. It is called *Jataveshtitaka* or the twining creeper, and implies merely a brief touch now and then. The *Vridkshadhirudhaka* or climbing tree is when you can use your touch to tell him what you feel by getting all over him. Then there is the *Tila-Tandulaka* or the mixture of sesame seed with rice, and the *Krshiranirака* or milk and water embrace.

Finger nails can also be used to convey the emotion your togetherness invokes in you. Pressing and nail marks are the sign language lovers use to remind, share and amuse each other with.

The love of a woman who sees the marks of nails on the private parts of the body, even though they are old and almost worn out, becomes again fresh and new. If there be no marks of nails to remind a person of the passage of love, then love is lessened in the same way as when no union takes place for a long time. *(Kama Sutra, Book II)*

It is said that if kissing kindles the fire of love, then pierc-

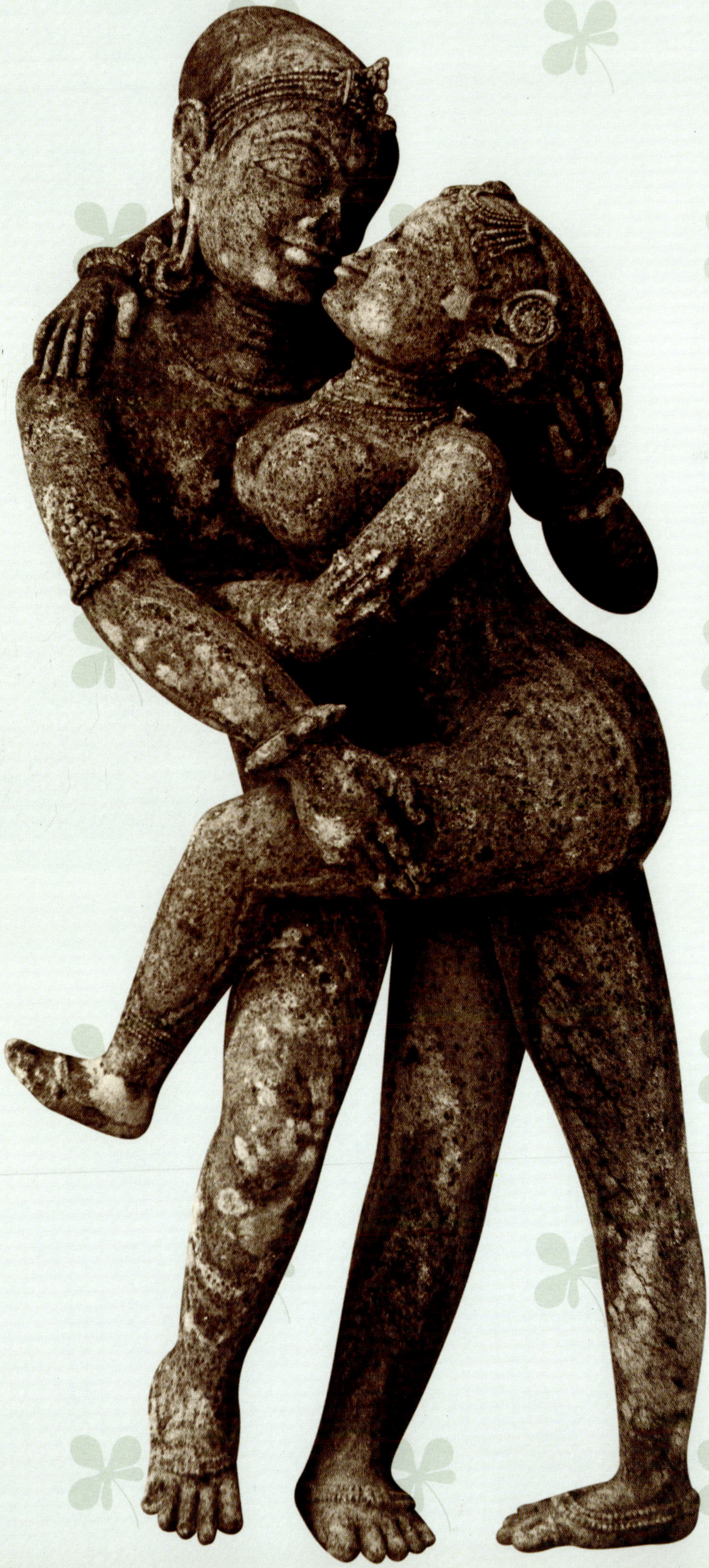

The Sun temple at Konark: Dedicated to *Surya*, the Sun God, the temple must surely be one of the most extraordinary temples in the world. Narasimha I of the Ganga dynasty started the construction in 1278 on an ancient site on the coast in Orissa but was unable to complete it. Massive in size, the temple is an interpolation of a *ratha*, chariot, drawn by the seven horses of *Surya*. The life-size figures in close union are in sync with nature's own union of plants. The learned *acharyas*, men of great knowledge, spoke of *vriksha dhirudhakam*, plant twining around a tree. This is immortalised in stone as the *nayika* climbs over her lover's body and clings to his shoulder, while his hands, similar to a vine clinging to a tree, grasp her. *Stone, Konark, 11-12th century.*

ing with nails acts like fuel for the fire. But nails should only be used when a degree of excitement has been attained.

THE MAGIC OF A KISS

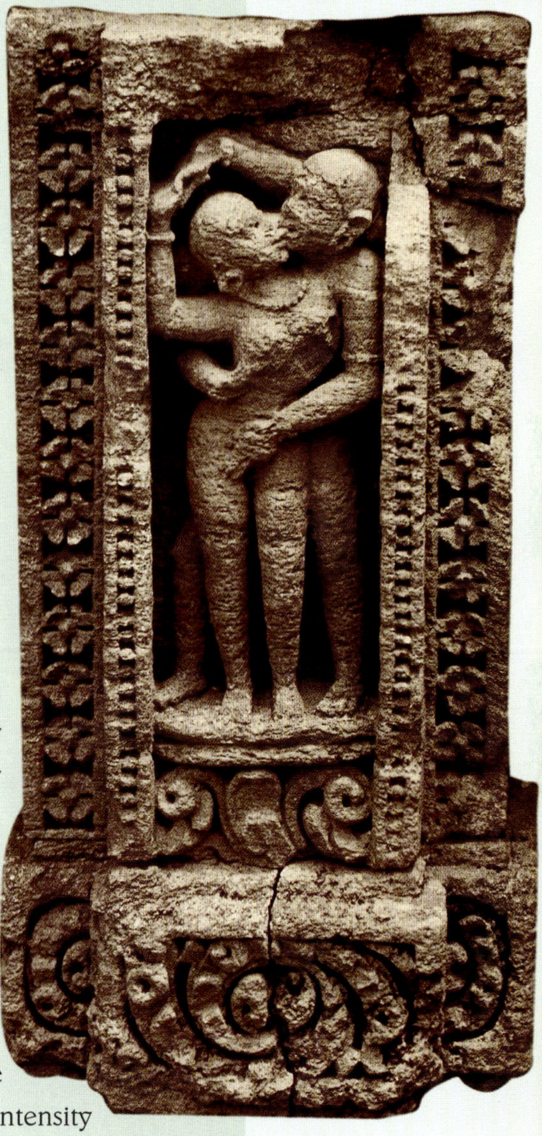

The most important act of foreplay is a kiss, a profound expression of love, faith and intimacy. Romeo and Juliet's parting kiss at the balcony and countless such moments remain with us, transcending time and location. But kissing too, is an art that requires practice and skill.

While kissing traditionally follows an embrace, it serves as a prompt accelerator. If you kiss your lover while he is asleep, you are expressing your desire to unite. Kisses vary in form and intensity. The most common form of the kiss is the *Samam*, the straight kiss, when your lips are in direct contact with those of your lover's. You can bend towards each other in the *Tiryak* or bent kiss. If one turns up the face of the other, holding the other's head and chin, it is the *Udbrantam* kiss. And during any of these, if one of you presses the lower lip of the other, it is *Piditakam* or the pressed kiss.

The most intense kissing takes place before actual coition and it raises the intensity of love, enabling lovers to unite at an emotional level. The female body is littered with points sensitive to kissing: the forehead, cheeks, eyes, breasts, lips, and palate inside the mouth. The *Kama Sutra* advises that these kisses should be reciprocated fittingly.

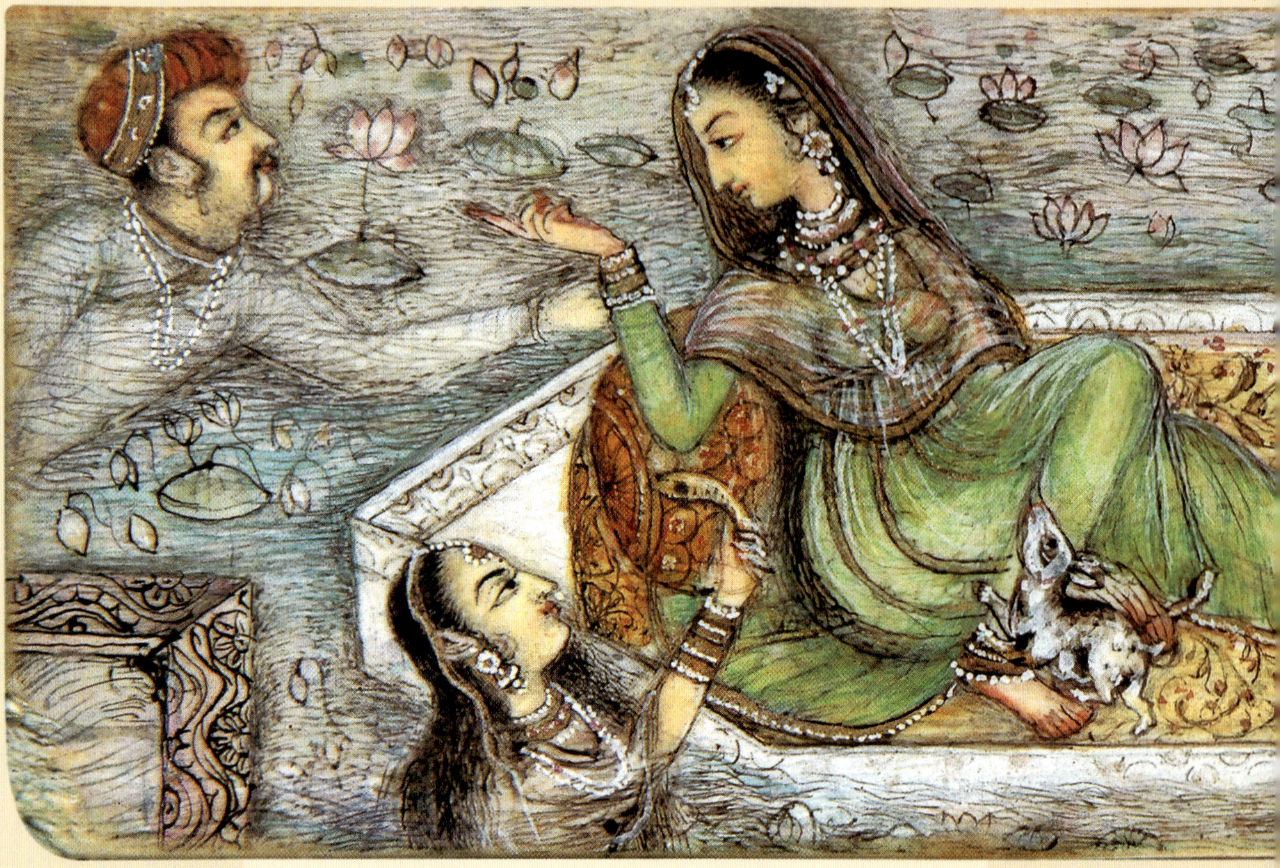

For a *kanya*, young girl, the *Kama Sutra* prescribes three kinds of kisses. When a girl touches the mouth of her lover with her own, but does not do anything herself, it is a nominal kiss called *Nimikatam*. If a girl sets aside her bashfulness a little, touches the lip pressed upon her mouth, and with it moves only her lower lip, it is a throbbing kiss termed *Sphuritakam*. Then there is *Ghattiitakam* or the touching kiss, when the girl touches her lover's lip with her tongue, shuts her eyes and places her hands on those of her lover.

The acts of kissing, embracing and biting are mostly thought of in relation to foreplay. There is no harm, and in fact, it is encouraged that these be performed in isolation, on their own for initiating a relationship. A passionate embrace before parting as the day beckons or a tender kiss while in a 'public' place, eases the distance between lovers,

A meeting by chance: In the scene here, the hero is on the prowl. It is evening and his romantic feelings are lighting up his torch! By chance, a very beautiful young lady, in her garden, feels a sudden impulse and the artist draws us into their realm. *Painting on ivory, Jaipur, Rajasthan, 20th century.*

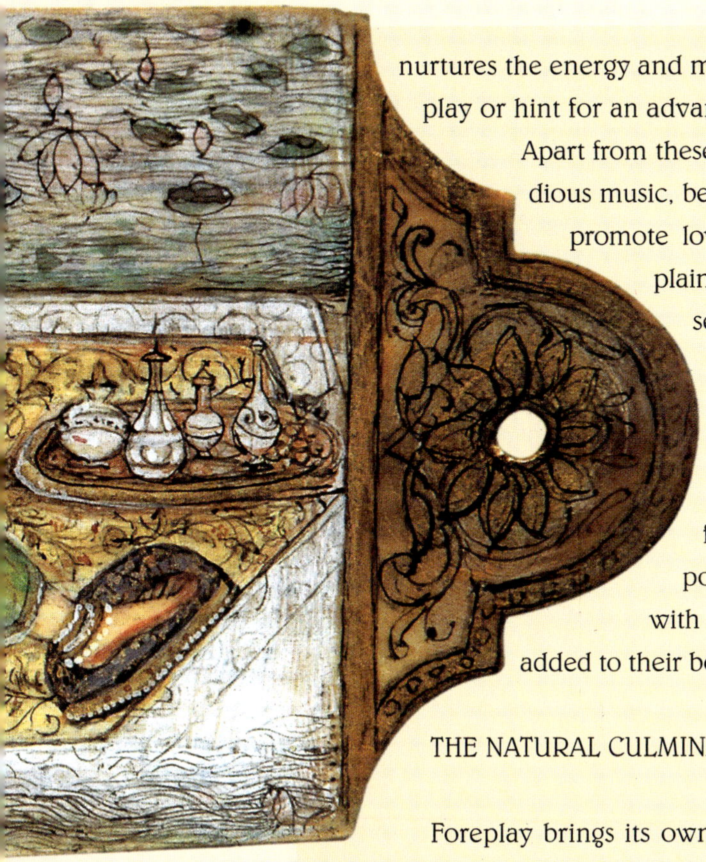

nurtures the energy and makes for an extended foreplay or hint for an advance in the relationship.

Apart from these, ingredients such as melodious music, beautiful sights and fragrance promote love. Some women may be plain, but they win men by their seductive voices and skill in music. There are some who combine beauty with intellect like the Salonnières of France or the courtesans from medieval India whose poise and grace combined with wit and poetic expression added to their bodily charm.

THE NATURAL CULMINATION

Foreplay brings its own pleasure and arouses the passions of both man and woman to a point where sexual union is a natural culmination. As women become more outspoken and move more freely in society, they are active players in the game of pleasure.

Once two lovers are overcome with love and desire, intercourse is the natural result. The *Kama Sutra* categorises sex types by the size of the *linga* (male organ), endurance and passion. Men are classified as one of three types: *Shasha*, the hare man; *Vrisha*, the bull man; *Ashwa*, the horse man. Women too are grouped according to the depth of the *yoni* (the vagina), as: *Mrigi*, female deer; *Vadava*, a mare; *Hastini*, female elephant.

It is generally believed that men attain climax faster than women. But Auddalaki states: 'Females do not emit as males do. Males simply remove their desire, while females, from their conscious desire, feel a certain kind of pleasure,

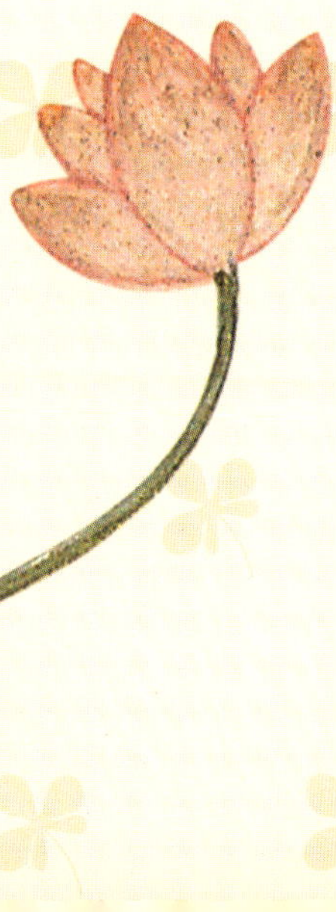

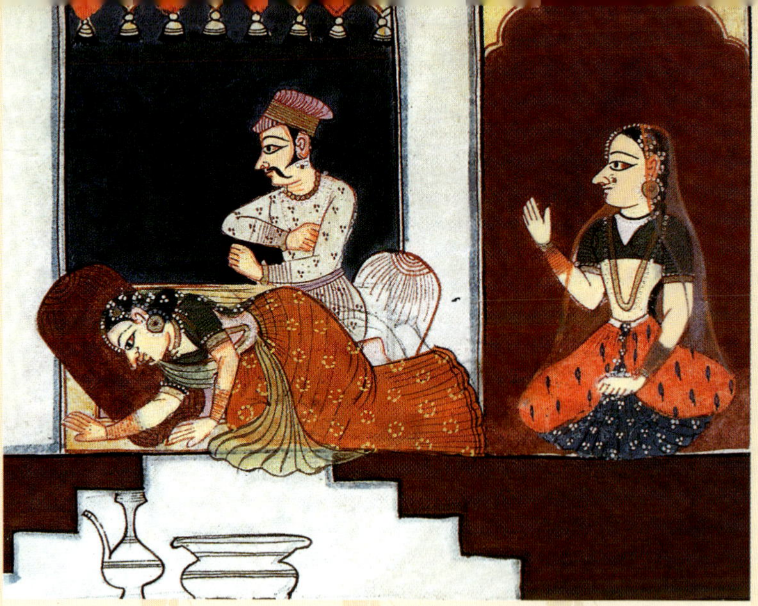

Erotic paintings of Sirohi: In the painting on the facing page, the posture shows the *nayika*, love struck, swooning with passion, loosing control, falling backwards and kissing the hero, as the hero is caught by surprise. The quality of the erotic paintings of Sirohi was influenced by the taste of the royal rulers, who commissioned a team of talented artists, who occupied a place of pride in the palace atelier. This painting is a fine example, and is recognisable as an invaluable part of an important rare series, which instructs in the erotica as well as excites. They, therefore, fall into a category of a work that provides a deep understanding of the human penchant for erotica, pleasure, delight, love and desire. Vatsyayana has taken in full measure, the value and effects of the love play that gradually arouses the sexual passions and stirs up hot blood into the vital parts. When this takes place, a life of love is assured. *Miniature painting, Sirohi, Rajasthan, early 19th century. Private collection.*

which gives them satisfaction, but it is impossible for them to tell you what kind of pleasure they feel. The fact from which this becomes evident is, that males when engaged in coition, cease themselves after emission and are satisfied, but not so with the females.' But this is more a matter of the mind and chemistry shared between the two partners. It is commendable to be sensitive to the needs of one's partner for a mutually fulfilling experience.

The *Kama Sutra* describes sixty-four positions at the time of congress. Some are simple, such as the *Veshtitakam*, the twining position, when you place one of your thighs over that of your lover's. There is also *Vadavakam*, the mare's position, when the woman forcibly holds in her *yoni* the *linga* after it is in. Others such as the *Shoolachitakam* and *Paravrittakam* are more physically complex and require practice.

All these positions are purely indicative as the guiding text itself clarifies - once the fire of passion is stoked, there are no strict rules. A compatible partner, understanding, communication and most of all, love, are the ingredients for a smooth and enduring relationship.

The sexual act is punctuated with actions such as kissing and scratching. Biting, striking, grunting and hissing are other actions during the congress that intensify *raga* or *vega*, the love that fills the soul and overflows in union. Biting either accompanies, or follows the piercing act. It makes the heat of exchange with your partner increase. All the kissing points except the upper lip, tongue and eyes are suitable for

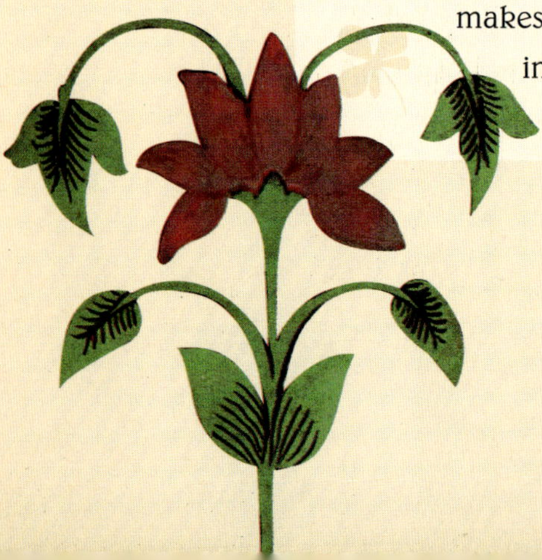

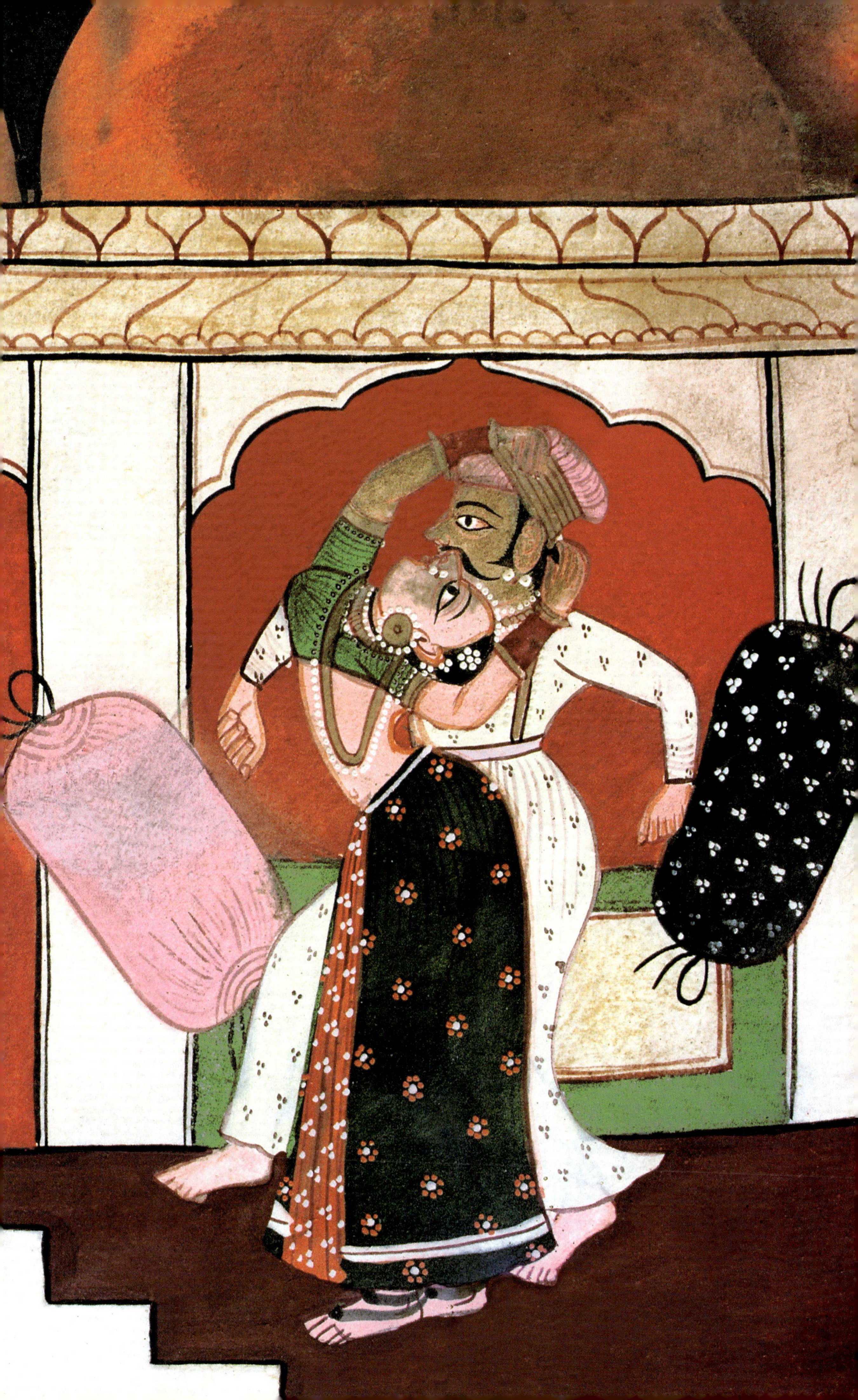

biting. The neck, armpits, thighs and breasts are the ideal spots. Of the bite, the *Kama Sutra* says:

When a man bites a woman forcibly, she should angrily do the same to him with double force. Thus a dot should be returned with a line of dots and a line of dots with a broken cloud, and if she is excessively chafed, she should begin to quarrel with him at once.

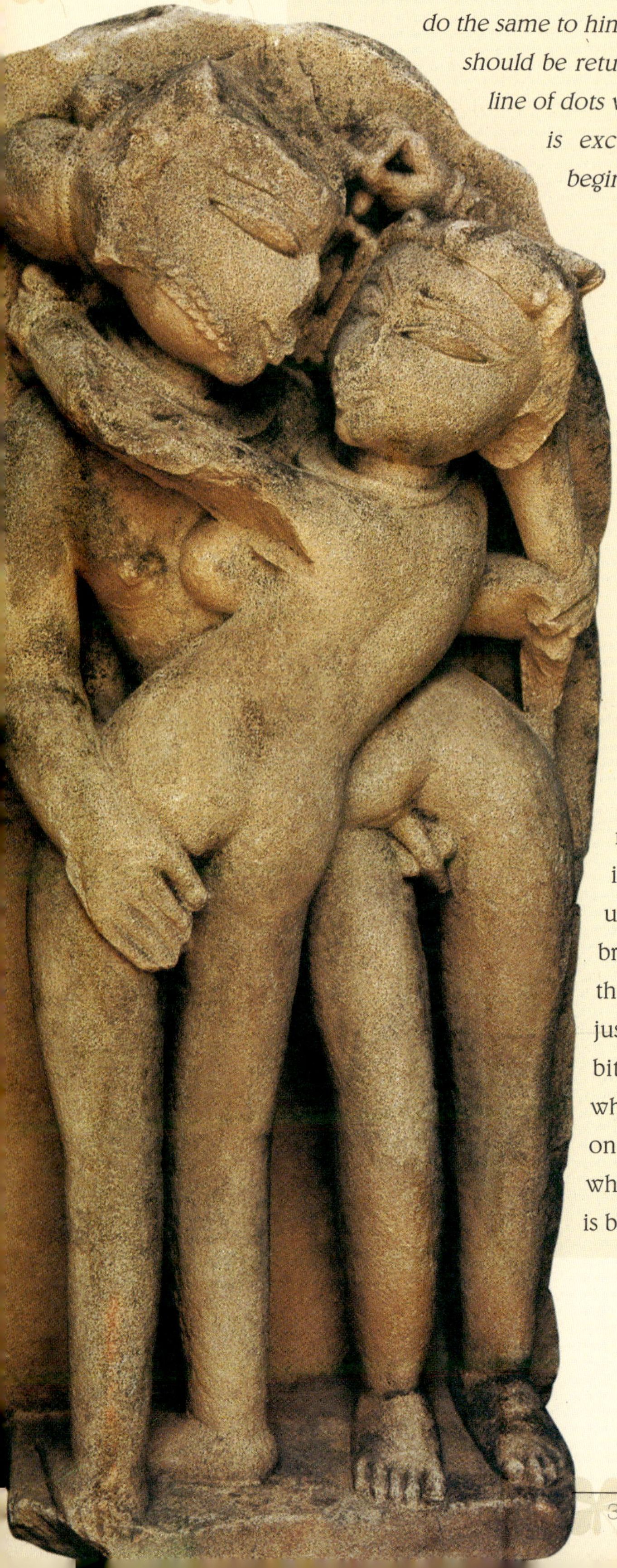

The *Kama Sutra* also offers a more refined typology of bites. Some of the more explicit bites are the *coral and jewel*, where both lips and teeth are used. When biting is done with all the teeth, it is called *a line of jewels*. When biting consists of unequal risings, it is a *garland*, and when it comes from the space between the teeth, it is called the *broken cloud*. This is best impressed on the breasts. *Biting of a wild boar* consists of many broad rows of dots near one another with red intervals in between. This is usually impressed on the breasts and the shoulders. Then there is the *hidden bite*, which is just an excessive redness of the bitten skin, the *swollen bite*, where the skin is pressed down on both sides, and *the point*, when a small portion of the skin is bitten with two teeth only.

Mithuna couple- lovers.
It is all in all, a very vigorous game of seduction, to attract and to charm him with all her alluring gestures. Her motions are full of suggestion, getting bolder all the time. Very exciting and flirtatious, her desirable body brushes against him, throwing him into an uncontrollable forceful embrace, drawing her so tightly into his grasp that her breath gasps at such lustfulness. A flash of anger and her sharp claws are ready to strike as she flutters her seductive eyelashes, coated with kohl. *Stone, Khajuraho, Chandella, 12-13th century. Private collection.*

Love play: The loving look accompanies the playful embrace of her hands and feet, and her whole body. He is encouraged and squeezes her busts. *Wood carving from temple chariot, Tamil Nadu, 20th century. Private collection.*

Following pages:
Kinds of union according to size: The folio on the right side illustrates two men describing the different classifications of the male *linga*, phallus into three distinct sizes: the *shasha*, hare man, whose *linga* is six fingers long; the *vrisha*, bull man, whose *linga* is eight fingers long; and *ashwa*, horse man, whose *linga* is 12 fingers long. Unusually, the artist has drawn models seen in the foreground of the animals to emphasise these points. The hero and heroine exchange the comparative depth of the female *yoni*, vagina, which is also classified as the *mrigi*, female deer; *vadava*, a mare; and *hastini*, female elephant. Vatsyayana states scientifically that there are, therefore, three equal unions, between corresponding couples, and six unequal unions when the dimensions do not correspond, making nine kinds of unions in all. Erotic satisfaction is assured, provided the hero is aware of his heroine's peculiarities, prior to commencing the seduction. Noticeable are the flowing *jamas*, long flowing coat and stylish *pugrees*, headwear, a particularly long cloth tied in the manner of this region. *Miniature painting,* Kokashastra *bound manuscript, Deogarh, Rajasthan, mid 18th century. Lance Dane collection.*

If biting does not appeal to your senses, you can express the spurt of energy by hissing and striking. These actions release the heightened passion of intercourse. Striking gives rise to *Sitkrita* or the pain of passion, and is usually accompanied by hissing or various other sounds like *hinkara* (nasal); *koojita* (cooing); and *rudita* (whimpering).

FULFILLMENT IN MARRIAGE

Marriage is a sensitive issue that demands clarity and conviction between the couple before sanction from others is sought. There are numerous suggestions in the *Kama Sutra* for a man to gain a woman in marriage. He may approach her family; he may disparage a potential husband in the minds of the girl's family. There is no definite way to act though.

The *Kama Sutra* also lists different types of marriages of which the most pertinent in our times is the *Gandharva Vivaha*. Literally, this translates into Love Marriage.

A girl who is much sought after should marry the man that she likes, who she thinks would be obedient to her, and capable of giving her pleasure. But when from the desire of wealth, a girl is married by her parents to a rich man without

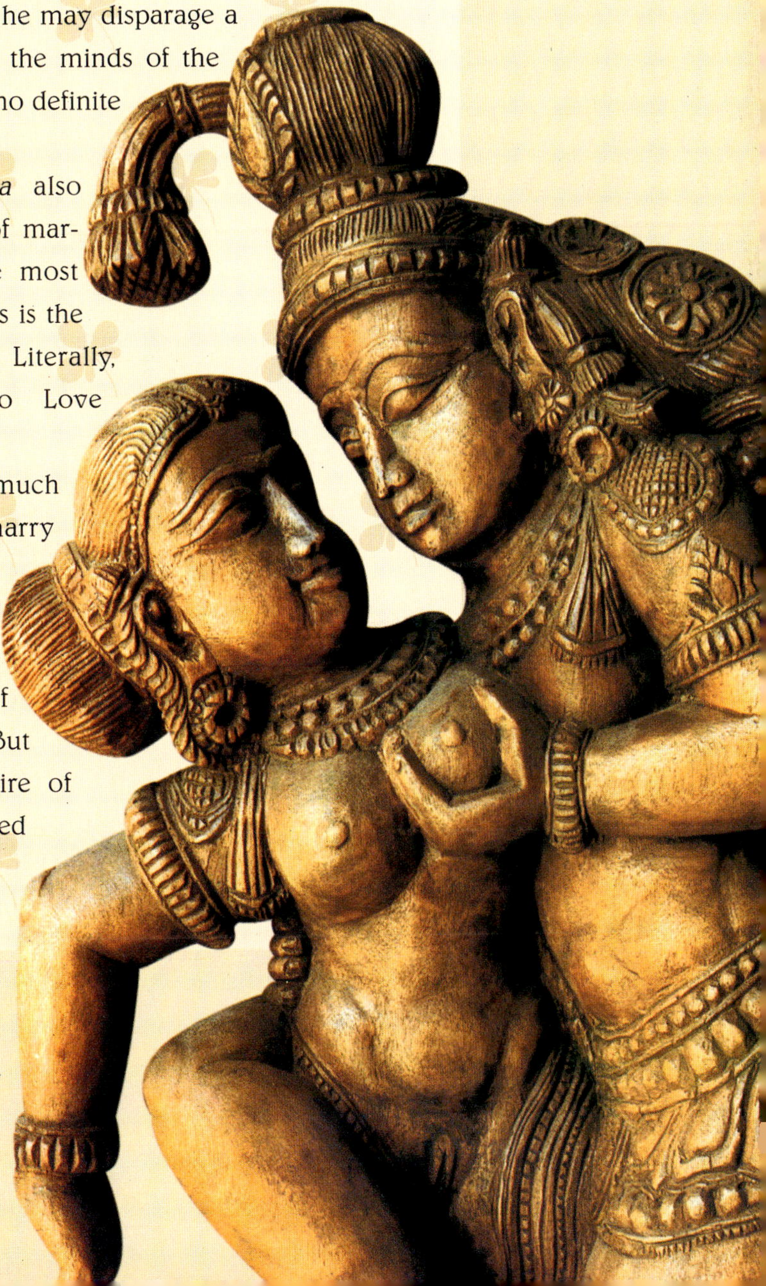

पषनिसुनीयोवतडी ॥ मोसोंपेलोनोक । ज्यानिथमोहिव
तादेदे ॥ २२ दोहा ॥ तबपषनिमुषऋायनै ॥ सातमदईवना
य ॥ निरतैजपकरऋाईयो ॥ ऋोबैऋमलवनाय ॥ २३ ॥
वारता ॥ तबकोकपषणीनैकदे ॥ जिणदिनथरोनांममोने
वताय । जिणदिनसामगरीतयारकरावां । तदपषनीक

कोकनैपषणीवानांकरैबै:

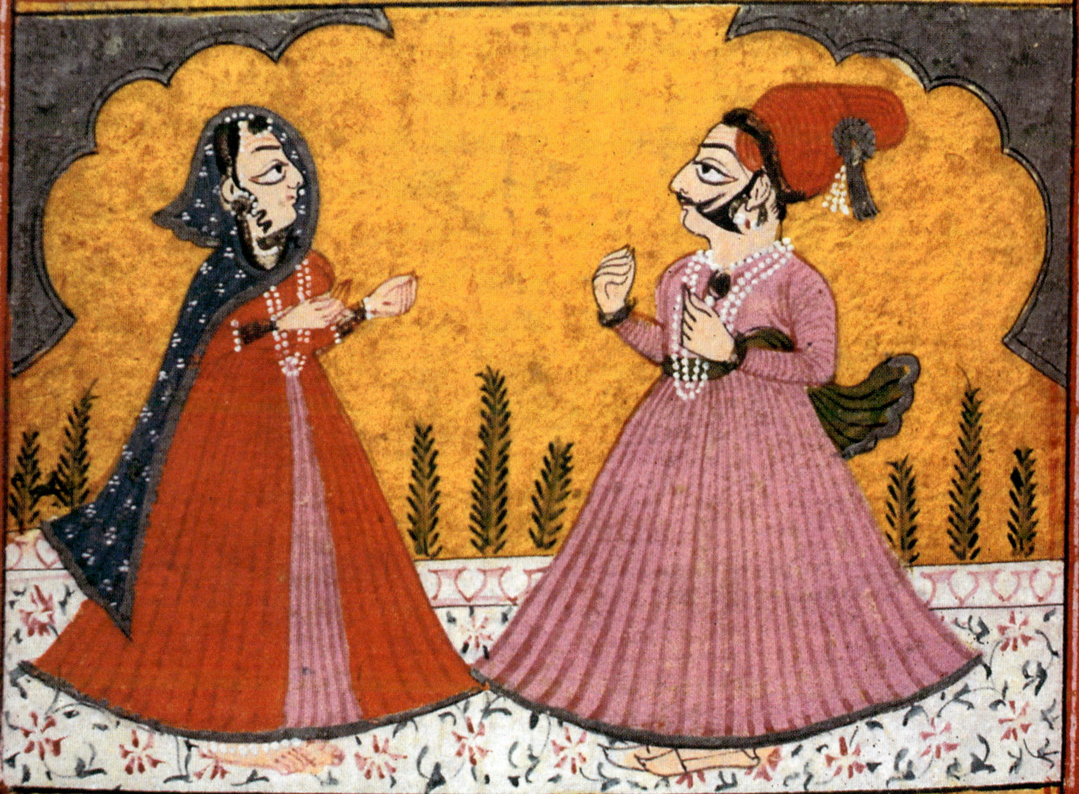

ह्या । सातमरैदिनश्रीदेवाजीरीहूजाकरथारैसुहऋागल
तयारहुं ॥ कातोम्हंमनैजोपैबै ॥ काम्हारीटांगतलैतनैका
हूंबू ॥ तदसातमरैदिनऋायो ॥ तबकोकपषणीनैकहायो
ऋाजसमसमीछे । तुमताबवणावकरनैवेगीपरवारजे । ऋ

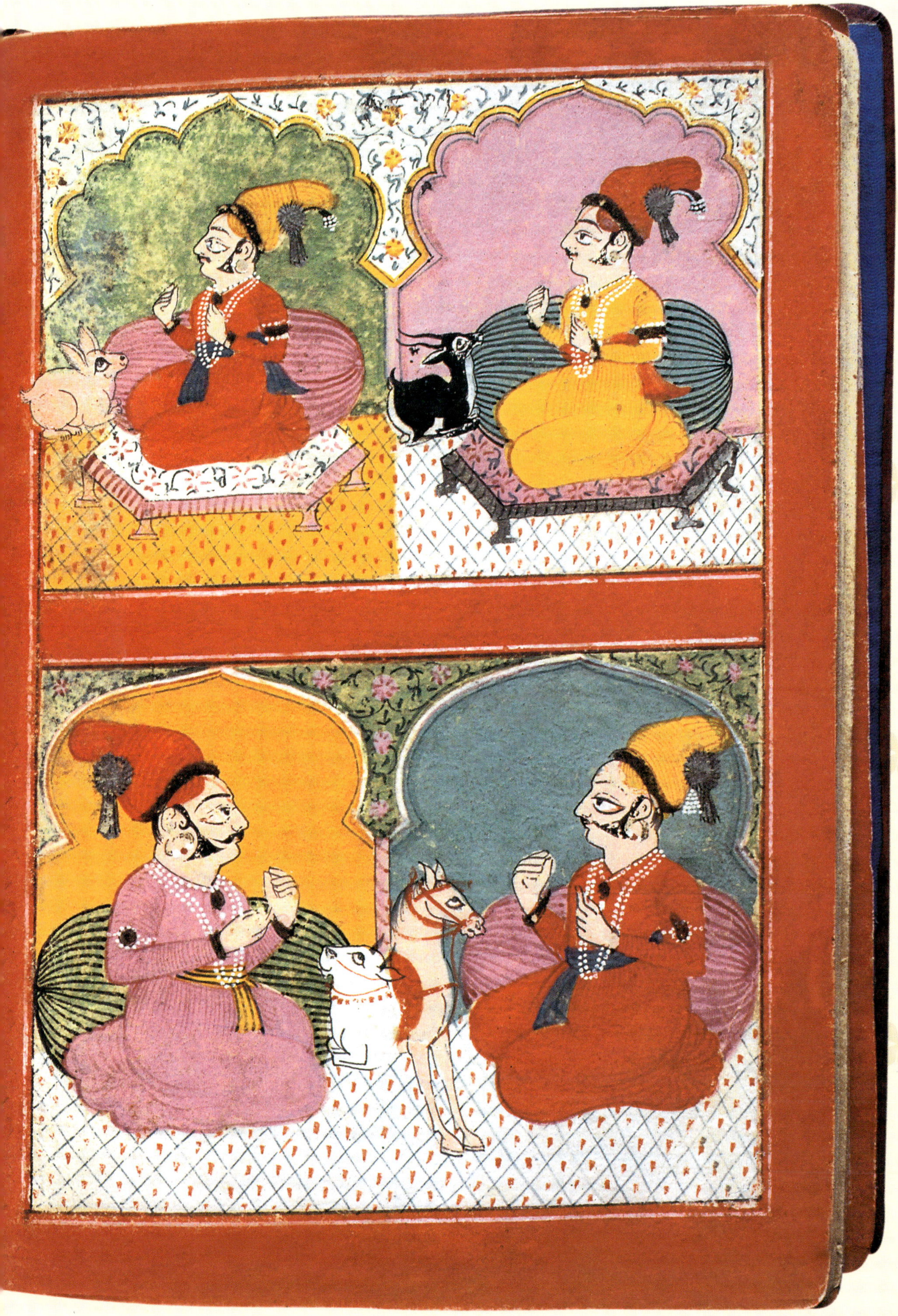

taking into consideration the character or looks of the bridegroom, or when given to a man who has several wives, she never becomes attached to the man, even though he be endowed with good qualities, obedient to her will, active, strong and healthy, and anxious to please her in any way.

IT QUALIFIES THAT:

A man who is of a low mind, who has fallen from his social position, an old man or a man who is much given to travelling, does not deserve to be married; neither does one, who has many wives and children, or one who is devoted to sport and gambling, and who comes to his wife only when he likes. Of all the lovers of a girl, he only is her true husband who possesses the qualities that are liked by her, and such a husband only enjoys real superiority over her, because he is the husband of love.

After marriage, every effort should be made to cushion the experience of a new home for the woman. Time spent in togetherness is vital to ease the changes a newly wed bride encounters. Sexual intercourse, too, should be experienced comfortably. There is no harm in abstaining should either not be in a receptive mood. In fact, the *Kama Sutra* advises abstention from sex for the first three nights altogether. Then the husband should make advances with soft embraces, reassuring conversations, dining together, till such time that sex becomes a natural culmination.

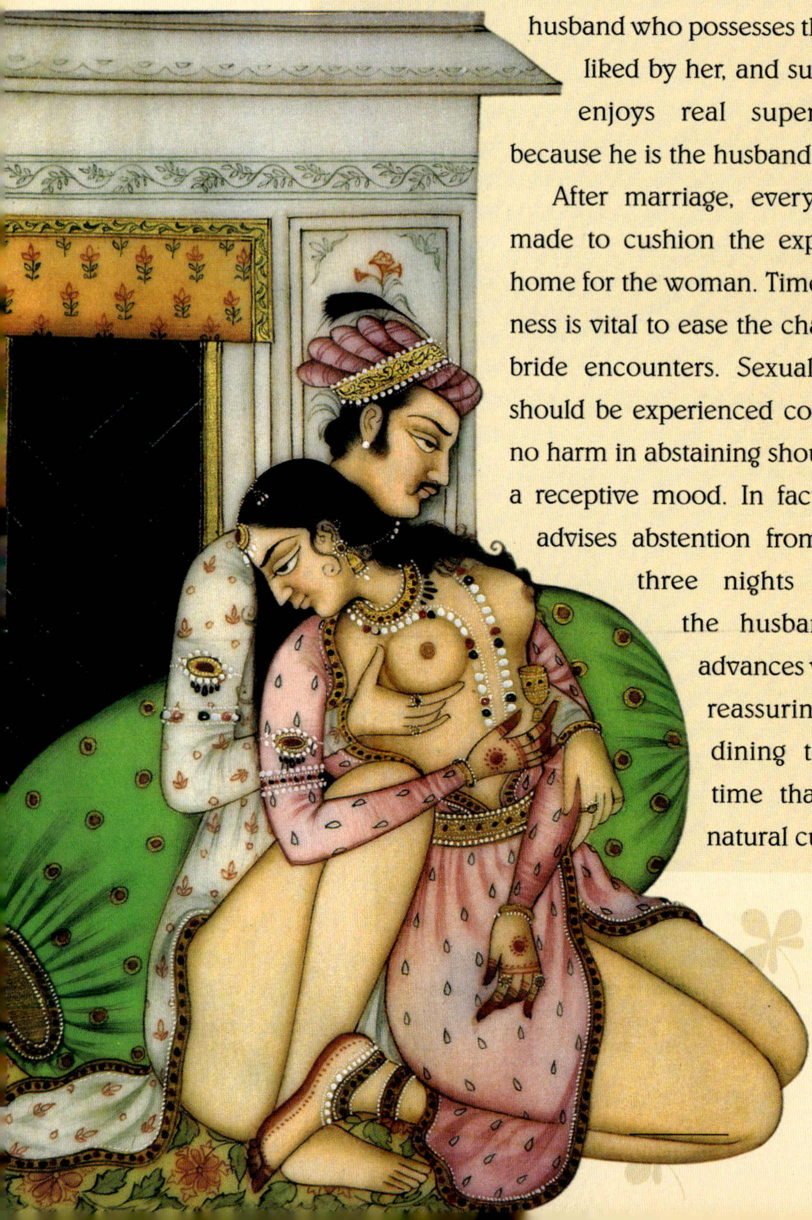

Painting on ivory: The medium of ivory innovates an additional feel for the posture, in the decorative surrounding of palatial splendour. Many of the princely palaces in Rajasthan have been converted into hotels and the splendour enhanced to benefit the visitors. *Miniature on ivory, Jaipur, 20th century. Private collection.*
Facing page: **The Kiss:** "So long as lips shall kiss and the eyes shall see, so long lives this and this gives life to thee." *Wood, Tamil Nadu, 20th century, Late Dr. Mulkraj Anand collection.*
Following page: **The begining of love:** A young man, his touch so delicate and gentle, plucks the cord of his lover's lower garment. She is pleased and accedes to his suggestion. The *Kamasastras* are a storehouse of information on the knowledge of erotica, a collection of learning on sexual well-being, as expounded by historical Hindi writers. They were sought out for study by Vatsyayana, whose *Kama Sutra* was a masterful compilation as also was the *Rati-Rahassya*, where Koka Pandit recorded his personal experiences with a nymphomaniac. His handbook classifies females into different categories. However the *Rati-Rahassya* did not enjoy the same popularity as the *Kama Sutra. Miniature painting on ivory, Jodhpur, Rajasthan, 20th century. Private collection.*

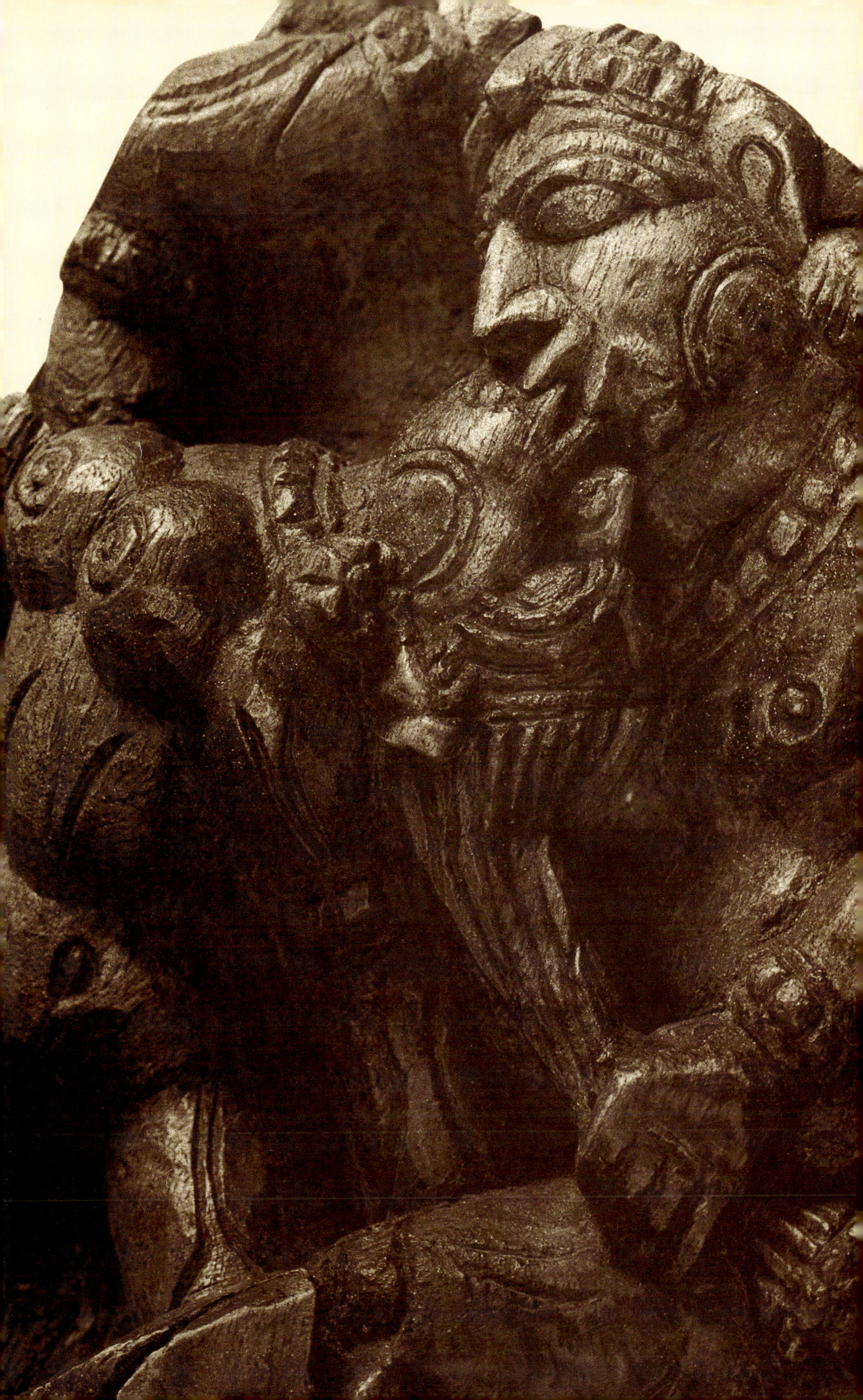

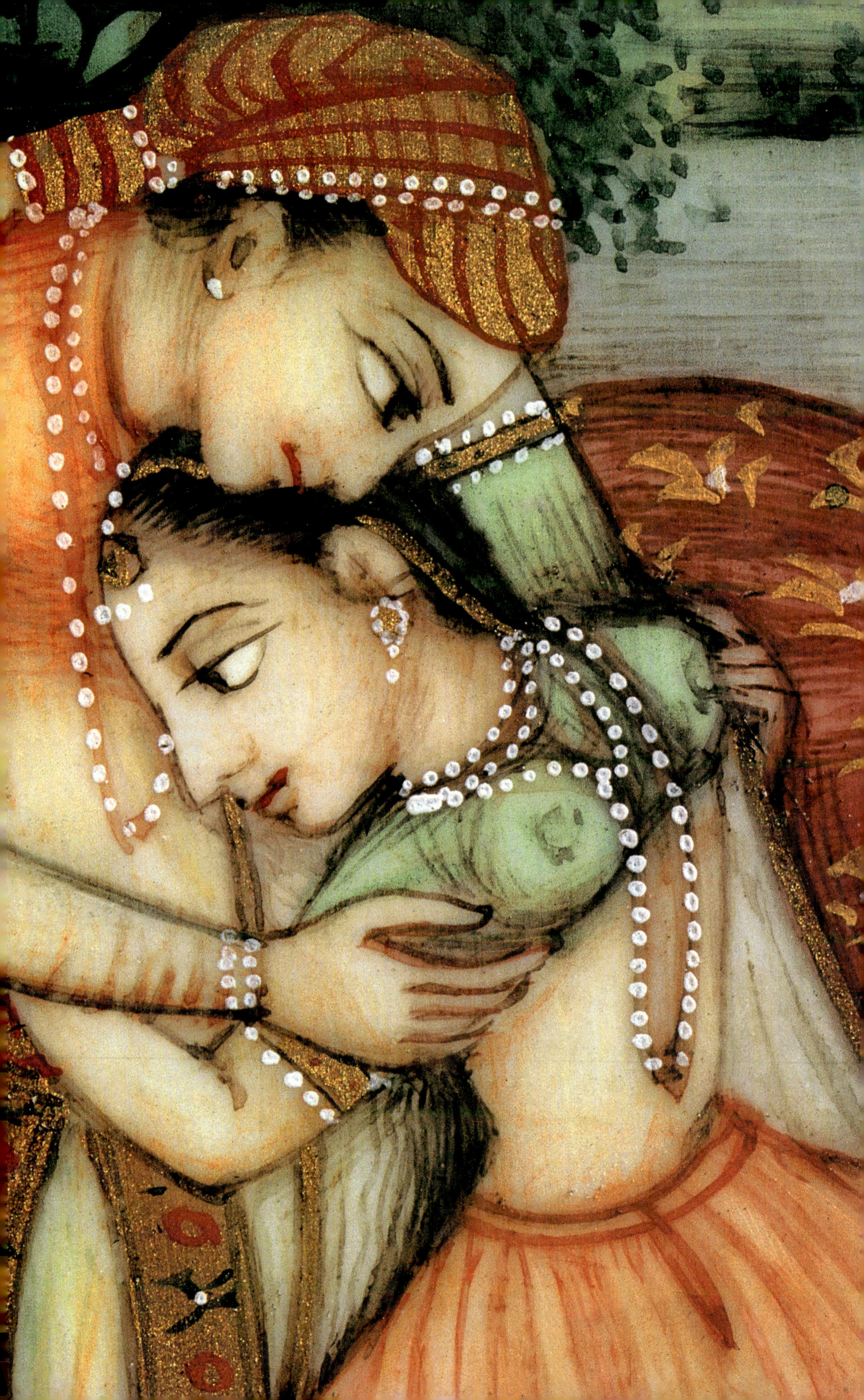

Thus a man practising Dharma, Artha and Kama enjoys happiness both in this world and the world to come. The good perform those actions in which there is no fear as to what is to result from them in the next world, and in which there is no danger to their welfare. Any action which conduces to the practice of Dharma, Artha and Kama together, or any of two, or even one of them, should be performed, but an action which conduces to the practice of one of them at the expense of the remaining two should not be performed

Kama Sutra

leading a well-ordered LIFE

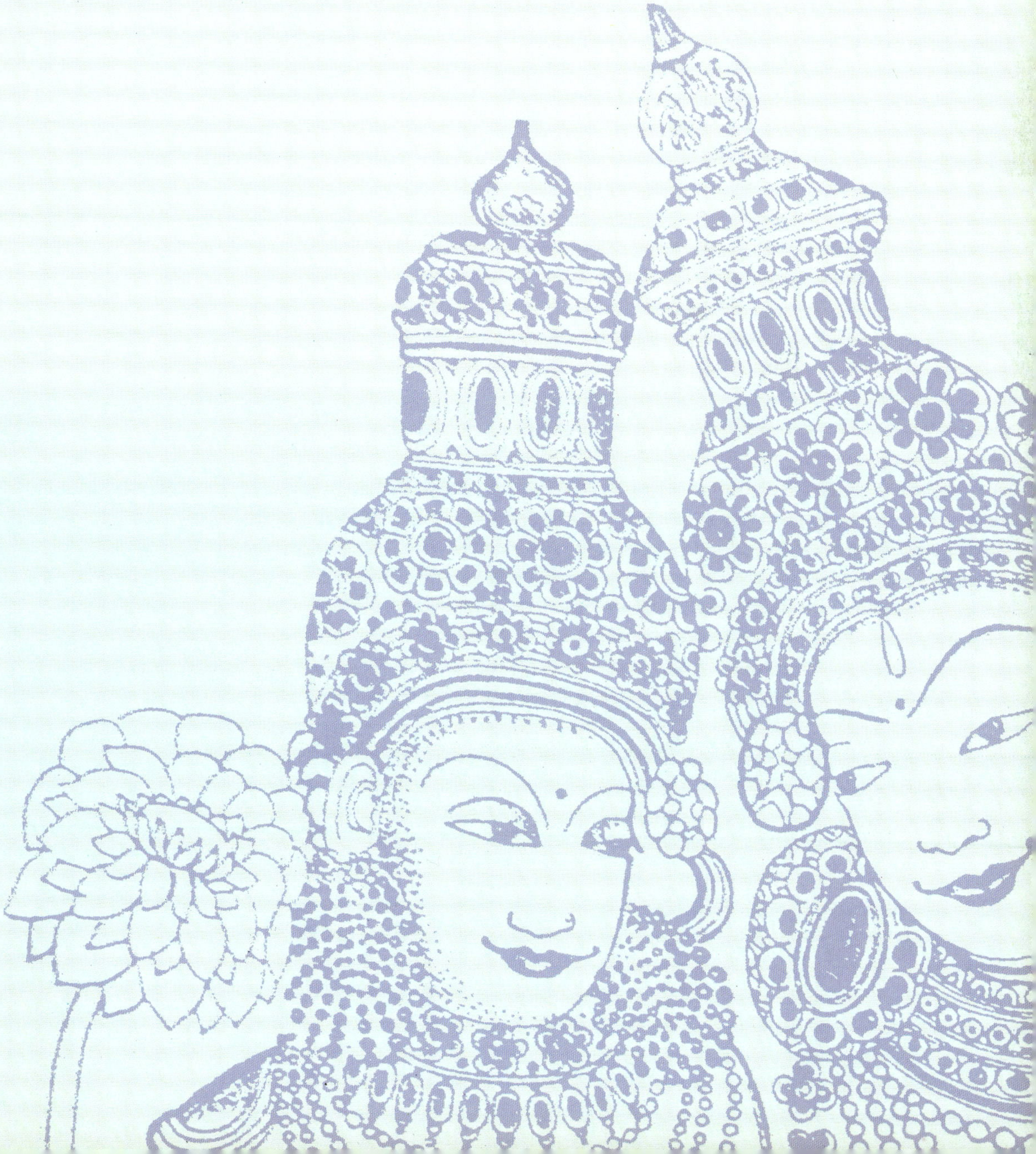

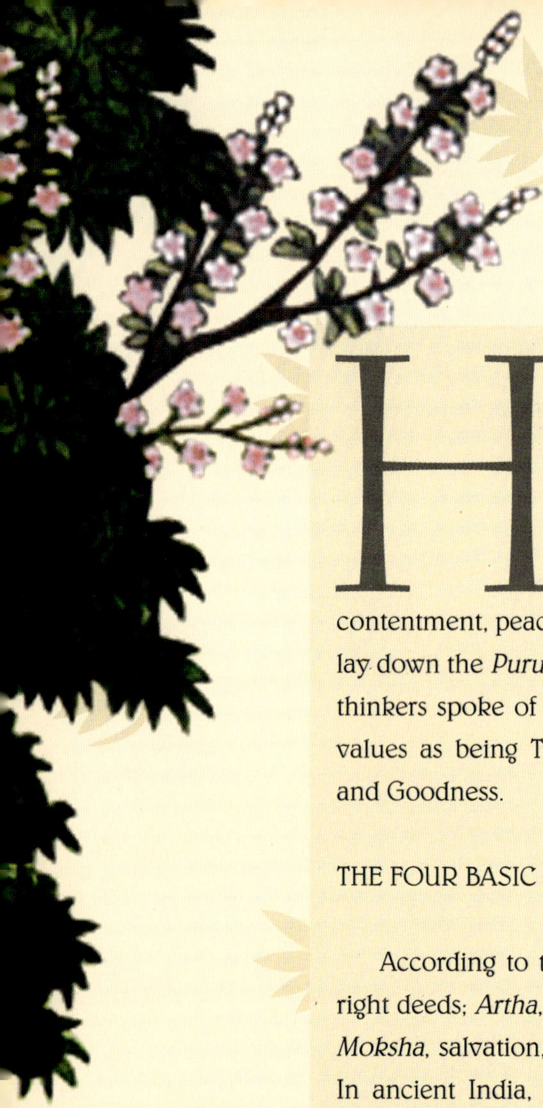

Human beings long for pure joy and everlasting happiness, free from the least trace of pain and misery. Every culture and religion has laid down its own framework as guidelines to be followed for the purpose of achieving contentment, peace and salvation. Hindu saints proceeded to lay down the *Purushartha*, aims and purposes of life. Western thinkers spoke of the ultimate values as being Truth, Beauty and Goodness.

THE FOUR BASIC GOALS

According to the *Agni Purana*, *Dharma*, right deeds; *Artha*, power; *Kama*, pleasure and *Moksha*, salvation, are the primary goals of life. In ancient India, the study of the *Kama Shastra*, Erotic Science, was at par with the study of the *Dharma Shastra* or Religious and Social Law and the *Artha Shastra* or Economic and Political Science. *Dharma* includes piety, duty, morality, social obligations and justice. *Artha* signifies material success and power and can also be translated as profit or gain. *Kama* represents love, pleasure and sex, and more broadly, encompasses the entire sensual experience of the arts and music. The *Kama Sutra* provides detailed advice on love and passion, within the social and moral context of the times in which it was written. In fact, some later commentators, including Devadatta Shastri (in 1964) stated that though the *Kama Sutra* deals with such topics as adultery, it does not appear to favour its practice. It was advised that the *Purusharthas*

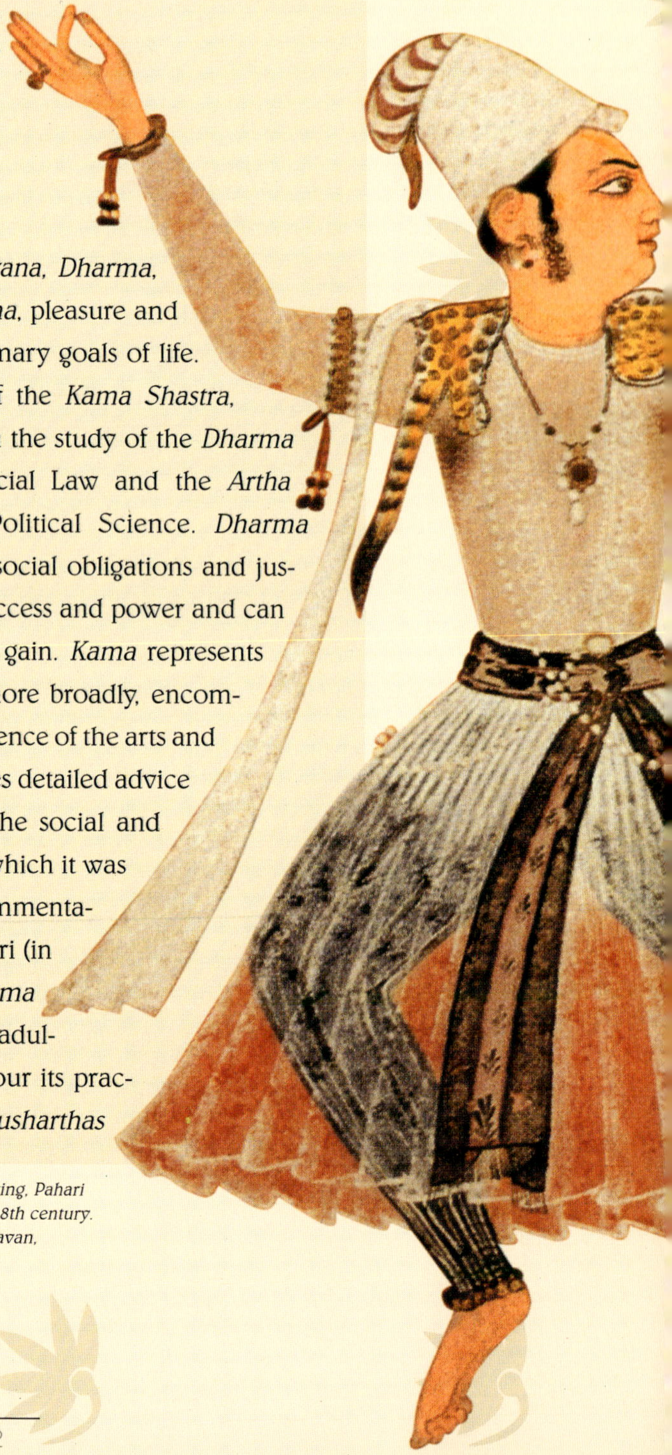

Celebrations: The tradition of calling music parties to celebrate household functions enables the social gathering to thoroughly enjoy the ceremonies.

Miniature painting, Pahari Hills, Mankot, 18th century. Bharat Kala Bhavan, Varanasi.

were followed in the correct manner prescribed, else, their scope, content and importance could be altered.

Dharma means the stability of society, the maintenance of social order, and the general welfare of mankind. Whatever is conducive to the fulfillment of this purpose is called *Dharma*. *Artha* is the acquisition of arts, land, gold, cattle, wealth, equipages and friends. Further, it is the protection of what is acquired, and the increase of what is protected. *Artha* is the foundation upon which the whole structure of life has been built, and all the other *Purusharthas* can be achieved only by the fulfillment of this primary goal. *Kama* was recognised in ancient Indian thought as the stimulus of action, and personified as the god of erotic love. *Kama* implies enjoyment of appropriate objects through the five senses of hearing, feeling, seeing, tasting and smelling, assisted by the mind and soul. It is from *Dharma* that *Artha* and *Kama* result. *Artha* and *Kama* form the two fundamental aspirations of man. *Moksha* literally means deliverance, that is deliverance of the soul from bondage. Our great philosophers argue that so long as the soul is imprisoned in the body, subject to the shackles of human tendencies and inclinations, and is enmeshed in materialism, it will never be free from the taint of misery, pain and suffering. *Moksha* results from the

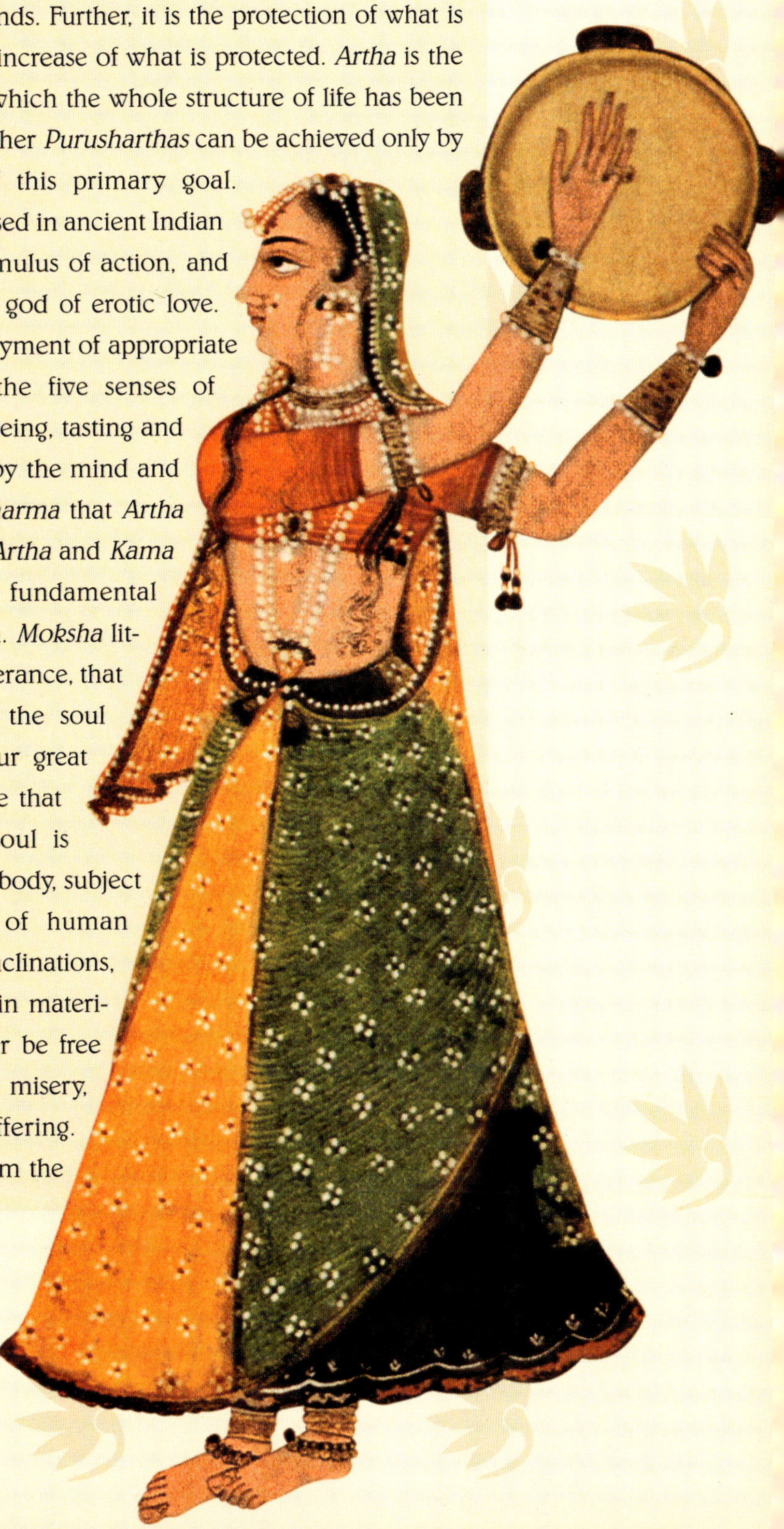

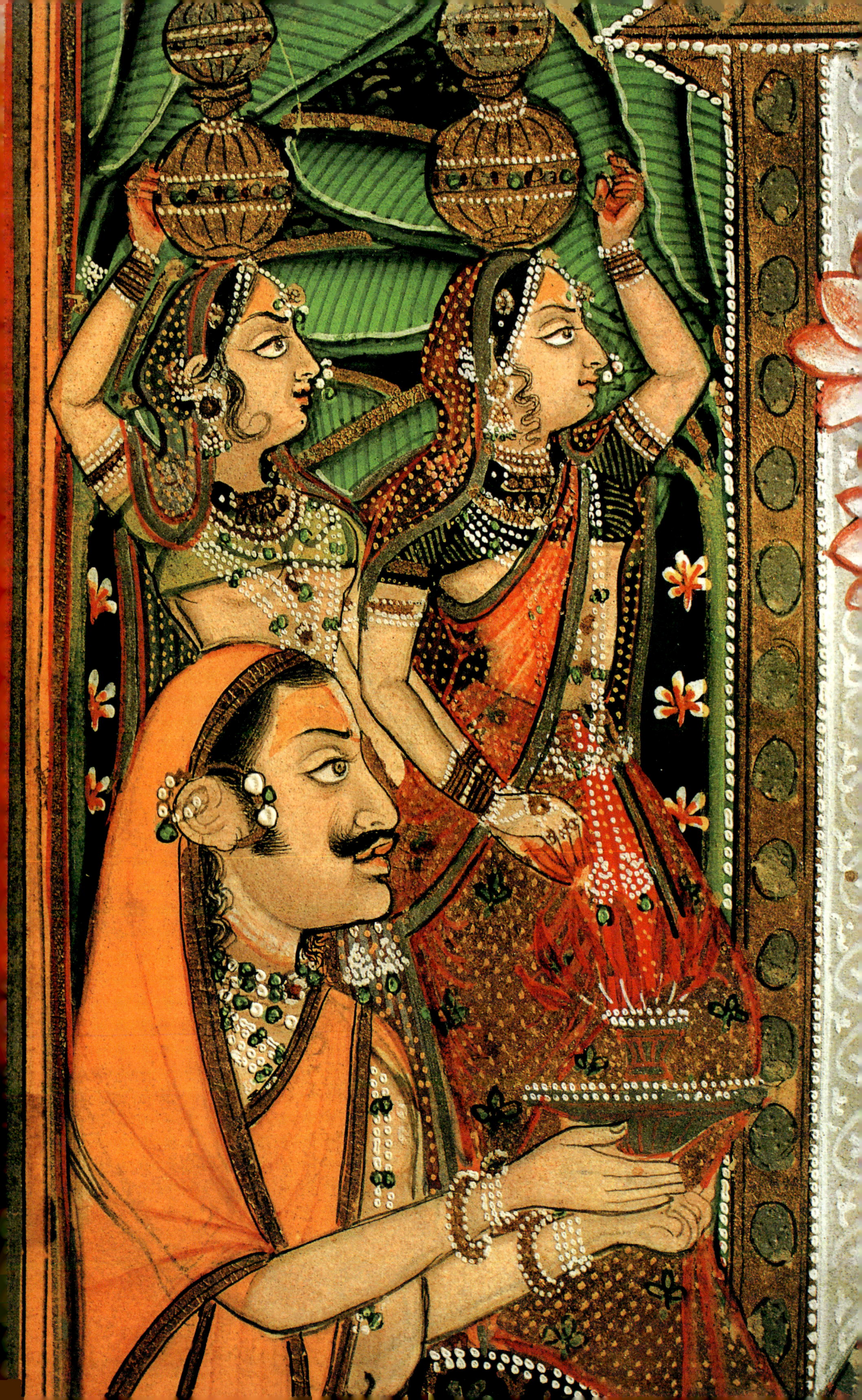

extinction of false knowledge, which causes the extinction of lust and hate, which extinguishes all *karmas*, which again results in cessation of all births. When the cycle of births and deaths is at an end, sorrow ceases and *Moksha*, the perfect state of bliss, is attained.

Sexuality and erotica are seen as being important, integrated elements of human existence - the same as eating - and apart from serving sensual pleasures, they also help mankind to propagate. The sensual pleasures of erotica and sexuality not only serve to increase the joys of life and maintain psychological balance, they aid the further development of the mental-spiritual spheres. The senses are perceived as being a refinement of the physical on a higher plane of consciousness. In short, sexuality and erotica contain the secret of life within them.

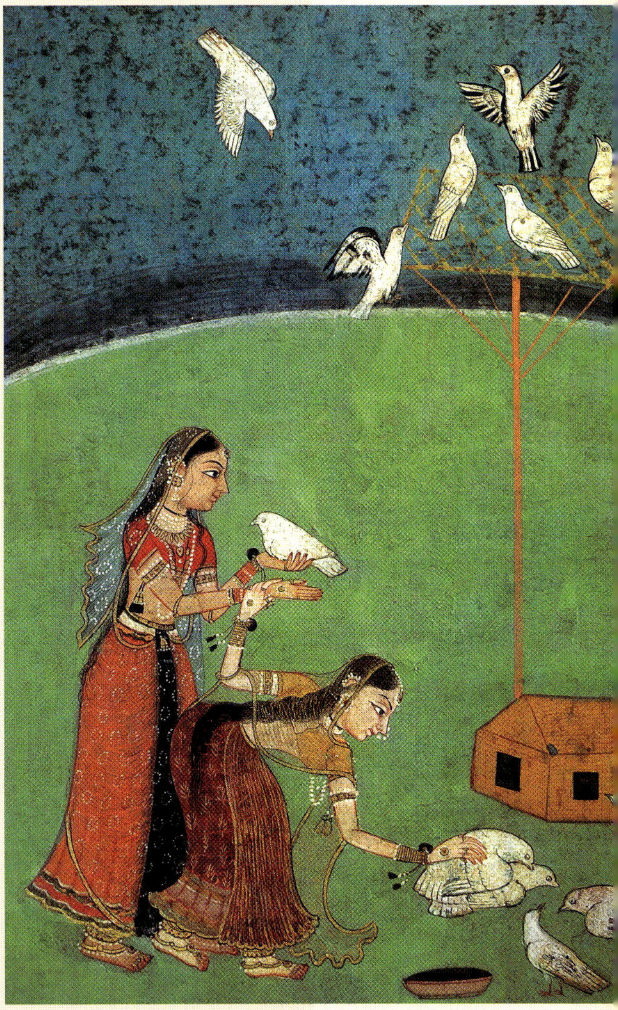

THE ROLE OF THE *NAYAK* AND THE *NAYIKA*

From 500 B. C. to A. D. 500 Indian society was largely suffused with the pleasure principle. A man's prime concern was to keep his beloved happy and he spend his wealth and resources on gold and jewels so that she could adorn herself. Even in the figurative arts, the treatment of the female was opulent - ornate jewellery bedecked her. However, by A. D. 600, the heavy bosomed, voluptuous figure of a woman was

Daily Domestic life: The home stead is the place where the whole family finds the time to be together, and enjoy the performance of all those tasks, which ensure tranquillity. Such aspects find a place in the artistic menu, and they abound with paintings depicting the woman, enjoying in her home as the caretaker. These are two specific examples of elegance of home life, its peace and serenity depict scenes from the household *puja* and the garden. *Facing page:* Pichhvai, *Nathdwara, Rajasthan, 19th century. Above: Miniature painting, Jodhpur, Rajasthan, 18th century. Private collection.*

replaced by a slender, refined and stylised one. From the gracefully poised dancing girl of Mohenjo Daro through the sensuality of the Didarganj *yakshi*, to the *apsaras* at Ajanta and Ellora and Khajuraho, Indian visual culture is soaked in celebrating femininity. During Vatsyayana's time, sexual practice was an essential component in the education of a *nagarika*, citizen. The *nagarika* was adept in the sixty-four *kalas*, arts, in which the behavioural nuances of men and women were taught alongside other arts and sciences. A woman was a full participant in sexual life, an active player and not just the passive recipient of a man's lust.

Indian literature has explored the various aspects of love and classified its heroines in relation to their lovers based on the intensity of their love, depth of love, expression, maturity of age, experience and temperament into eight types or the *ashtanayikas*, eight heroines. Radha was considered the supreme *nayika* and Lord Krishna, the supreme *nayaka*.

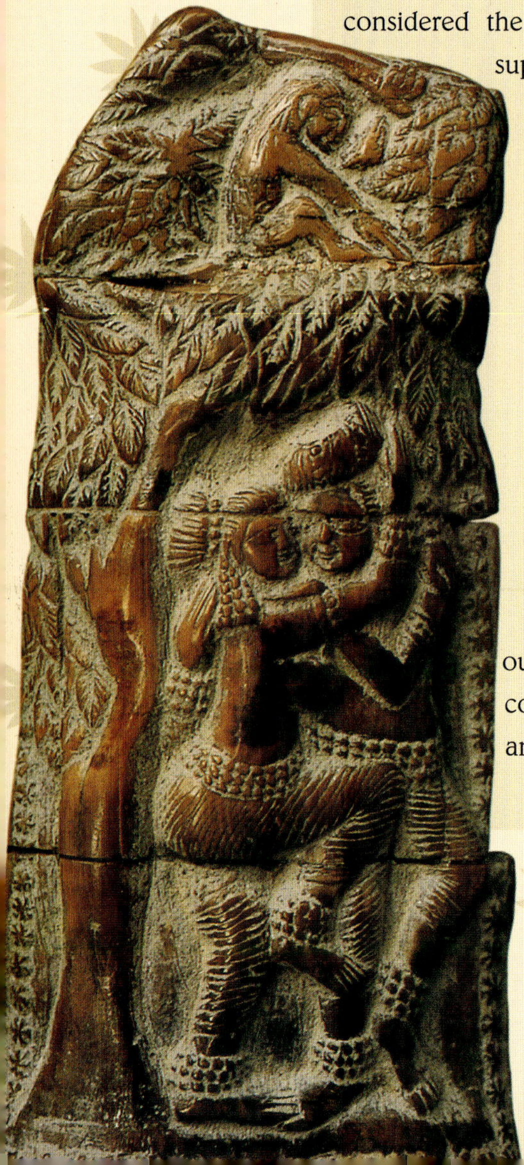

The cloud but comprises fire, smoke,
vapour and breeze,
And love's messenger is a mind
with wisdom sealed
Yet he realised it not and implores encore.
The amorous heart is irrational to all,
Animate and insentient alike.
Meghadoot, Kalidasa

A WOMAN'S HOME: HER HAVEN

From the very beginning, a wife endeavours to attract the comfort zones by showing continually her devotion, her good temper, and her wisdom.

Homemaking is an art, a science, a skill

Love unites: In recent times archaeological sites were excavated in handraketugarh (now West Bengal) revealing large numbers of terracotta objects of amazing artistic merit and extraordinary originality, also a few ivory and bone figurines. Seen here, a small masterpiece bespeaks the life and times of Kalidasa's play Malavika and Agnimitra, celebrating the beauty of Malvika.
The sculpture has a fine touch of artistic merit, a vision of amorous lovers under the wind blown tree. Costumes reveal the style of the period. Terracotta, *Chandraketugarh, Sunga, 1st century A.D., Private collection.*

Facing page: **Love bites:** In the elaborate palaces of the kings of Nayaka, Tamil Nadu, three hundred years ago, ivory decorative objects exquisitely carved by adept craftsmen, gave added pleasure to daily life. Such toiletry objects, like hair combs give expression of romantic love play to the love *sutras* of Vatsyanana's descriptions on love games, biting and pinching, which are fascinating. Biting as seen by excessive redness of the skin in a hidden place, is called the 'hidden bite'. The skin pressed down on both sides, is the 'swollen bite'. Small portions of skin, when bitten with two teeth only, is the 'point' and when such small portions of the skin are bitten with all teeth and lips, it is called the 'coral and the jewel'. If done with all the teeth, it is the 'line of jewels'. The biting, which consists of unequal rising in a circle, and which comes from the space between the teeth, is called the 'broken cloud'. Impressed on the breasts it is a 'talisman'. Gracefully, the artist has depicted the *nayika* biting her hero's toe, in return for his not too forceful tugs on her braided hair. *Ivory comb, Tamil Nadu, 18th century. Private collection.*

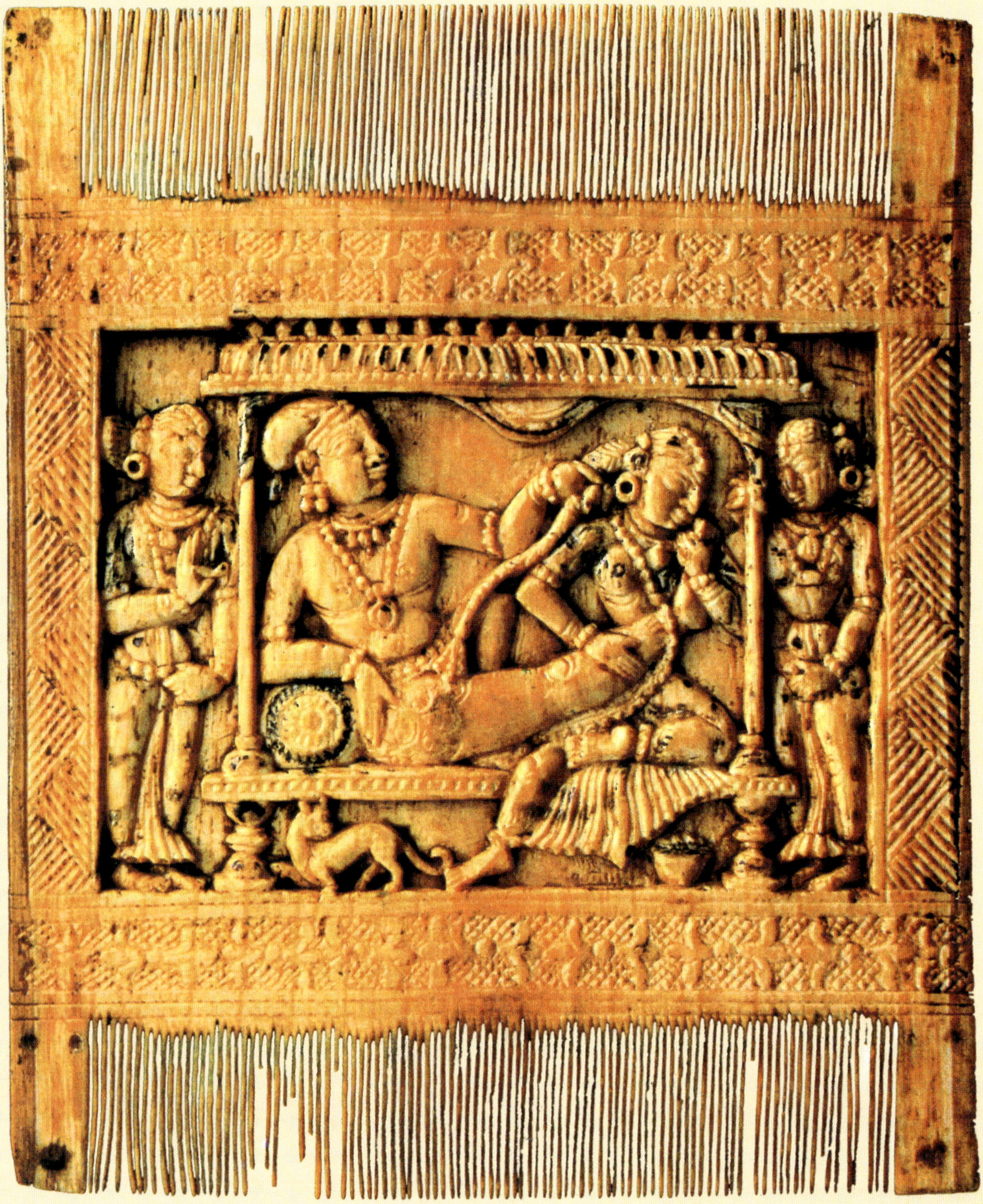

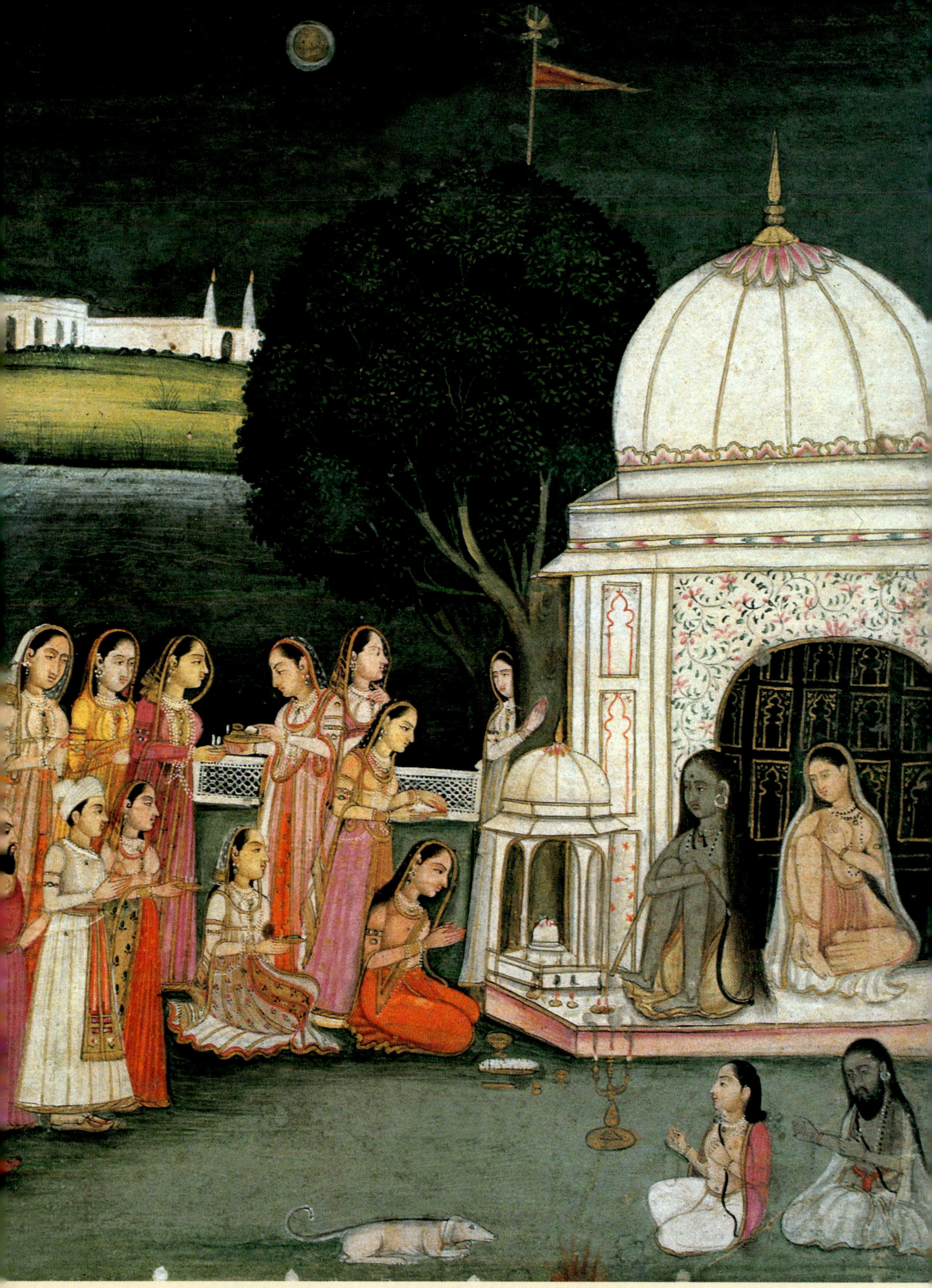

Shivalinga puja: The wonderful miniature paintings of Rajasthan also depicted their stoic and fearless womenfolk, who were beautiful and feminine, and devoted to the worship of their deities. The family is seen here in a private secluded pavilion, for rituals and the daily *puja*. The ambience is peaceful and calm as the princess is conducting worship of the *linga*, before a gathering of attendants and in the presence of a *yogini*, female *sadhu*. The garden area with the tree extending its leaf laden branches highlight the background palace monuments. *Miniature painting, Udaipur, Rajasthan, late 19th century.*

and most of all, an extremely emotional engagement. It is the primary theatre where the man-woman relationship is performed and materialises. While love is the foundation on which this unit is built, its edifice is made of more practical fare.

In olden times, the roles and duties of man and wife were clearly defined. Girls were trained in the fine nuances of homemaking since childhood. Functions were demarcated and performed smoothly. There was time for work, leisure, social engagements and intimacy. In many cases, the family unit comprised of two or more generations as the joint family system was prevalent.

Within the urban spaces and with an emphasis on tertiary occupations, the joint family system has fragmented. Nuclear families are the fast-growing norm of the day. Add to that the fact that the onus of running the home is now shared equally by both partners and the distinctions between their roles is no longer as sharp as before. There are certain codes of conduct intrinsic to the Indian tradition that have been handed down through the generations, which stand a woman in good stead no matter where she builds a house. *Kama Sutra's Book IV*, devoted to the institution of marriage, opens with the following remarks:

A virtuous woman, who has affection for her husband, should act in conformity with his wishes as if he were a divine being, and take upon herself the whole care of his family.

Expressing concern and a willingness to share in activities, will instill a confidence and strength in the bonds a woman develops with her husband's family. Some of the ancient modes are seeds of timeless wisdom, which stand the test of time, and are merely re-framed from era to era. They are the means by which a woman can preserve the facets, nature has endowed her with, and which will bring good cheer as she shares them with those around her.

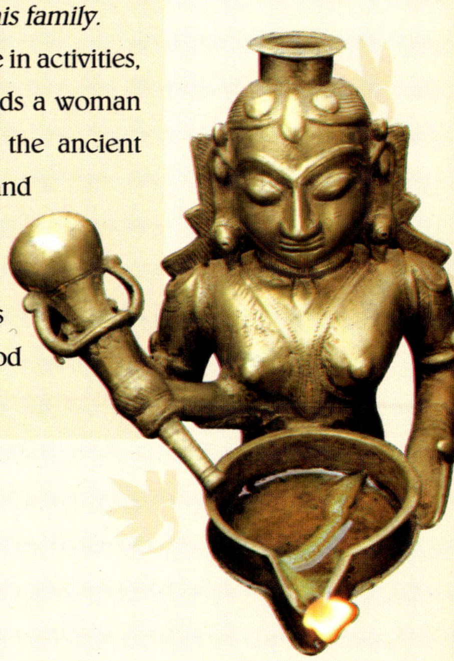

A brass *diya*: Oil lamp, from Tamil Nadu , with an interesting and unusual lamp holder. *Brass, late 18th century, Sanskriti Museum of Everyday Art, New Delhi.*

The offering: In the middle hours of the night , the hero and the heroine in reconciliation. Hero, a young noble man, enrobed in courtly fashion, listens attentively to his beloved and offers her *paan*, betel leaves. *Miniature painting, Udaipur, Rajasthan, 19th century. Private collection.*

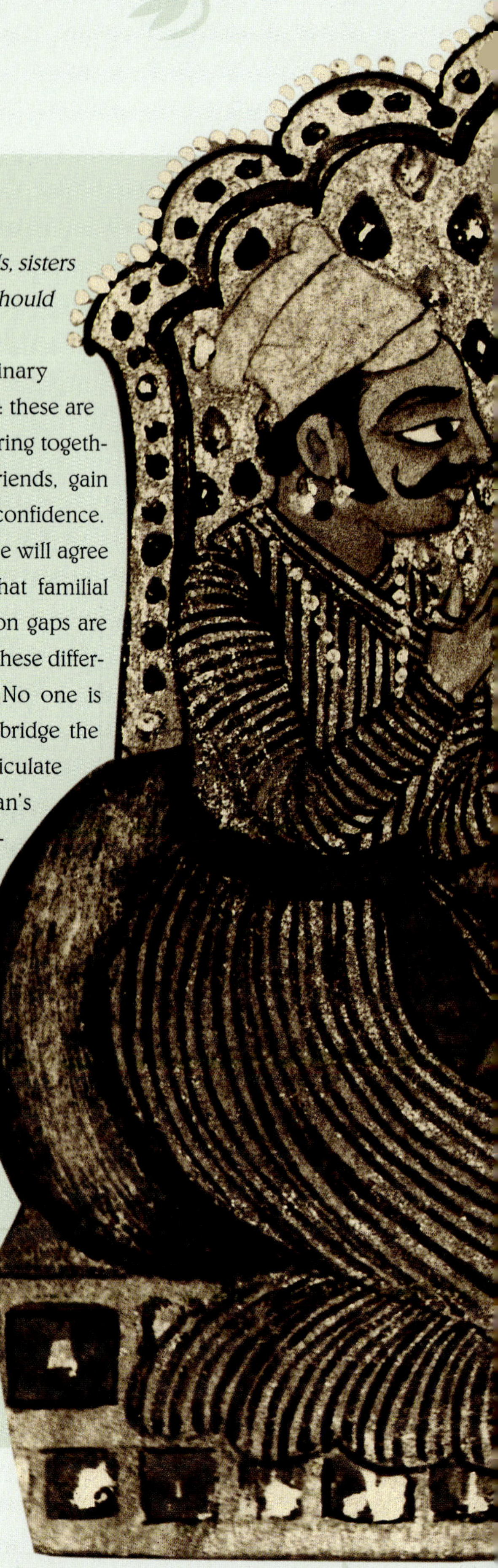

THE *KAMA SUTRA* STATES:

Towards parents, relations, friends, sisters and servants of her husband she should behave as they deserve.

Gifts, an outing, a special culinary feast , picnics, religious engagements: these are some ways in which a woman can bring together the larger body of family and friends, gain their affectation, and win her man's confidence.

Anyone with a familial experience will agree on the security, joy and comfort that familial bonds create. Even though generation gaps are more pronounced than ever before, these differences can be overcome with skill. No one is equipped better, than a woman, to bridge the gaps. Women have an invisible, inarticulate strength. When enraged, a woman's ferocity can border on destructiveness. She should make sure that her gestures of love and care are interpreted as such. In turn, the response should be one of compassion and concern.

The wife, whether she be a woman of noble family, or a virgin, widow remarried, or a concubine, should lead a chaste life, devoted to her husband. A woman acting thus will acquire *Dharma*, *Artha* and *Kama*, and keep her husband devoted to herself.

Even though there is a mild air of antiquity in this expression from the *Kama Sutra*, stay a while

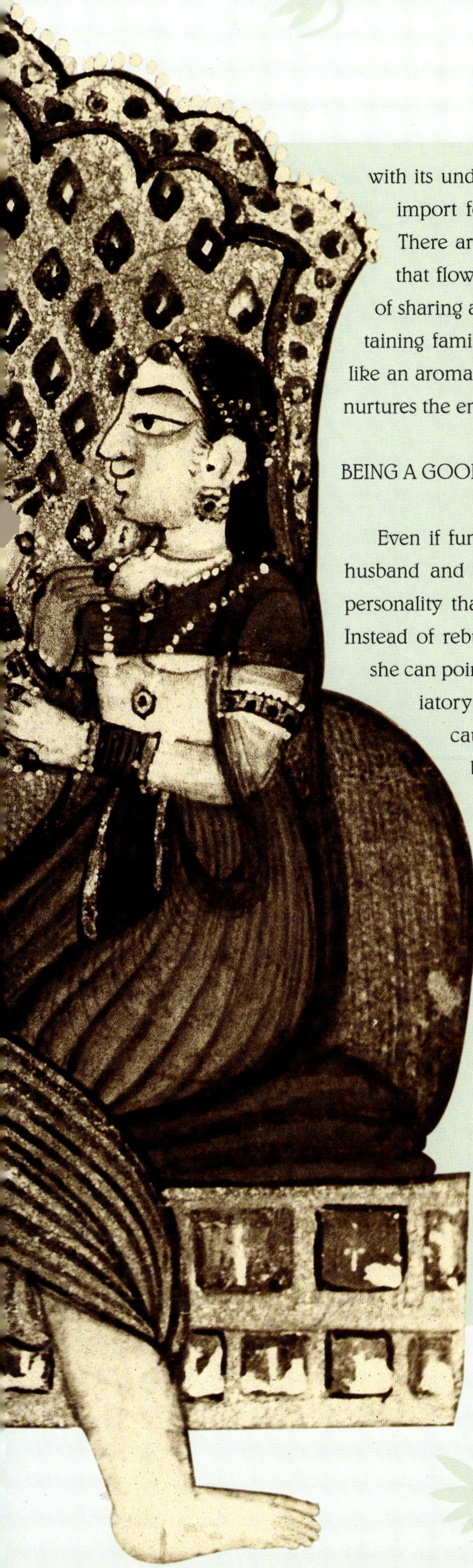

with its underlying thoughts, and one finds an import for the contemporary wife as well. There are some aspects of running a home that flow naturally from the feminine space of sharing and response. Similarly, while entertaining family and friends, a woman's touch is like an aromatic garnish on a delicacy. A woman nurtures the environment in a home.

BEING A GOOD WIFE

Even if functions are shared equally between husband and wife, it is the softness of a wife's personality that keeps the serenity in the house. Instead of rebuking and using abusive language, she can point out her husband's faults in conciliatory words. Says Gonardiya: 'There is no cause of dislike on the part of a husband so great as this (scolding) characteristic in a wife.' It is suggested that sulky expressions, muttering aside, and other mannerisms can be avoided when a wife is enraged with her other half. By carefully and sensitively negotiating disagreements, she will gain respect and affection.

Marriage changes the balance in a relationship from courtship to sharing of responsibilities. The difference in approach is encapsulated in language, both bodily and verbal, and through dress. The savvy wife is one who maintains the intimacy of her privacy with her husband within the confines of the bedroom.

Her everyday dress should be composed of thin, close-textured cloth, a few ornaments and flowers, and a little scent. She should also observe the fasts and vows of her husband, and when he tries to prevent her from doing this, she should persuade him to let her do so.

A husband needs attention and care. Small gestures are vital to strengthen the bond. Consider his likes and dislikes, avoid things that are not good for him, see him off and welcome him if schedules permit, and try to incorporate his tastes in the house even if they are different to yours. Not disturbing him while he is asleep, awakening him with gentle words, sounds or movements of the body, wearing ornaments of his liking while going anywhere with him - all these bring to the relationship a finesse, an identity and a sense of propriety. There are suggestions that hold equally for a man with respect to his beloved. Consent between partners for attending various social engagements makes participating in them more pleasant.

It is a folly that if both partners are working, their time of leisure is spent only in discussing their professional pursuits. This should be avoided with conscious effort. Conversations about the order of things at home are essential, but it is healthy to digress at times. The relaxation of togetherness can be perpetuated by talking about

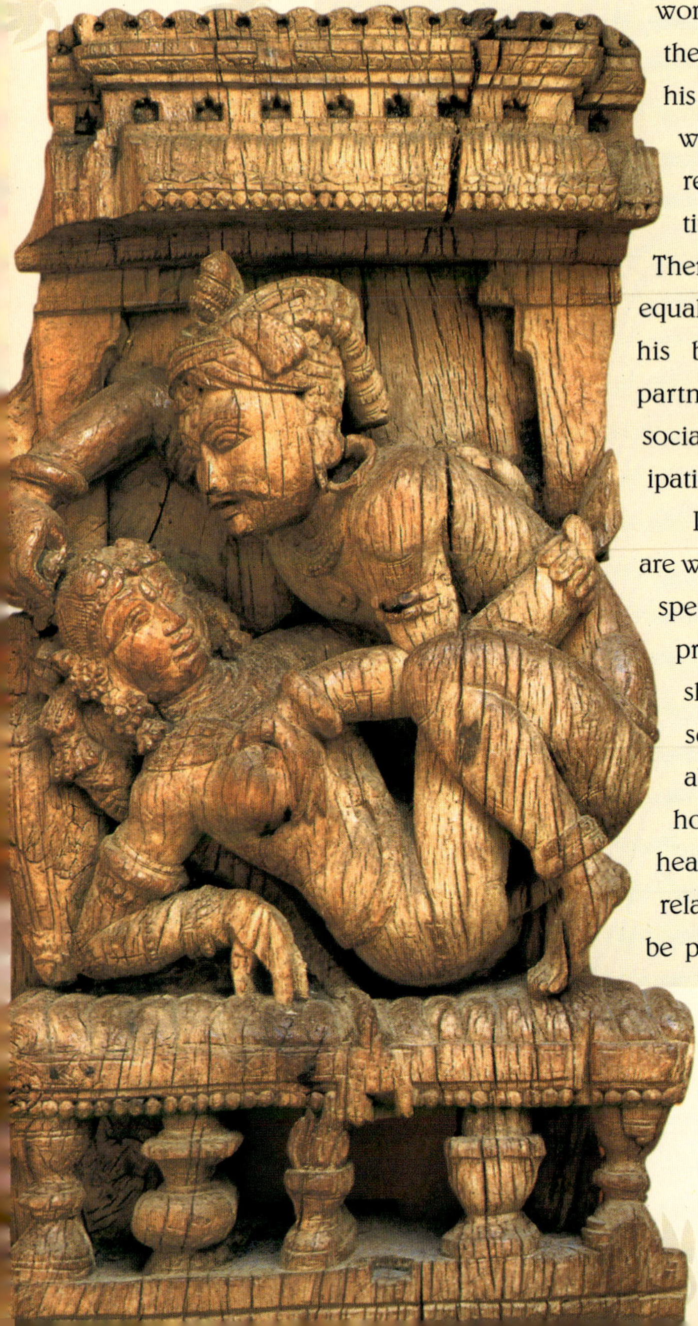

Ardhapiditakam Asana, (Mayurpadakam)
Making nail marks on the breast resembling the peacock's foot: One leg kept in an upward position, the sculptor has wrested a masterpiece from the natural wood, which climate and age have further embellished. The unknown *sthapati*, visualiser, has immortalised the delicate moment of the climax, the ecstasy of fulfilment, and has instilled *prana*, the breath of life, into these carved lovers.
Wood carving from a temple ratha, processional chariot. Tamil Nadu, Thanjavur district, late 19th century. Private collection.

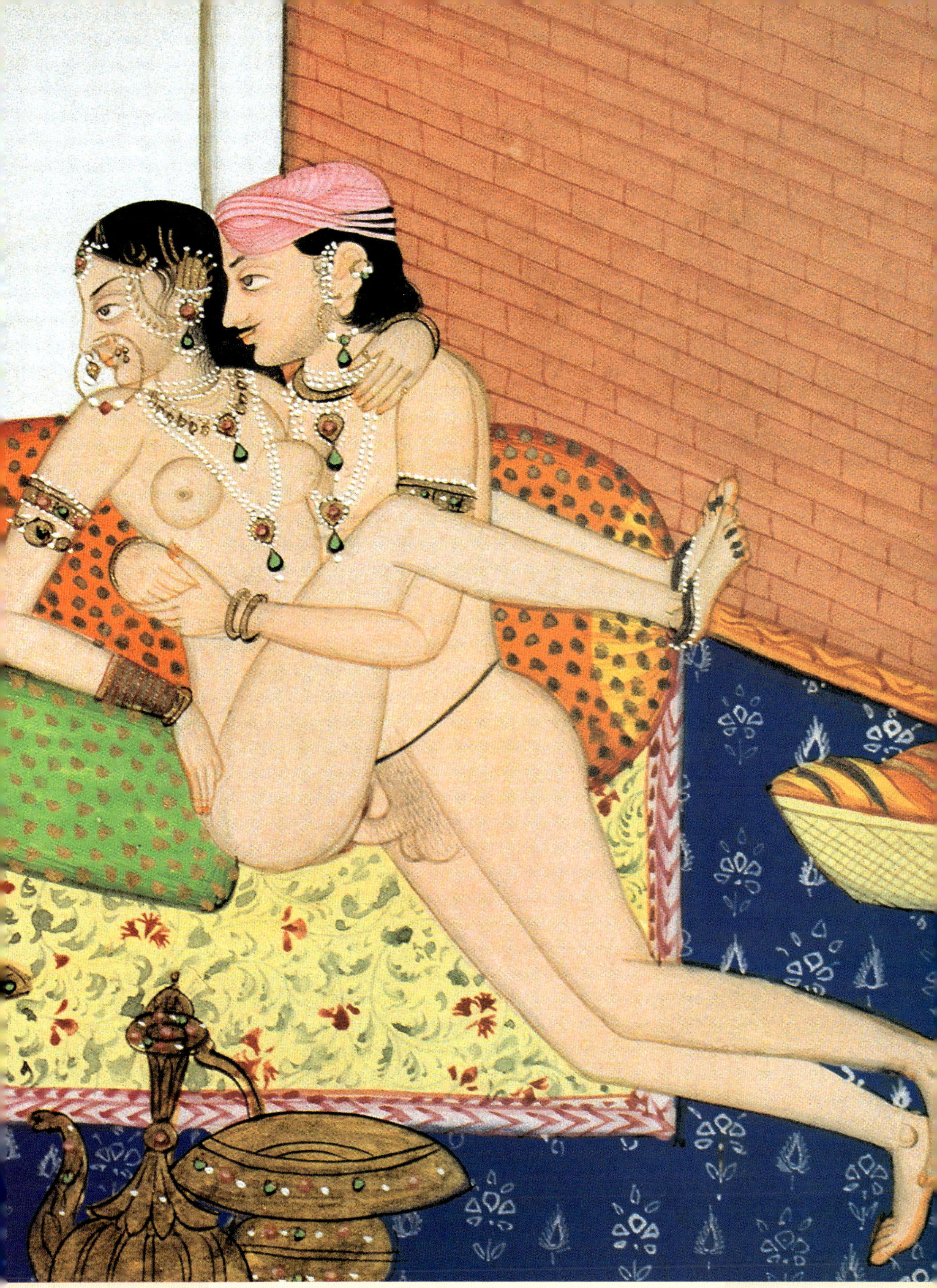

After a long night of love making: The lovers in the middle of their ardent and passionate love making, are distracted from their enjoyment, by the crow of the cock, announcing daybreak. The boy's turban and the girl's very large nose ring is typical of the Pahari school. *Miniature Painting, Pahari Hills, Kangra, Sikh Kalam, 19th century. Private collection.*

inconsequential subjects like nature, common interests, skills and traits, spirituality. These will provide a breath of fresh air to your association and provide rest too.

The *Kama Sutra* also advises:

The wife, moreover, should not tell strangers the amount of her wealth, nor the secrets which her husband has confided to her. She should surpass all the women of her own rank in life in her cleverness, her appearance, her knowledge of cookery, her pride, and her manner of serving her husband.

ON MARRIAGE AND REMARRIAGE

Causes for remarriage according to the *Kama Sutra* are folly or ill-temper of the wife, a husband's dislike towards his wife, the want of offspring, continual birth of daughters and the incontinence of the husband. While situations such as these seldom arise in the modern context, it is spectacular how people, years ago, conducted themselves with such grace, reflecting a high quotient of maturity within society. While the elder wife played mother to the younger ones, guiding and helping them, the younger ones treated the elders with deep respect such as due to an older sister.

With respect to widow remarriage, once again we encounter a high degree of liberalism combined with a profound sense of culture and belonging in ancient society. Vatsyayana felt strongly that a widow was entitled to marry any man she liked and considered suitable for herself.

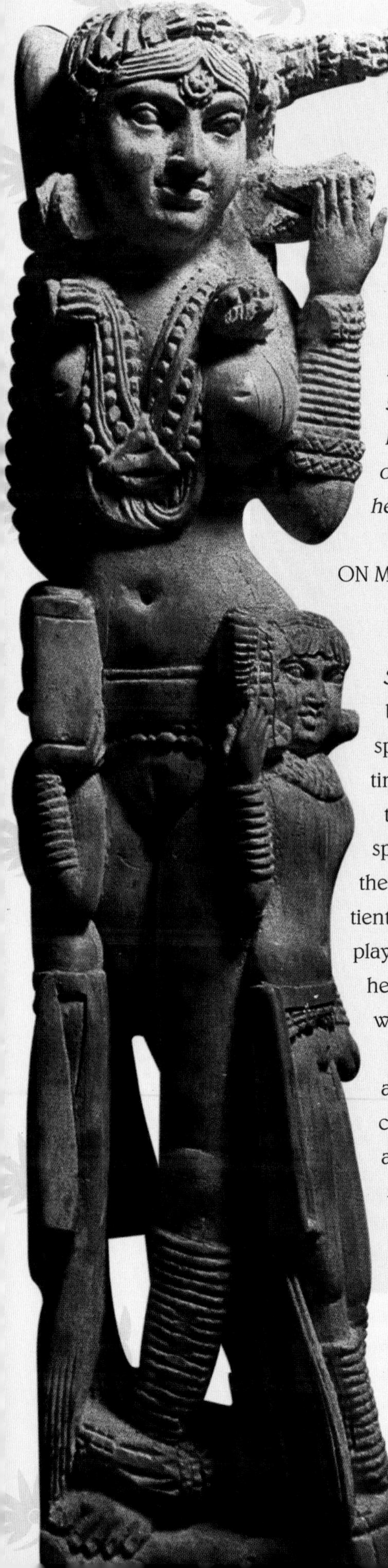

Ivory mirror handle: Inspired by the earliest beliefs of the Aryans, and then the great philosophy of Buddhism, Jainism and Hinduism, this vast sub-continent of India became a treasure trove of art. This masterpiece is probably crafted at the behest of a wealthy courtesan, who takes her responsibility and her livelihood seriously. Wealthy courtesans in those days enhanced communal life, particularly by making outlays for more gain from rich merchants, who preserved attractive and collectable artefacts, and also by buying rare accessories and jewellery from all the most famous and distant regions - like this wonderful ivory mirror handle, a rarity. *Ivory mirror handle, Satavahana Dynasty, Andhra Pradesh, 1st century.* By a miracle this article was recovered from ancient Pompeii, where it was fortunately buried in the volcanic ash of Mount Etna. *Now preserved in the Naples Museum.*

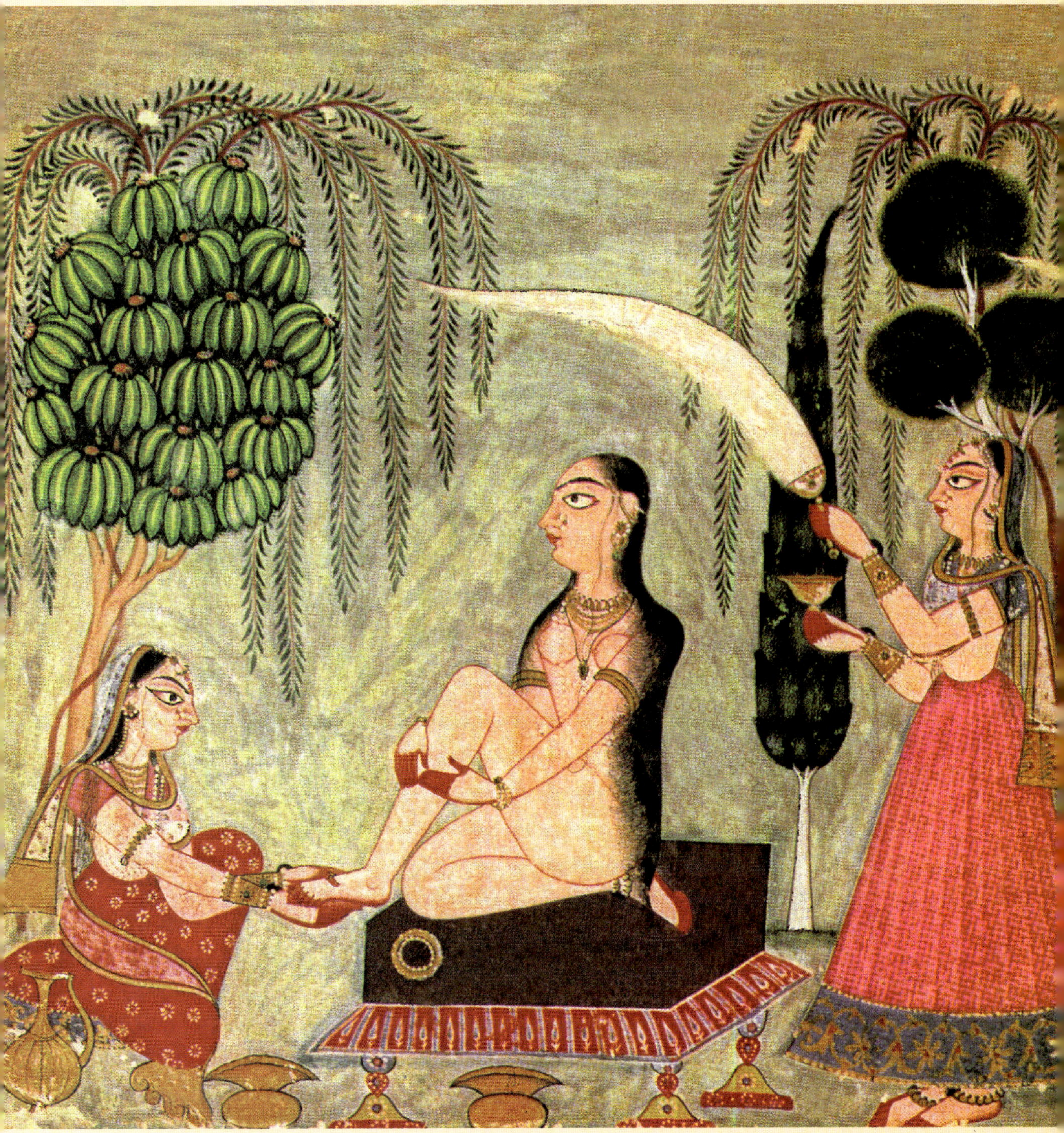

Cooling herself in the outdoors: Flora and Fauna find favour with the artistic community of the Himachal region, in particular the hilly regions of Kulu, Mandi and Basholi. Trees and bushes provide plenty of natural covers for the gorgeous *nayika*, heroine indulging in outdoor liberations from the nearby pool to cool her body. The composition is fascinating. Her companion, with delicate hands, paints *mehndi* on her feet, adding a distinctive charm. The stylistic trees are mind boggling. *Miniature painting, Pahari Hills, Kulu Valley, 18th century. Private collection.*

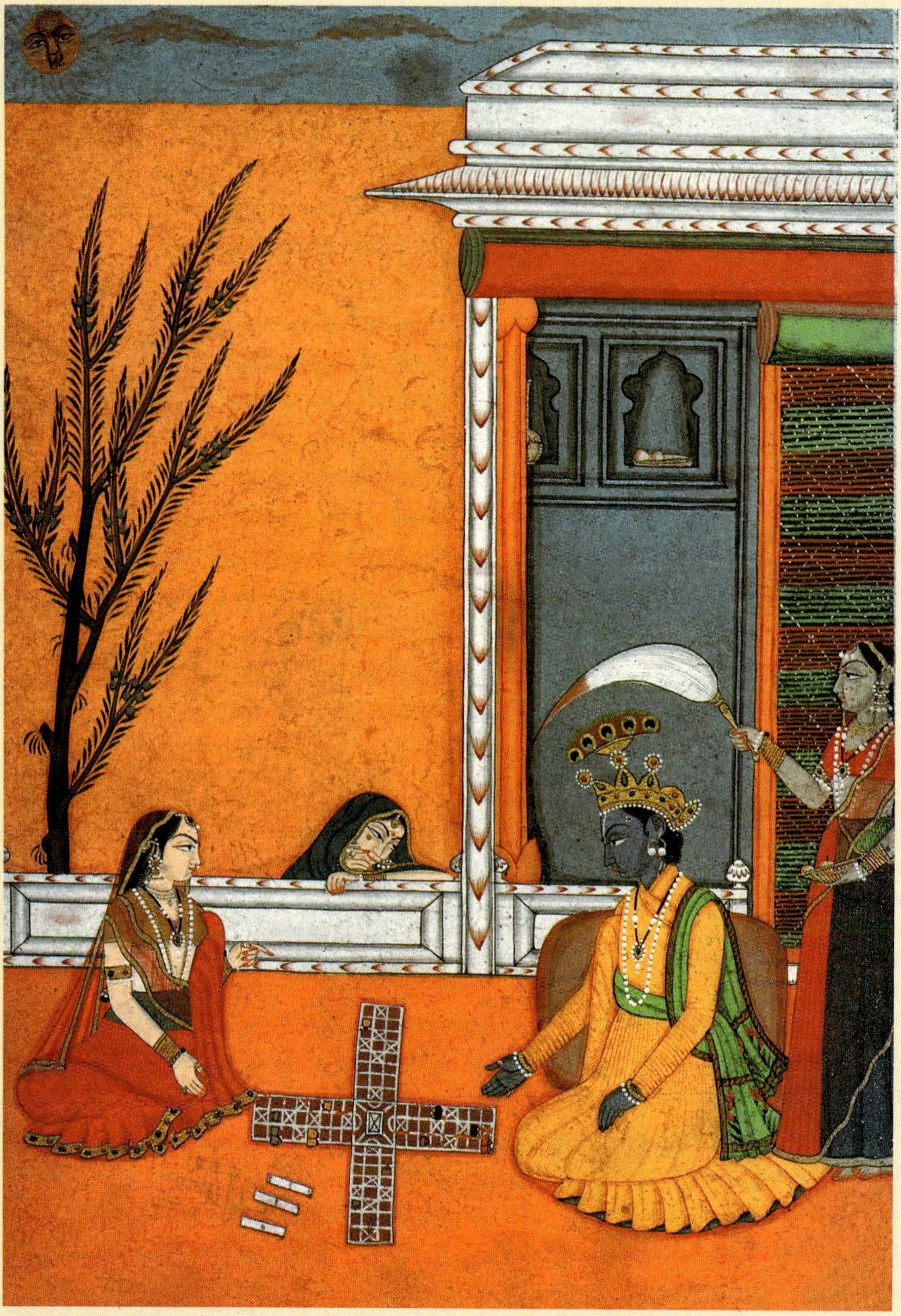

Facing page: **Floral *Dandia*, flowers on a wand:** With a wave of the wand, a special small stick, the magician performs an act to bring good fortune, and thereby pleasure. The outdoors, on a nice cool sunny day in spring, is indeed most pleasurable and it is good fortune for the young girl to be with her lover. Games, outdoor as well as indoor, are a delightful way to try out one's luck, and with the ware of a *Phool Dandia* one can assure not just luck, but good fortune. *Miniature painting, Lucknow, late Mughal style, early 18th century. Private collection.*

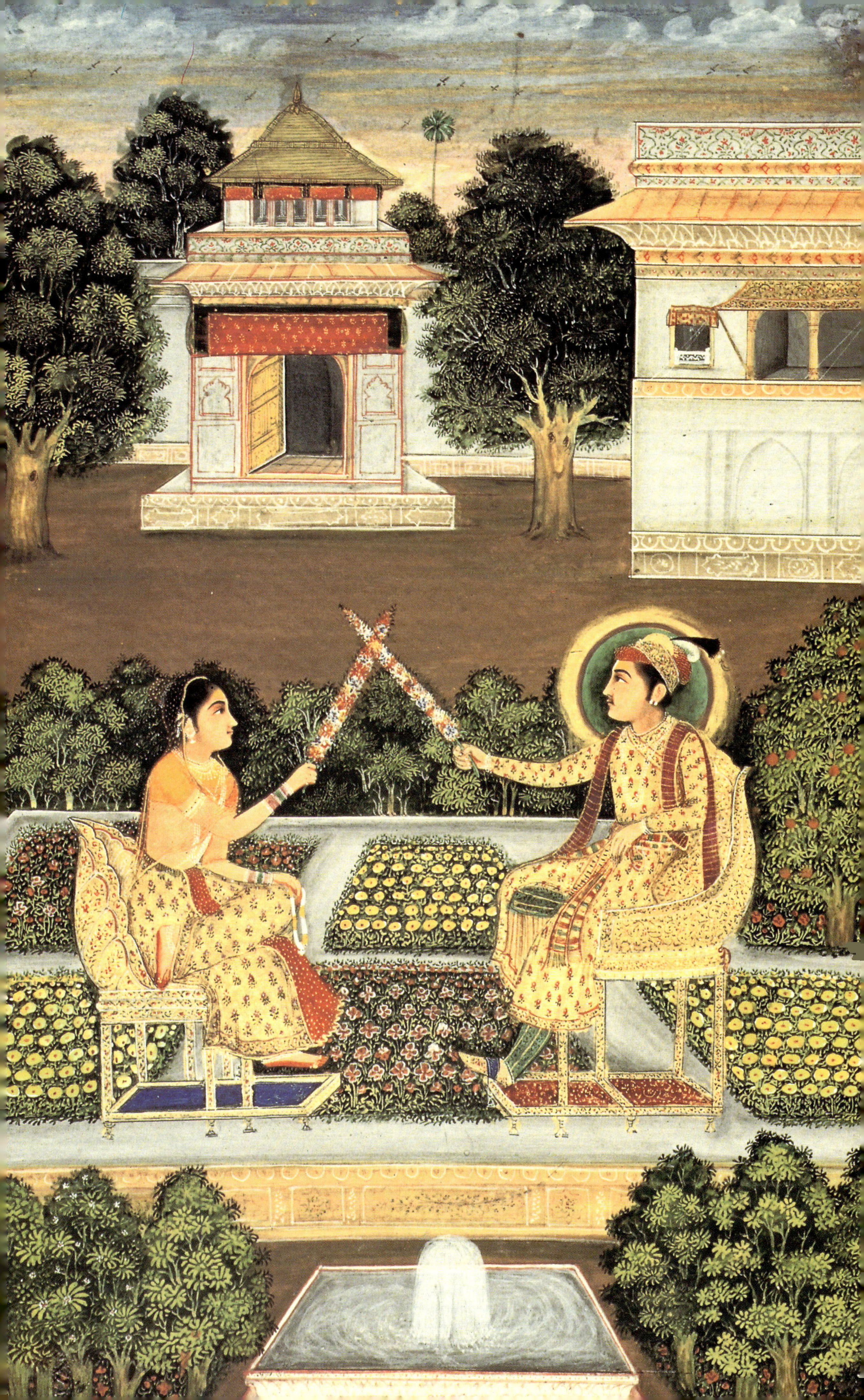

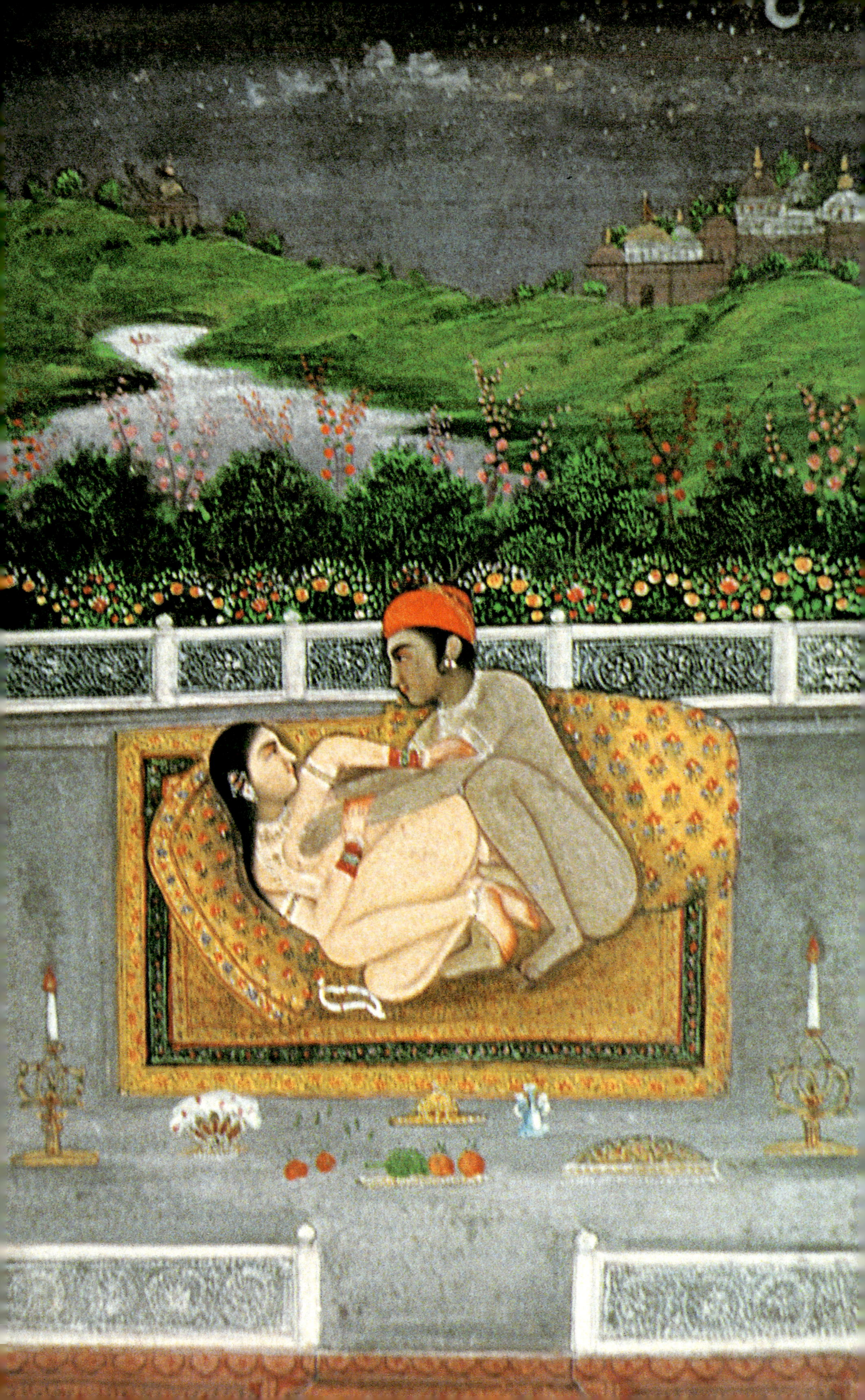

Facing page: **Love tickles and fancies:** The artistic mannerism of love and sex, in all their glory, are told by Vatsyayana in a manner, which revealed he was a devoted connoisseur. Noticeable is the manner in which the heroine tickles his privates with her feet, making the moment all the more pleasurable for him, while he ably enjoys her charms. The posture requires considerable physical ability as far as the woman is concerned. *Miniature painting, Lucknow, Late Mughal style, early 18th century. Private collection.*
Previous page left: **Gains in love, and in competition:** Enjoying *Chaupad*, a game of dice, with her present lover, a clever move by her, displays her attitude for the game, and she is the winner. *Miniature painting, Bundi, Rajasthan, mid 17th century. Private collection.*

Further, codes of conduct after remarriage are described in detail in the *Kama Sutra*. The rules favour the strengthening and maintenance of a woman's dignity within the relationship. So it is advised that if a woman is driven out of the house by her husband, she need not return anything to him. If, however, she leaves her husband of her own accord, she should restore to him whatever he may have given her, with the exception of mutual presents. Upon marriage she is encouraged to live in her husband's home as one of its chief members and she should 'treat all other ladies of the family with kindness, the servants with generosity, and all the friends of the house with familiarity and good temper.' She should not hesitate from expressing and making use of the sixty-four ways of enjoyment.

Underpinning the liberal attitude of the ancients is a sense of harmony and belongingness as shared among all members of society. And though our times do not facilitate leisurely social interactions, but some aspects, such as the approach to remarriage can be imbibed into our lives as well. Of course, the attitudes of ancient thinkers will have to be reframed within the contemporary context, but we can still preserve their essence to strengthen the values of contemporary society.

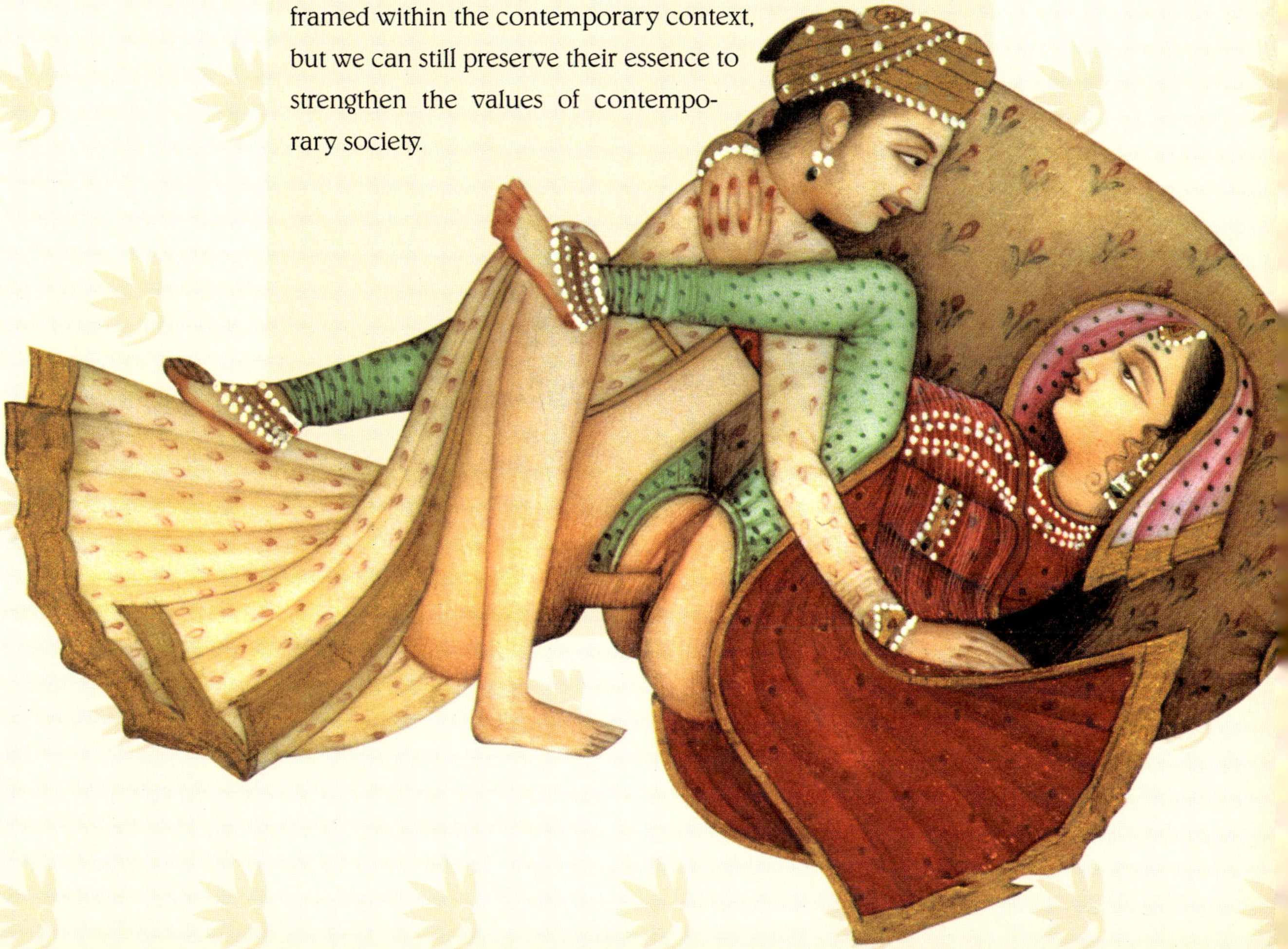

A flexible move: The figure is a good example of flexibility and physicality, as the *nayika* raises one of her legs to rest on his shoulder. The move promises to provide the deepest penetration possible, to her over excited lover. *Miniature painting, Rajasthan, 19th century. Private collection.*

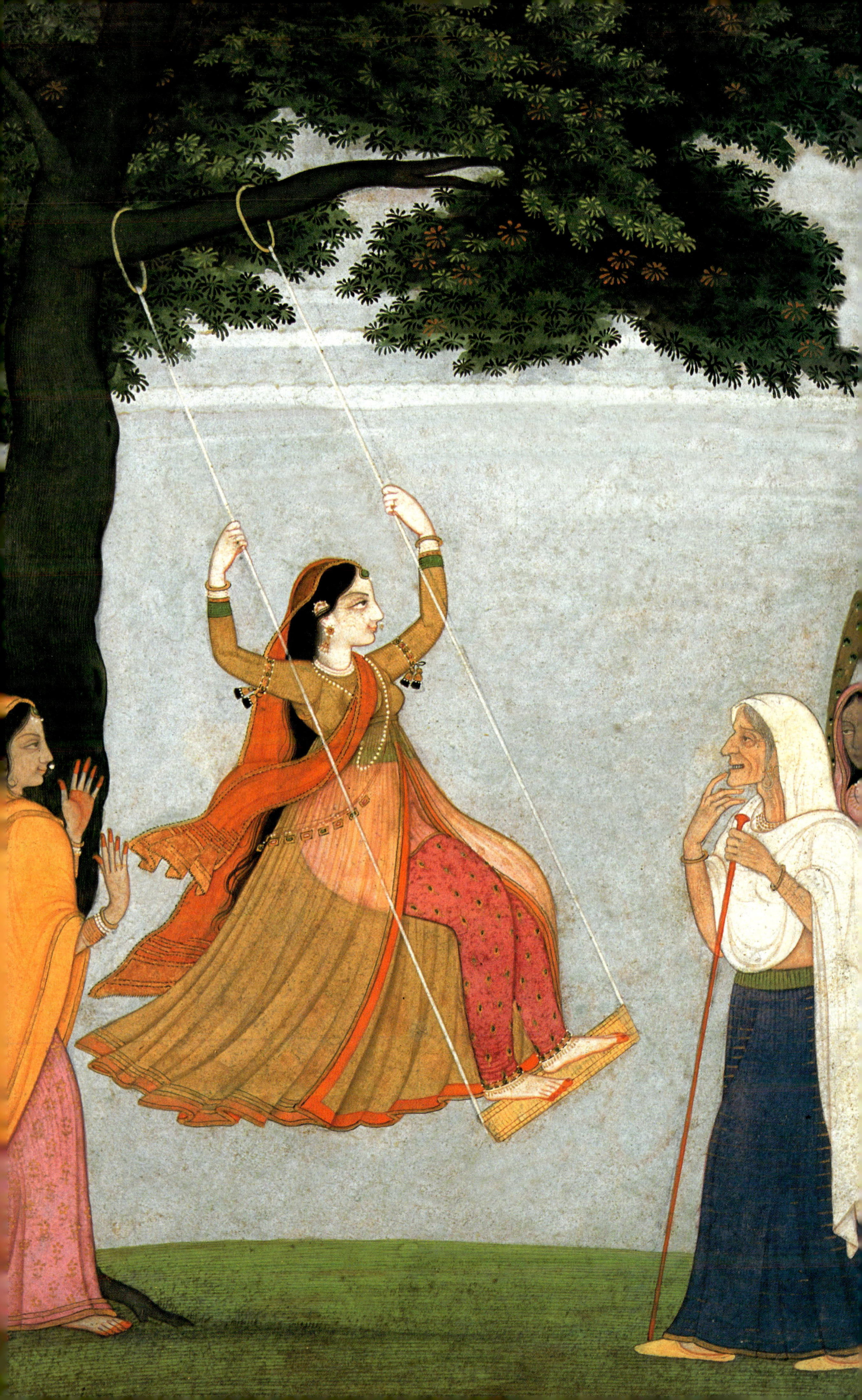

*Desire, which springs from nature and which is increased by art,
and from which all danger is taken away by wisdom, becomes firm and secure.
A clever man, depending on his own ability and observing carefully
the meaningful signs and gestures of women, and removing the causes of their
turning away from men, is generally successful with them*

Kama Sutra, Book V

love and PLEASURE

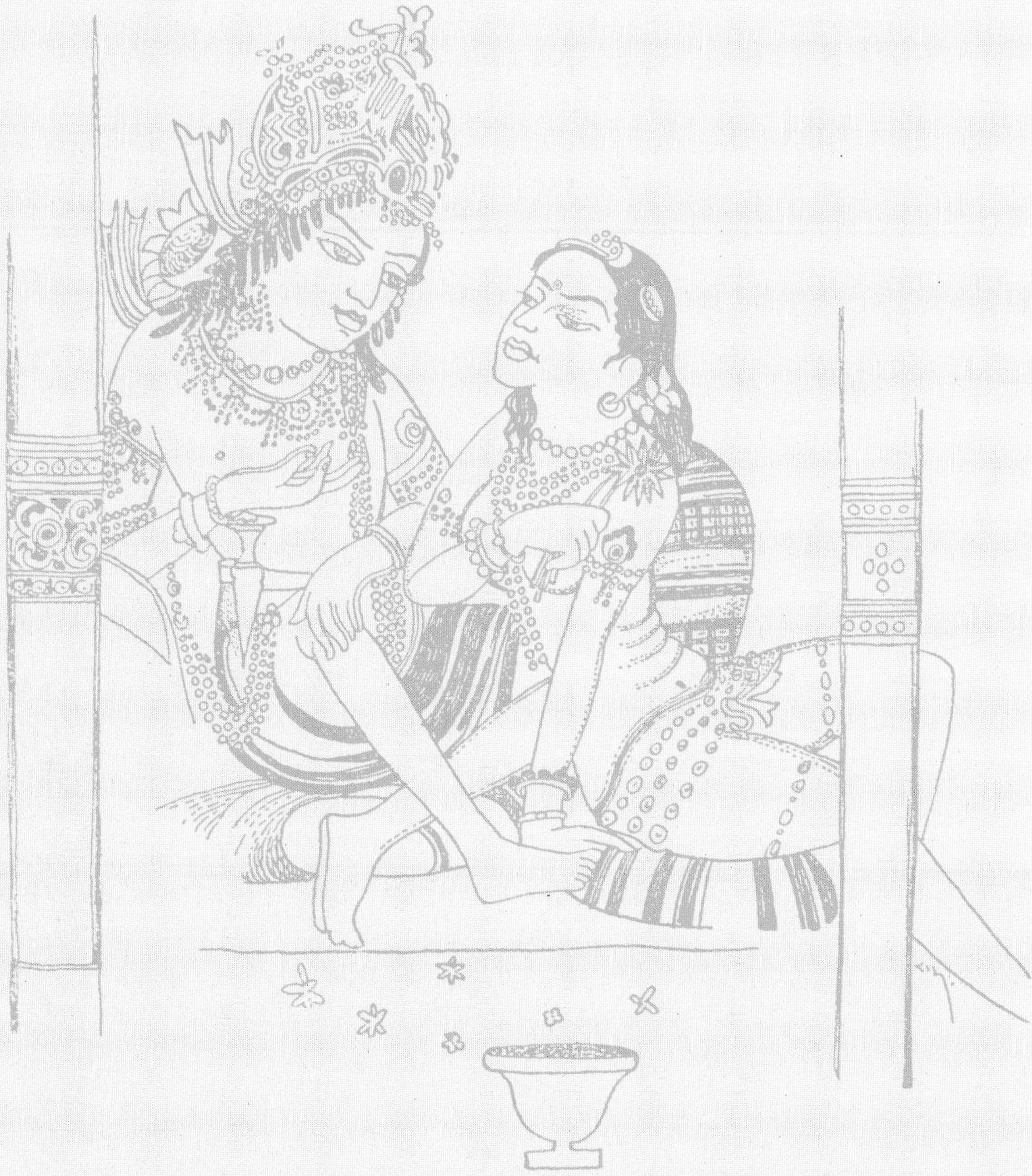

Sex is the earliest desire of man. It is the starting point of creation. The male and female involvement is not only a human factor but relates to material objects too. There is soft wood and hard wood, soft stone (like soap stone) and hard stone (like granite). The Moon is considered female and the Sun, male. Such sexual identification is seen in many cultures and countries.

In Indian spiritualism, sex is placed at a very high altar. It is seen not just as a sensual play, an intercourse between man and woman of lust and satisfaction; it is a means towards spiritual achievement. The *Rig Veda* and the *Atharva Veda* contain references to the male and female. The *Atharva Veda* speaks of herbs and charms to be used in the art of sex. The *Upanishads* highlight the sexual act as a sacred act. As a subject of study, sex was considered a science. Even prostitution had a high status. Women who engaged in this age-old profession were not just ordinary, not just those who provided satisfaction to the body. They indulged in sexual art as artistes and led their partners to a state of ecstasy and bliss. They were respected members of society. It was acknowledged that prudent indulgence in eroticism would help overcome deficiencies of mind and body. Certain sexual acts were suggested to maintain body-mind equilibrium. Medicines and herbs, applications and gadgets were recommended to overcome sexual deficiency. Sex was

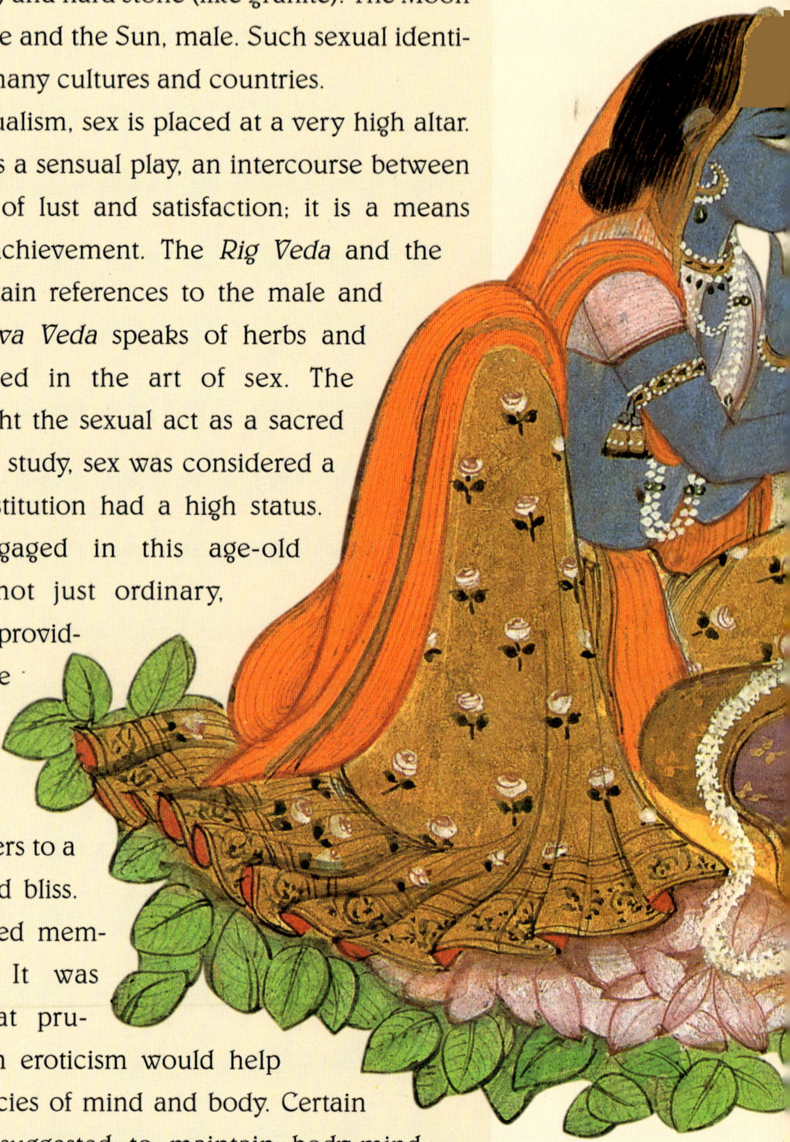

Previous page: **The swing:** The *nayika* enjoying a flight of fancy, an attainment, which opens up vistas of the motion to fly through the air. The elderly woman encourages her ward and is watchful for her safety. *Miniature painting, Kangra, Pahari Hills, 20th century. National Museum.*

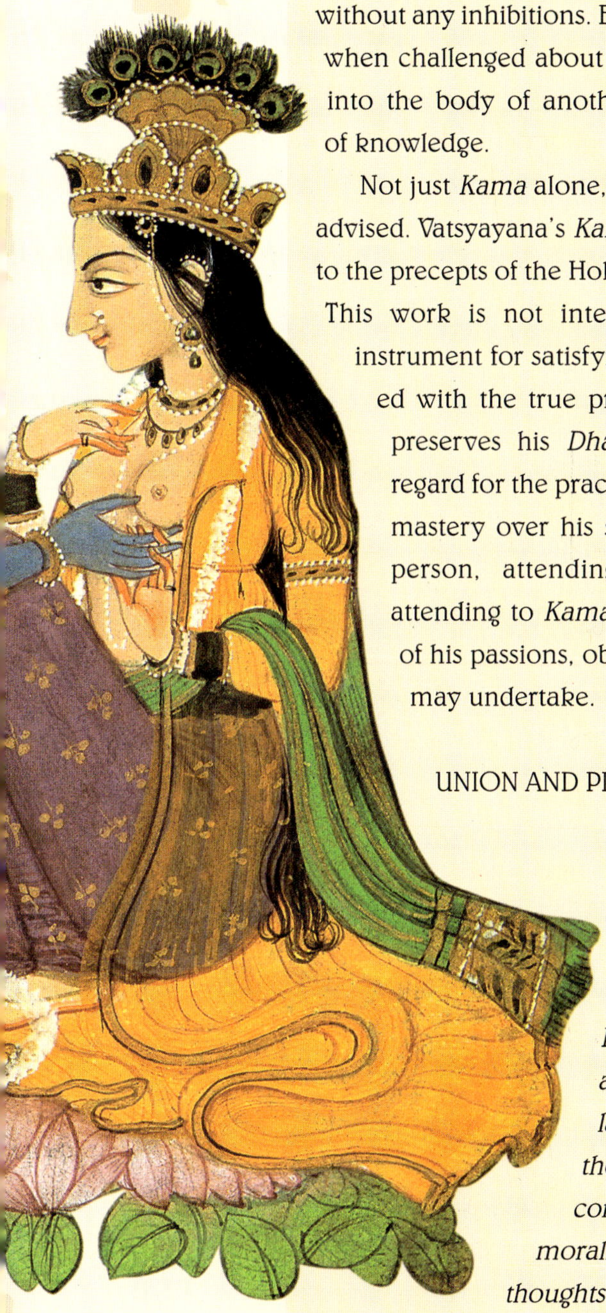

considered one of the sixty-four subjects of study. The *Kama Shastra* was studied as a subject with an open mind and without any inhibitions. Even the great saint Sankaracharya, when challenged about what he knew of women, entered into the body of another person and learnt this branch of knowledge.

Not just *Kama* alone, but *Kama* along with *Dharma* was advised. Vatsyayana's *Kama Sutra* was produced 'according to the precepts of the Holy Writ', for the benefit of the world. This work is not intended to be used merely as an instrument for satisfying our desires. A person acquainted with the true principles of this science, and who preserves his *Dharma, Artha* and *Kama*, and has regard for the practices of the people, is sure to obtain mastery over his senses. An intelligent and prudent person, attending to *Dharma* and *Artha*, and attending to *Kama* also, without becoming the slave of his passions, obtains success in everything that he may undertake.

UNION AND PLEASURE

When a man first makes up to her, she naturally shrinks from him, even though she may be willing to unite herself with him. But when the attempts to gain her are repeated and renewed, she at last consents. But with a man, even though he may have begun to love, he conquers his feelings from a regard for morality and wisdom, and although his thoughts are often on the woman, he does not yield, even though an attempt be made to gain him over. He sometimes makes an attempt or effort to win the object of

Cross-dressing: The heroine and first among all of Krishna's *gopis* is Radha, adored and much favoured by him. She was married to Ayanaghosha, and lured away from him by Krishna. Romantic adventures are full of stories about them, the games they played, the idyllic raptures of the divine lovers, sporting under Kadamba blossoms or dallying in the Tamal groves of the Yamuna, where after a swim, they would redress, she in his clothes and he in hers. Radha was living only for Krishna, yearning for him, burning with insatiable desire and ever longing to be merged with him - limb to limb, soul to soul. Their love is legendry - never, never ending. *Miniature painting, Kangra, Pahari Hills, 19th century. Private collection.*

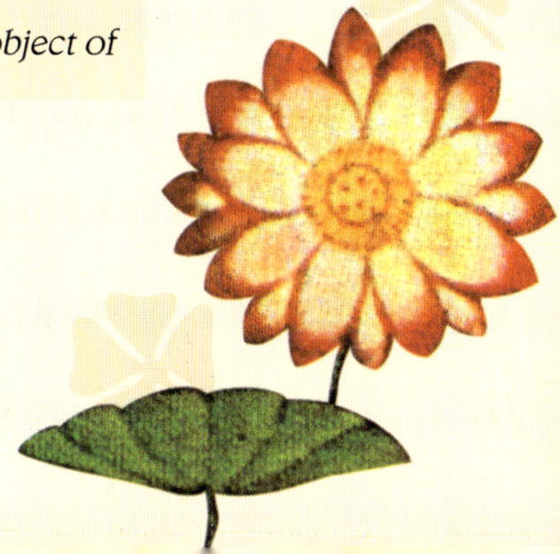

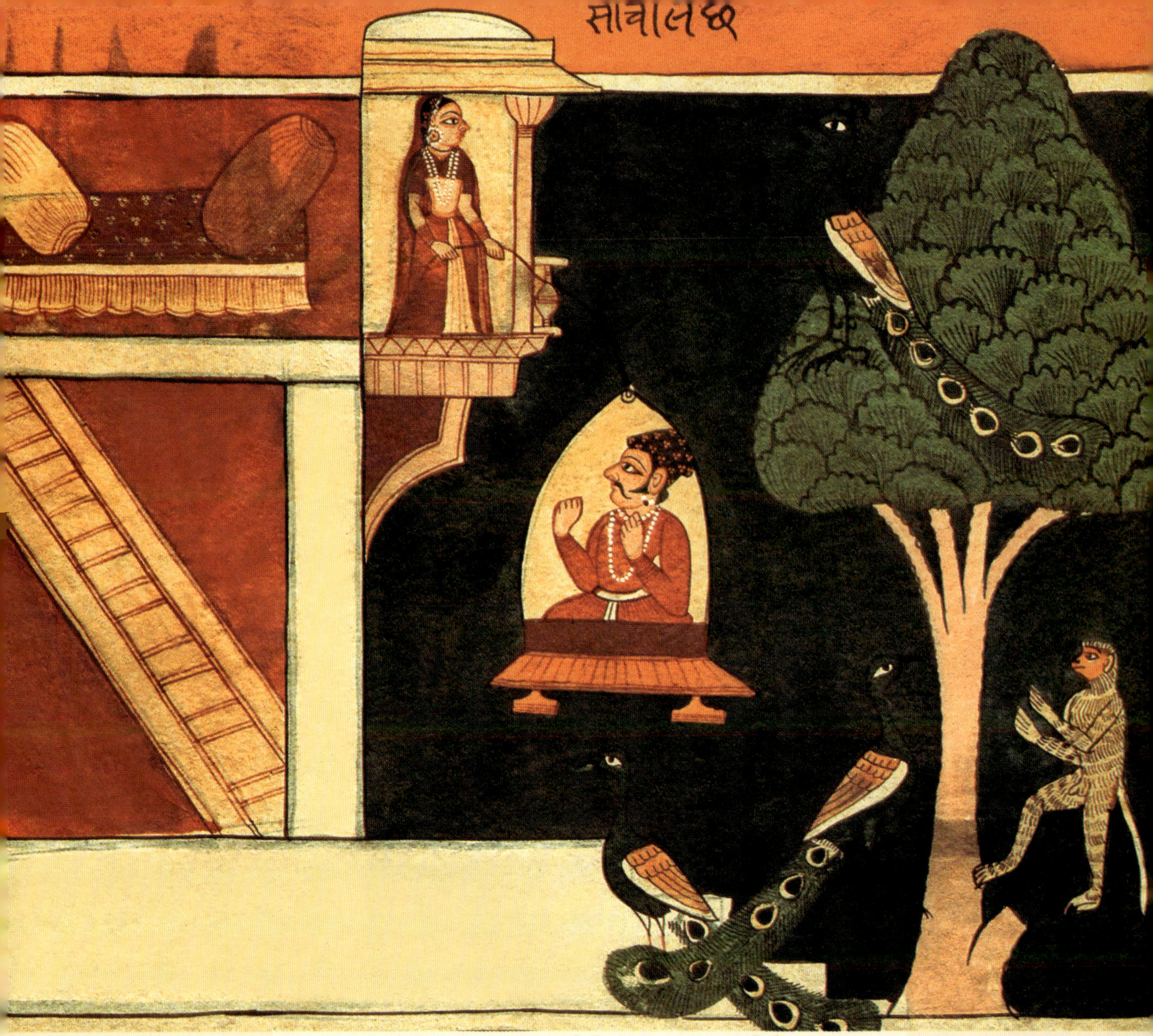

his affections, and having failed, he leaves her alone for the future. In the same way, when a woman is once gained, he often becomes indifferent about her. As for the saying that a man does not care for what is easily gained, and only desires a thing which cannot be obtained without difficulty, it is only a matter of talk.

KAMA SUTRA, BOOK V

Attraction can strike at any time, even after marriage. And as much as the *Kama Sutra* acknowledges this reality, it has considered issues about propriety. It states how sexual attraction and desire can be harnessed for the betterment of existing situations and for furthering one's own interests.

An Elopement: The excitement is seized upon by the artist, when he takes the opportunity to indulge in flights of fancy. The scene is full of drama, the actors conforming to a pre-arranged plan. The lovers are disposed by the artist in his presentation with a theatrical air. The young man has arrived and his lady love has lowered a cage, perhaps, an adaptation of some household need for filling things. It obviously works, for he is on his way up to her private quarters. Caution has been thrown to the winds. She could be a desperate housewife, enchanted by the young fresh cool hero ready to risk everything. *Miniature painting, Sirohi style, Rajasthan, early 19th century. Private collection.*

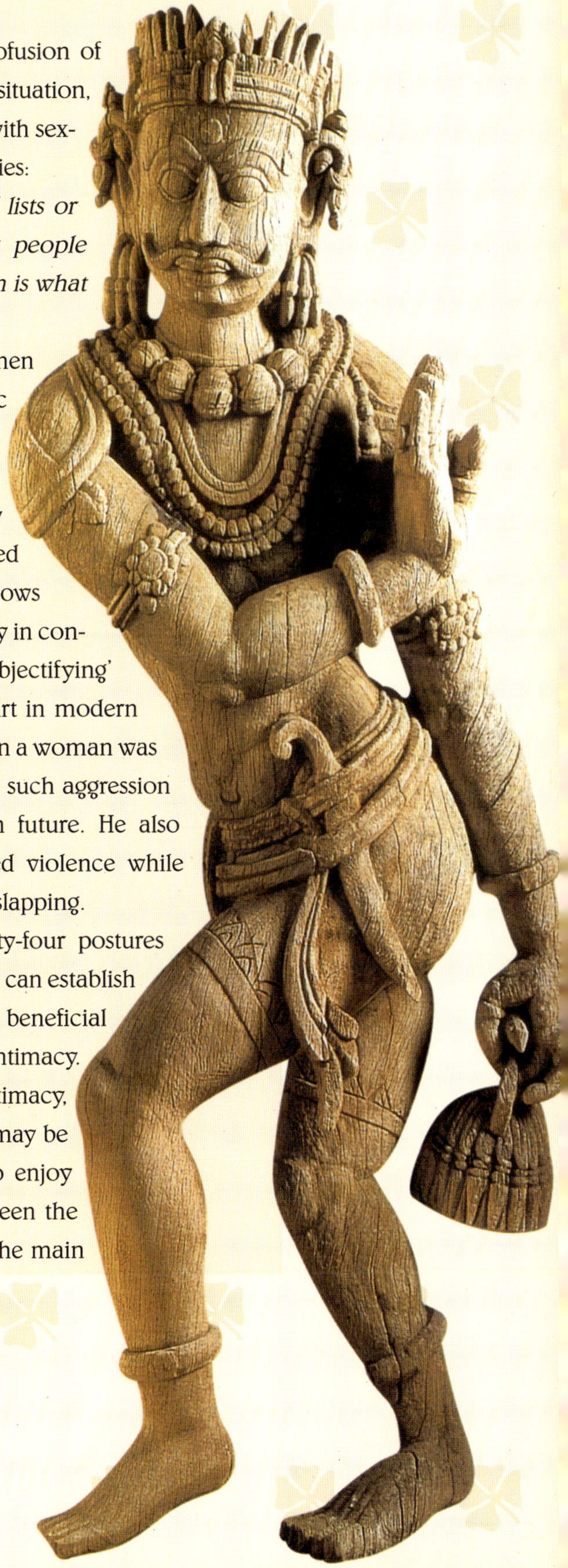

Man of the world: Young men, who are of the age, aim to take every opportunity to attract the opposite sex, and when preparing for a tryst, go through a lot of trouble to dress accordingly. This young man is identifiable in particular by his demeanour, his coiffure and his ornaments. His appearance is very handsome, and we can observe, he was in his day a very accomplished young fellow. *Wood, Temple chariot decoration, South India, 19th century. Private collection.*
Following page left: ***Samarata*, equal union:** Vatsyayana describes nine kinds of different unions. The artist has painted an *asana*, posture that is possible for an equal union - that is between a couple of corresponding dimensions. *Miniature painting, Jodhpur, Rajasthan, late 18th century. Private collection.*

Without patronising out-of-marriage affairs, it qualifies that other men's wives should only be seduced after thoughtful consideration.

The *Kama Sutra* contains a profusion of lists and categories for every type of situation, condition and position connected with sexual love. However, Vatsyayana clarifies:

This is no matter of numerical lists or textbook tables of contents. For people joined in the sexual ecstasy, passion is what makes things happen.

He emphasises the need for women to read the text and learn the erotic skills prescribed. Indeed, there are sections devoted to instructions to wives and advice to virgins. Many modern commentators have noted the fact that the *Kama Sutra* shows respect for women's sexuality starkly in contrast to the usual insulting and 'objectifying' attitudes prevalent for the most part in modern times. For example, forcing sex upon a woman was strongly to be discouraged because such aggression could interfere with her desire in future. He also warns of the dangers of unbridled violence while indulging in scratching, biting and slapping.

The *Kama Sutra* describes sixty-four postures through which a man and a woman can establish physical contact. These posture are beneficial to both. Joy is the first objective of intimacy. If a couple fails to enjoy this intimacy, there is no meaning to sex. There may be many reasons for a couple not to enjoy physical intimacy. Imbalance between the physical stature of the partners is the main

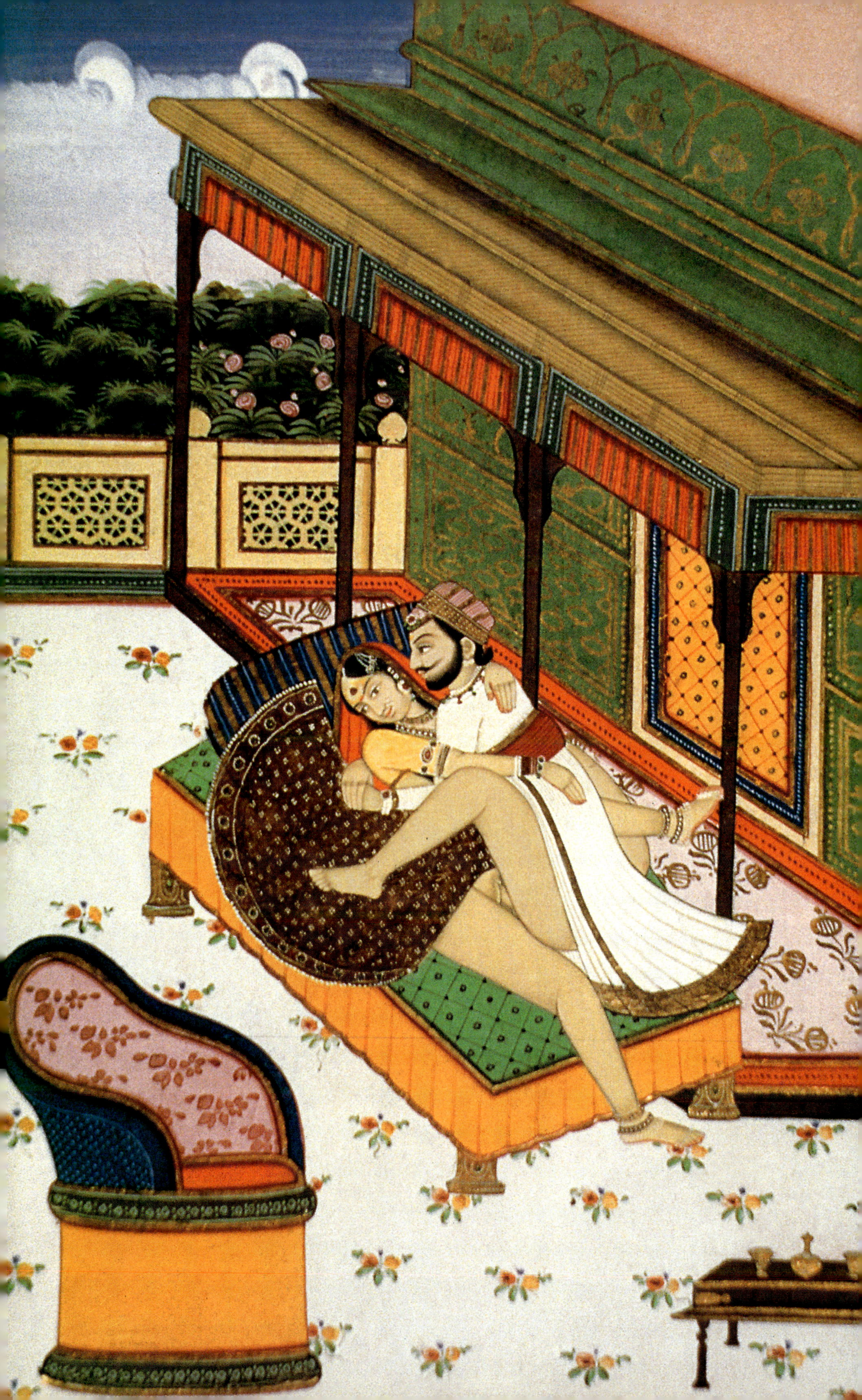

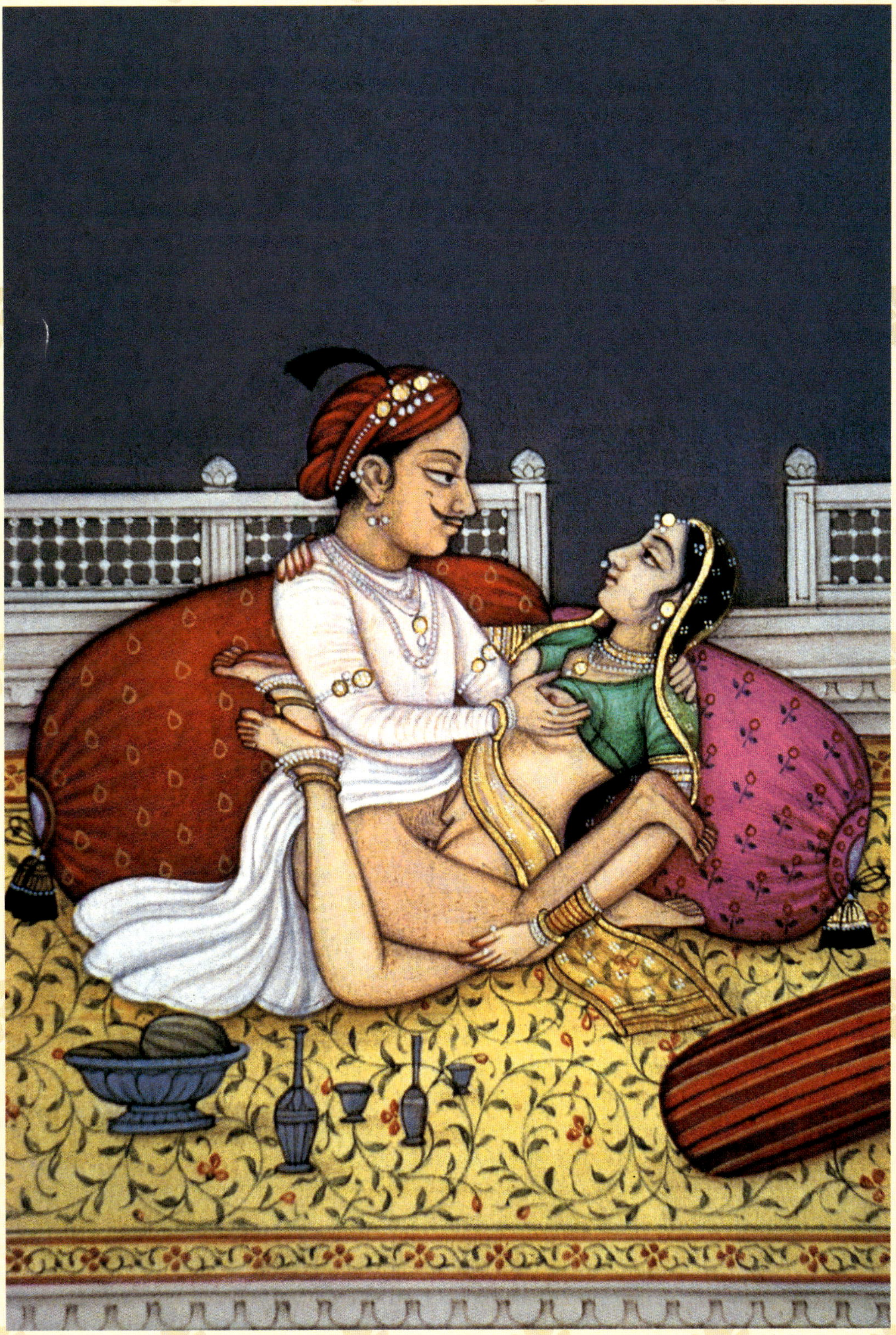

***Padmasana*, petals of a lotus:** The ambience is idealistic, *ghau-takia*, large round pillows, lend support to the couple as well as decorate the palatial setting. This is a leaf from an original album, which had a large number of paintings, depicting many different *asanas*. The couple here are comfortably embracing each other in the manner of the lotus flower on full blossom.

Miniature painting, Jaipur, Rajasthan, late 18th century. Private collection.

Ball of Flame: A famous artistic invention was first discovered in Pune, Maharashtra by the renowned Dinkar Kelkar, whose passion was to establish a collection of arts and crafts, concerned with everyday activities from dawn to dusk. He wanted to highlight each aspect of a woman, for it was she who was the heroine of the collection. His collection of different artist lamps from all over India is unique, and one of most rare and unusual highlight is this spherical-globular brass ball made into two halves with hinges to open and close. Cast in metal, the decor is a lively composition of loving couples in various love postures. The technique allowed for suitable gaps, open spaces, its purpose to illuminate the *zenana*, womens qaurters. Since it is a rotatable oil lamp, it throws light in many directions. *A metal cast ball, early 19th century. Raja Dinkar Kelkar Museum, Pune, Maharashtra.*

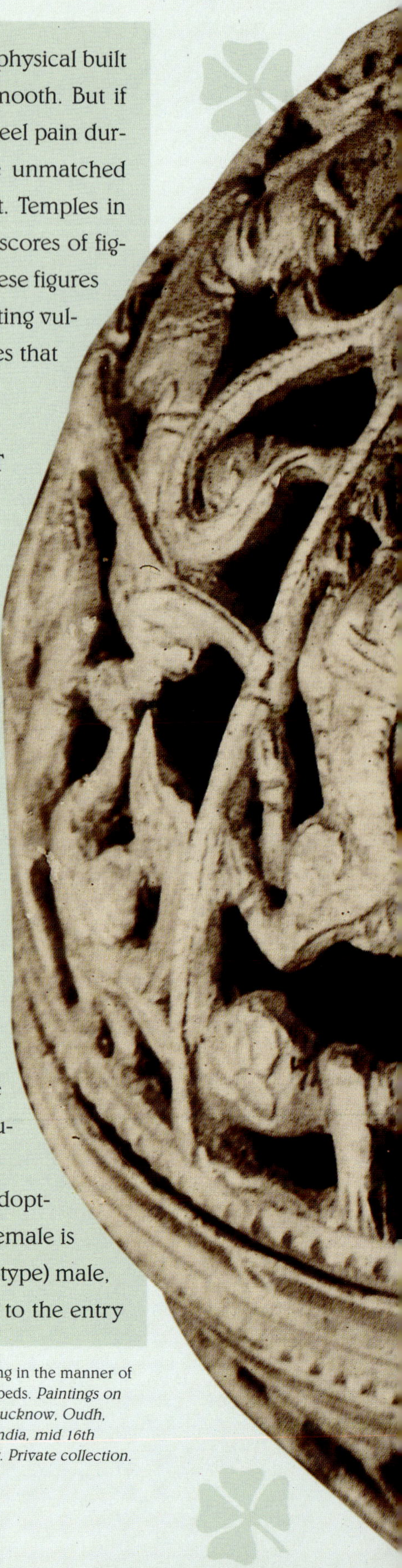

reason. If the partners are well matched in their physical built and age, the physical relationship should be smooth. But if they are not well matched, either of them may feel pain during intercourse. Postures, in this, case, tell the unmatched partners how to establish intimacy and enjoy it. Temples in Khajuraho and Konark, among others, contain scores of figures that depict posture from the *Kama Sutra*. These figures were not chiselled with the objective of propagating vulgarity. They depict the vital states of life-processes that beget life.

SOME OF THE MOST PREVALENT AND EASIEST POSTURES ARE:

***Mrigi* (Doe posture):** This is regarded as the most civilised posture. As a coy doe spreads both her hind legs to facilitate the entry of the male, similarly a woman with a small vagina spreads her legs apart. In this posture, the phallus of even a horse-type of male can have an easy entry.

***Hastini Asana* (She-elephant posture):** This posture is adopted by a *Hastini* (she-elephant) type of female, who has a large vagina. If the male partner is small, (rabbit type or bull type), such a woman should cuddle up to conform to the size of her partner.

***Samarati* (Equally matched):** If the male and female partners are well matched as per the size of their bodies, they may stretch their bodies naturally for maximum enjoyment.

***Badava Asana* (Cow posture):** This posture is adopted by a female of normal stature. If a cow-type female is having an intercourse with an *Ashva* type (horse-type) male, she must spread her legs as far apart as possible to the entry

Following page right: ***Dhenukam*, the congress of a quadruped:** When the couple adopt the stance and copy the actions of animals. Vatsyayana says, "A man can similarly adopt the postures peculiar to the cat, the dog, the tiger, the elephant, the horse and so on." *Mughal, painting on ivory, from a set of ganjifa, playing cards, style of Akbar, A.D. 1556 to 1605.*
Varikriditaka, elephants' love-play: elephants copulating in the manner of quadrupeds. *Paintings on ivory, Lucknow, Oudh, North India, mid 16th century. Private collection.*

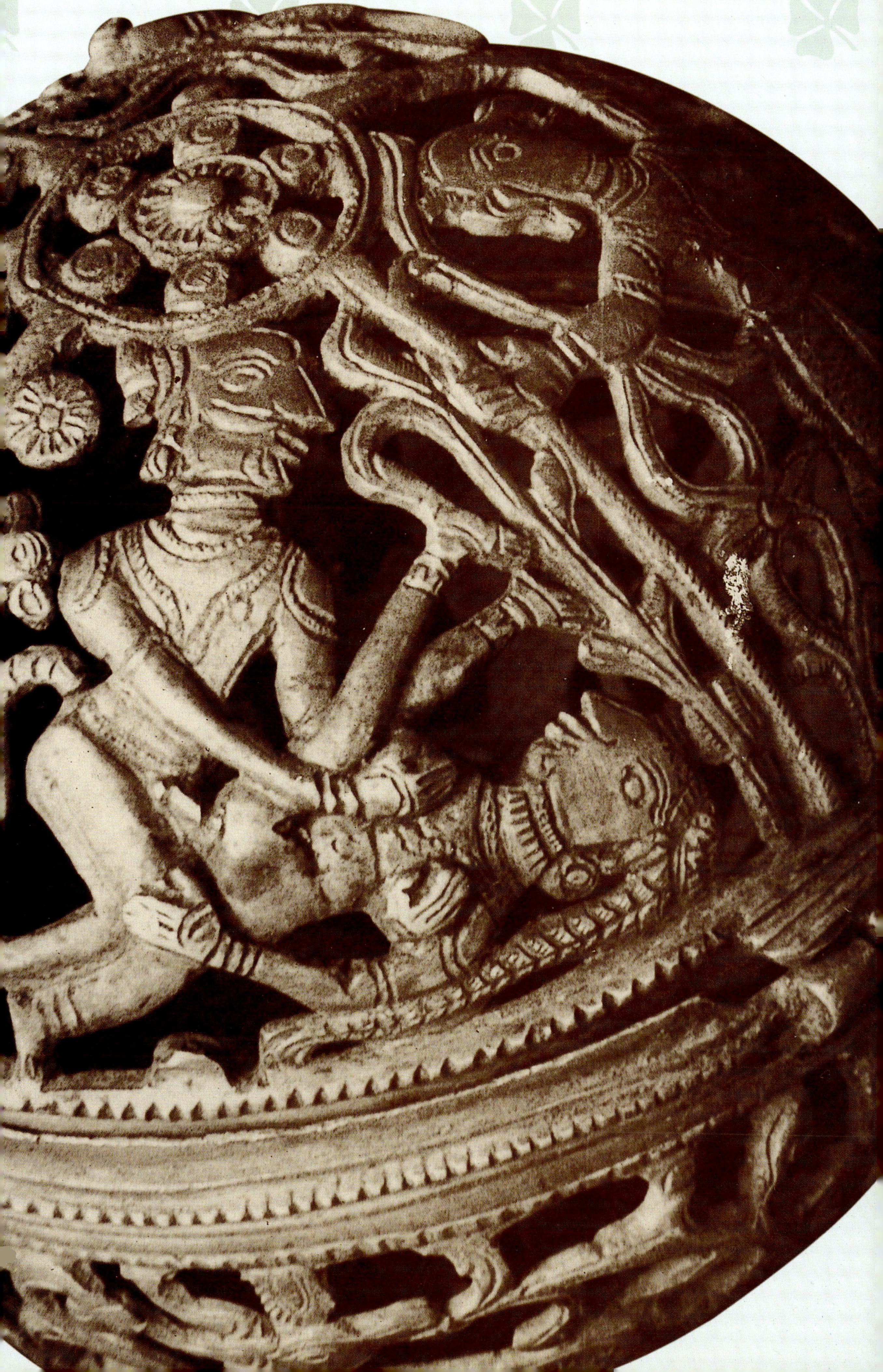

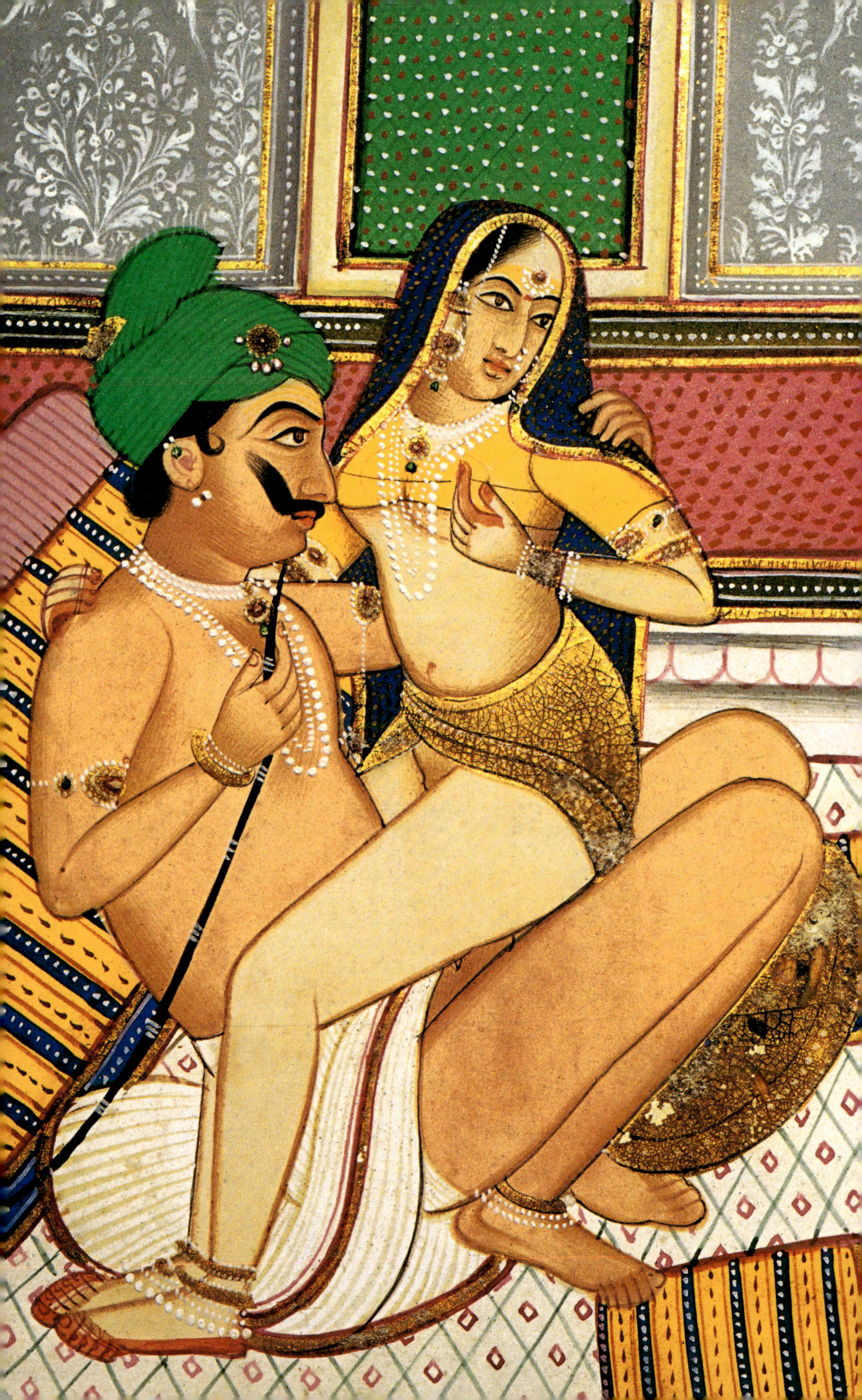

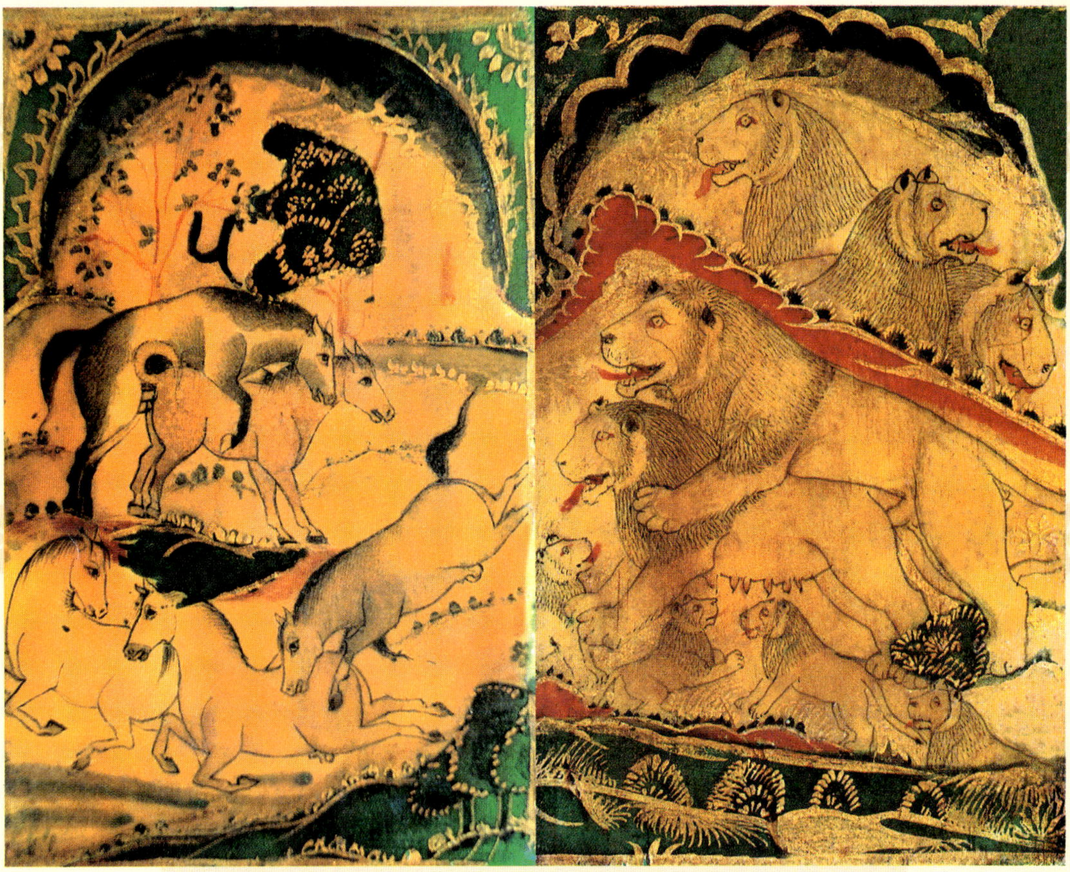

of a large phallus. If she is being mated by a *Shashak* type (rabbit-type) male, she should contract her body to the size of her partner. If the partner is a bull type, they may both spread and stretch their bodies normally to enjoy the union. But in either case, the female partner must allow the entry of the male organ only when her organ has achieved enough lubrication through the secretion of fluid.

Supine: Lying down supine on the bed is a facilitating posture for a female to enjoy intercourse.

Samputak: Both the male and female spread their legs straight during mating. This posture is useful when the partners are well matched.

Piritak: This implies hitting of the groin with the genital organ. This leads to tremendous excitement in both partners.

Vadava: This means contraction and tightening of the female genital organ. In this posture, a she-elephant type of female can please even a rabbit-type male who feels an extraordinary enlargement in his organ. It is common among women in Andhra Pradesh in India to adopt this posture.

Facing page: **The other man's wife:** The attraction felt for the wife of another presents insurmountable difficulties. Elders advise caution in strong terms to avoid the risk of injudicious relationships. Even so, there are special circumstances, in which event the preliminaries can be worked upon, beginning with a sort of middling acquaintance, before planning a move to the next stage is advisable. The connived arrangement of a surreptitious meeting looking like a natural chance is clever. Think in terms of dropping by her house, or get your best friend to invite her, or get the help of a very important person, who is under some obligation. When at last you manage a few friendly brushes, and get closer, you can test her weaknesses - a little trinket, or flowery praise of her attractions, a sip of wine from your flask, and of course, persistence. *Miniature painting, Udaipur, Rajasthan, 19th century. Private collection.*

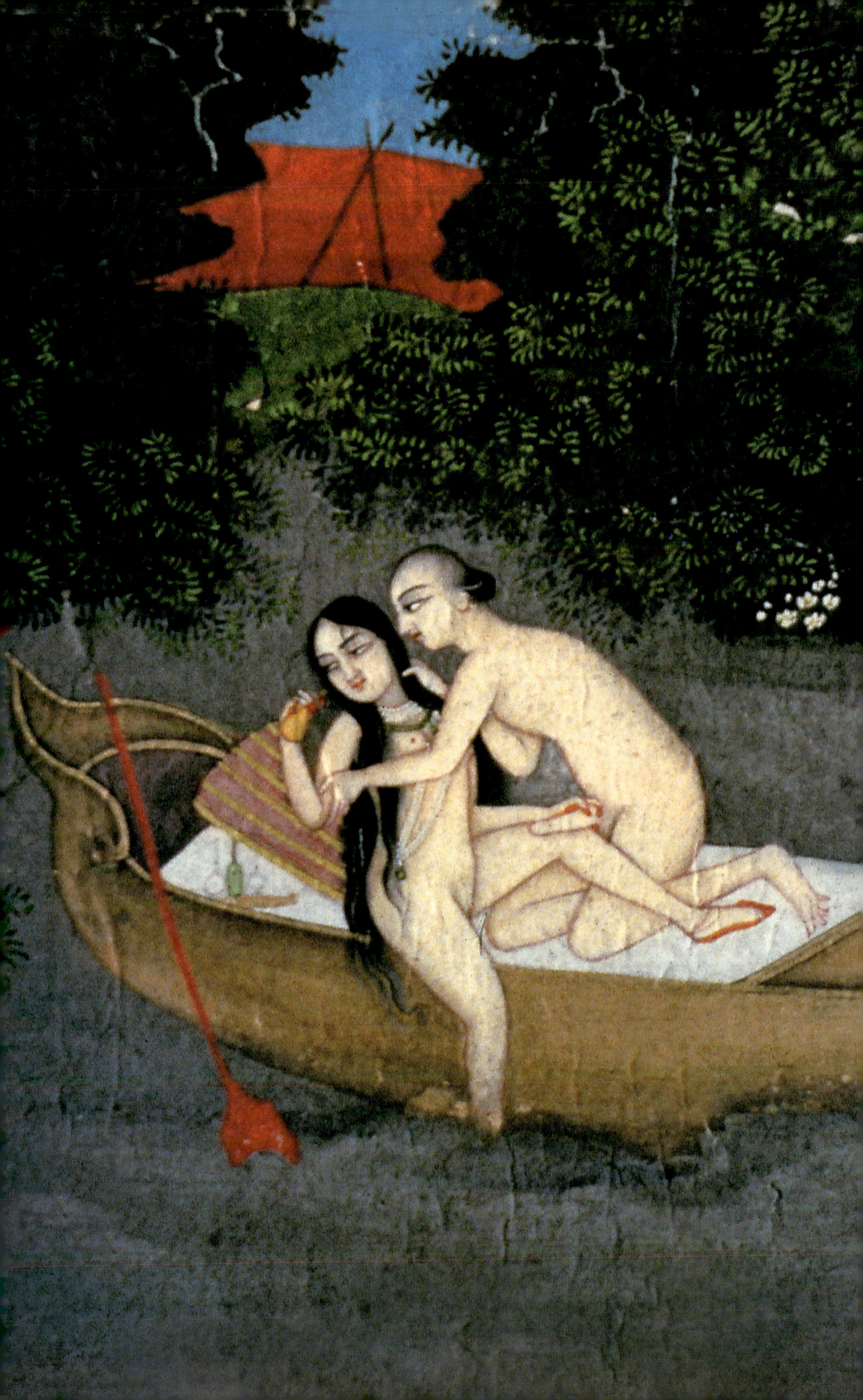

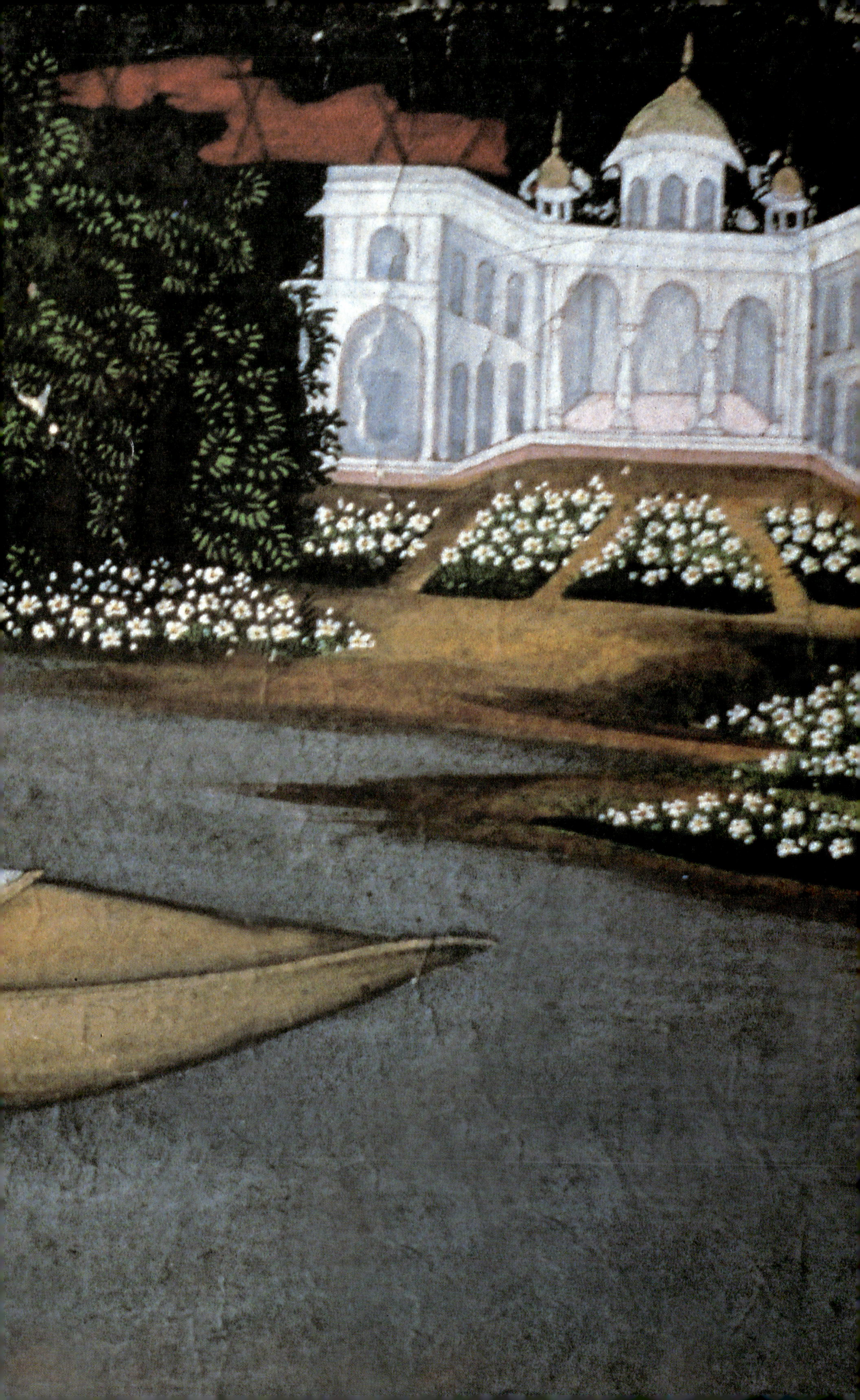

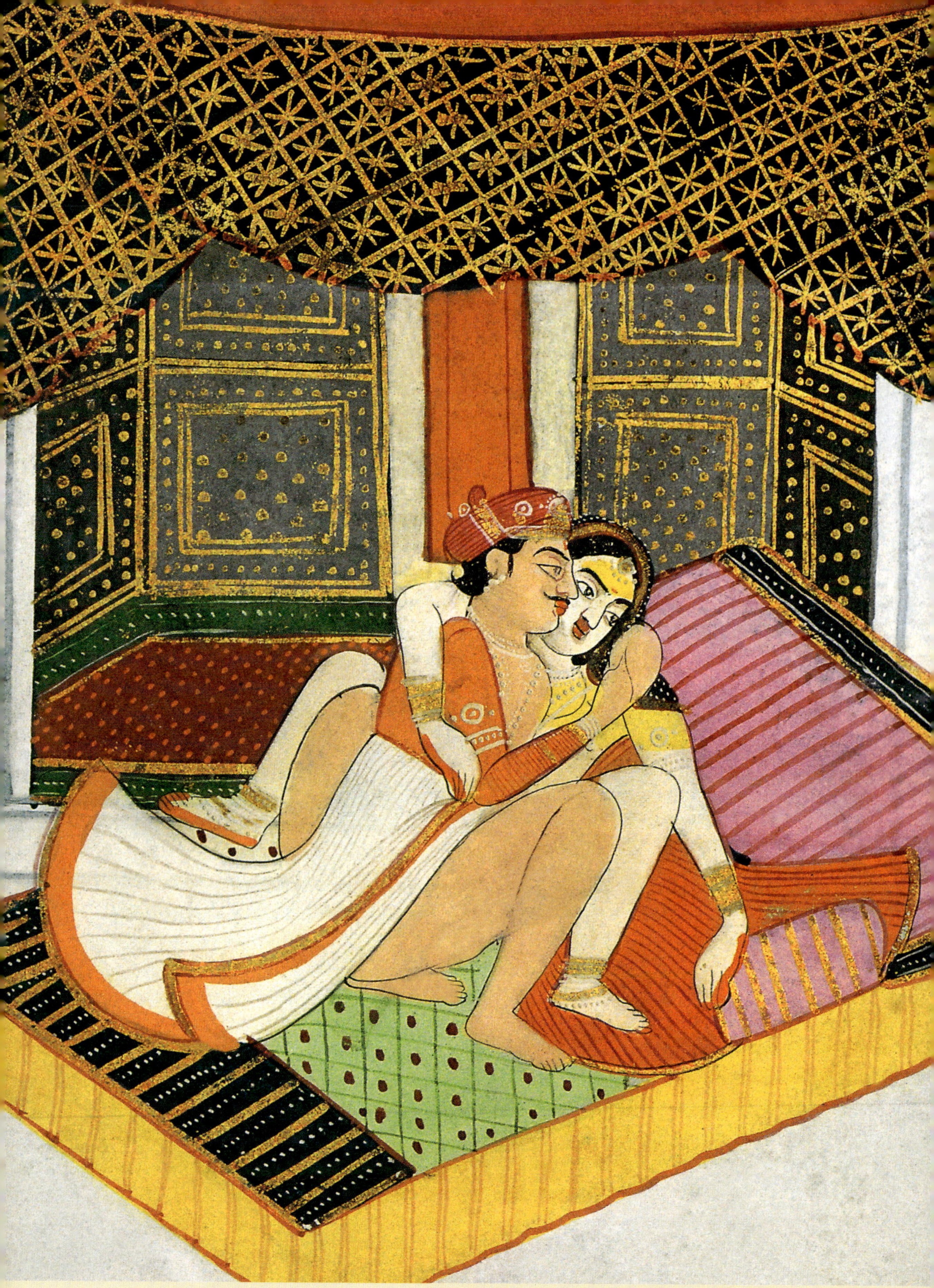

Young lovers: The ambience of the private quarters, richly decorated with fittings, curtains and tapestries woven with gold threads, are an ideal setting for the young noble couple, still experimenting on their love making. They probably started out in a lying posture and are moving around, to add more thrills. Interestingly, both are wrapped around in a squatting pose initially, and then move to the marble floor, with the *divan* for comfort, as he tries to enter her from behind.
Miniature painting, Jaipur, Rajasthan, 19th century. Private collection.

Bhugnak: This posture is when a female lying supine folds her legs at the knees and raises her thighs, but does not spread her legs apart. Instead she rests her knees against the chest of her mate who then enters the female in a half-sitting position.

Jrimbhitak: The female raises her legs and puts them on the shoulders of the male. The male also adopts a sitting posture with his knees up to the level of his partner's shoulders. Such a posture leads to a contraction of the female organ.

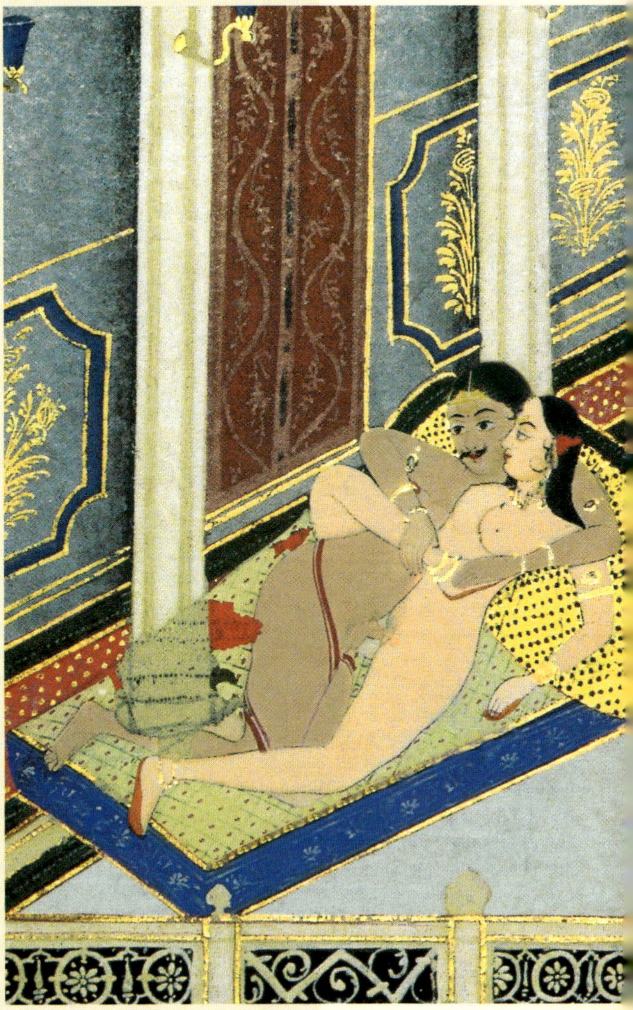

Utpiritaka: Folding her legs, the female rests them against the chest of her partner. The male spreads his legs around the shoulders of the female. All through the mating, the legs of the female are supported on the male's chest. Such a posture causes a peculiar thumping sensation in the hearts of both the partners.

Padmasana: The female adopts the *Padmasana* pose while lying supine and raises her thighs without undoing the *asana*. The male puts his hands through the folds of her legs and holds her shoulders in order to mount her.

Imitation of animals: Every animal has a peculiar way of mating. Human beings observe their postures and adopt them in mating rituals. Cows, buffaloes, dogs, horses, goats and sheep are some tame animals that breed in human presence. Humans are also aware of the postures wild animals adopt for mating. They imitate these postures to add to the novelty of

Previous page: **The lovers' tryst on the lake:** The tingling warmth of their young bodies is enhanced by the bright red *shamiana*, its colour symbolic of ardent, passionate love. They drift on a boat beneath the canopy of the sky. The idyllic setting is enriched by the lake-side pavilion, surrounded by lush trees and flowers. The painting breathes an air of mystery and wonder, at the act of love.

Miniature painting, Jaipur, Rajasthan, 19th century. Private collection.

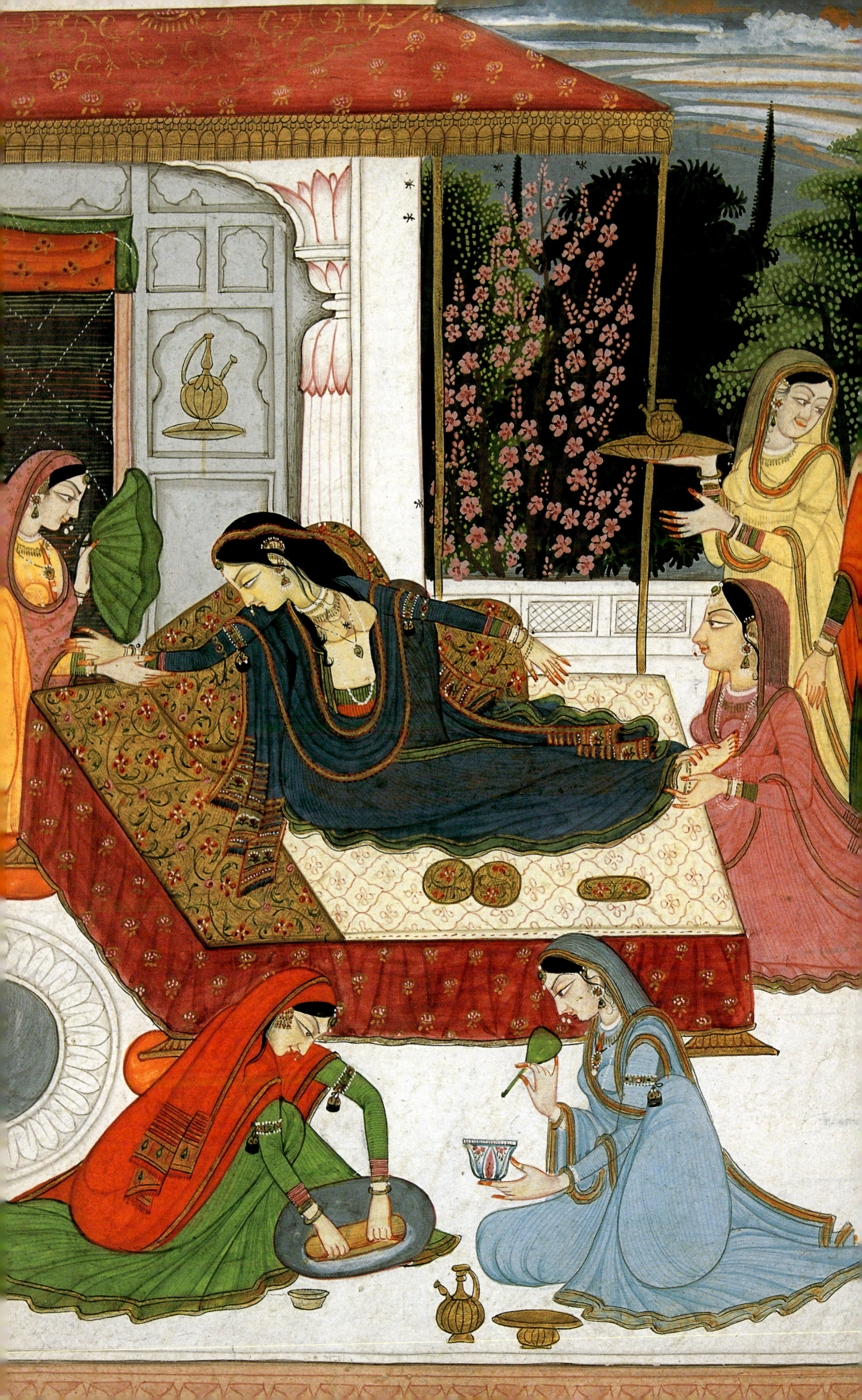

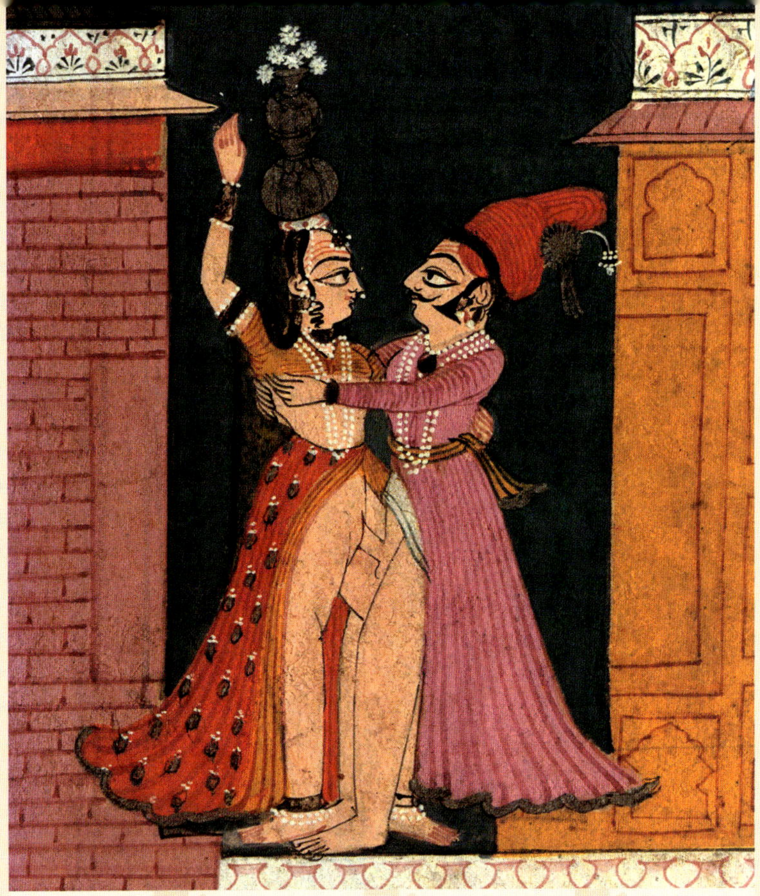

Standing posture: Another leaf from the Deogarh manuscript has a romantic persuasion. Water pots are balanced upon her head. They are full to the brim and pinned at the pinnacle by a bunch of blossoms. Underlying is the romantic village theme and its associations, enticing young village males into amorous pursuits, who could freely embrace girls carrying water pots, who afraid of the fall of their pots, and having no chance to escape or run away, would submit to the boy. The posture is *sthitarata*, upright stance. In folk and village dances, girls adept at this act, dance and sway to music, whilst balancing the pots and motioning their hips in a circular, very sexually attractive and stimulating revolution. *Miniature painting manuscript, mid 18th century, Deogarh, Rajasthan.*

the process, but these should only be used if they do not cause any pain to the female partner.

ROLE REVERSAL

At the end of the mating process, very often the partners exchange their roles. The main reason for this is to provide relief to the tired partner, and to rekindle his enthusiasm in the process. In the reversal of roles, obviously, the female partner plays the male role and vice versa. It is not necessary that the role reversal take place at the end of the process. It can be adopted for a change as a different experience for the main part of the coition. In the reversal of roles, the female mounts over the male and their genitals unite as usual. Experts say that when the role reversal is desired, the female must behave like the male from the beginning. She must take the initiative, start touching, embracing, kissing and indulge in all the fore-play first. Shivering of the hands is the first sign that shows that the woman has reached the height of excitement. At this stage, she shows deep love and does not allow her partner to withdraw even when he has ejaculated. All males must look out for this sign

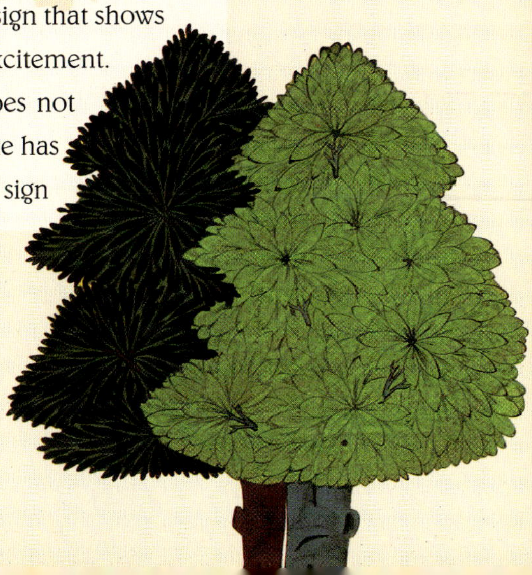

Facing page: **The heroine, waiting anxiously for her lover in her pavilion:** The atmosphere inclines to the view that the girl is feeling desperate, for any feeling of joy is completely absent. Yet she shows no signs of sorrow as her companions are full of smiles, suggesting that the lover may be just around the corner. *Miniature painting, Bundi, Rajasthan, mid 18th century. Private collection.*

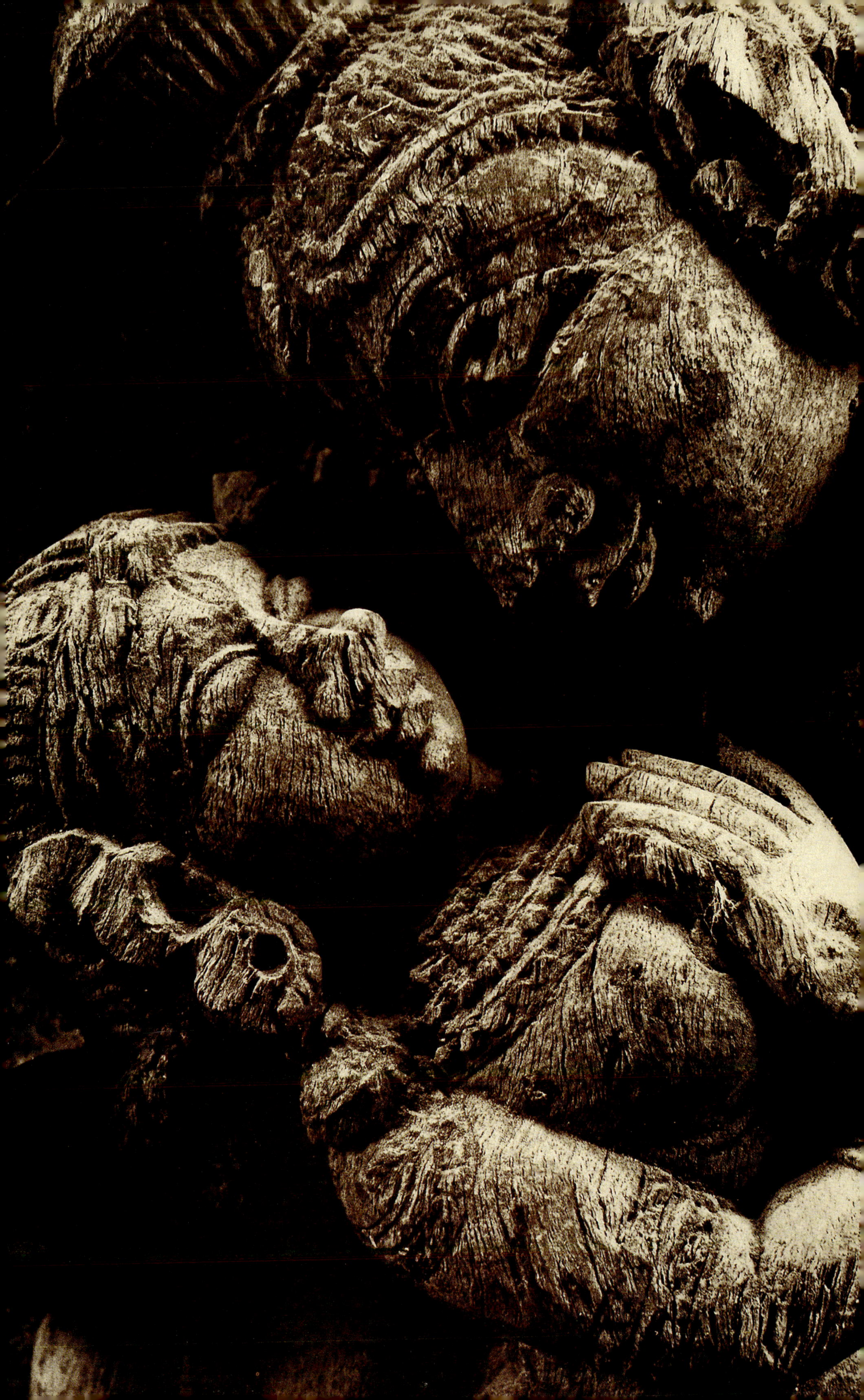

Below: **Amorous encounters of a village boy and girl, in a sitting posture:** The loving couple are a constant source of inspiration. They seem to get easily bored with the more simple aspects of love. *Miniature painting, Kulu style, mid 18th century. Lance Dane collection.*
Facing page: **Prahanana, striking:** An essential feature of the sex act, for though apparently painful, if conducted judiciously, it adds extra thrill to the sexual enjoyment. According to Vatsyayana, "Sexual union is by nature a combat between the two". *Wood carving from a temple ratha, processional chariot, Chidambaram, Tamil Nadu, late 19th century. Private collection.*
Following page: **The pranks of Krishna:** Krishna, the cowherd boy is in continuous narrative, displaying his amorous attainments with his *gopis*. In a most romantic incidence, Krishna purloined the *gopis'* clothes, as they bathed naked in the river. It provided an enviable opportunity for him to pinch their clothes, and hide them up a tree, refusing to return them unless they came to him! They are depicted here trying to shield their naked bodies in broad daylight. Krishna insisted that they lift their arms so that they stood bare before him. *Ettumaanoor murals, Kerala, 19th century.*

and see that they do not begin intercourse before that. They must wait till the female partner has achieved proper lubrication of her genitals and has acquired an open posture by leaving her body loose. There are certain manual ways to bring a woman to the height of excitement. Fondling of the female genitalia with skilful fingers is the most certain way. Some males force their partners to have oral sex. But the scriptures forbid this practice. They maintain that during intercourse, the mouth of a woman is a sacred thing and should not be defiled with oral sex.

THE BEGINNING AND THE END OF INTERCOURSE

Intercourse is a highly sensual activity to be enjoyed in privacy. That is why much significance is attached to the nuptial night and nuptial chamber. The ambience of the chamber should reflect the mood that needs to be created. It is recommended that soft cushions be placed on the bed and the air be perfumed. The male partner should occupy a place to the right of the bride, while talking gently to her. He should then hold her hands and caress them. At this stage, both of them may enjoy a mild intoxicating drink to do away with any shyness. Embracing, kissing, fondling, undressing and finally, intercourse, follow. After intercourse is over, the partners should not part with each other immediately. They must continue to feel each other's presence for some more time. This helps to maintain a close intimacy between them. Even after separation, they should sit together and talk lovingly, and partake of nutritious food and drink.

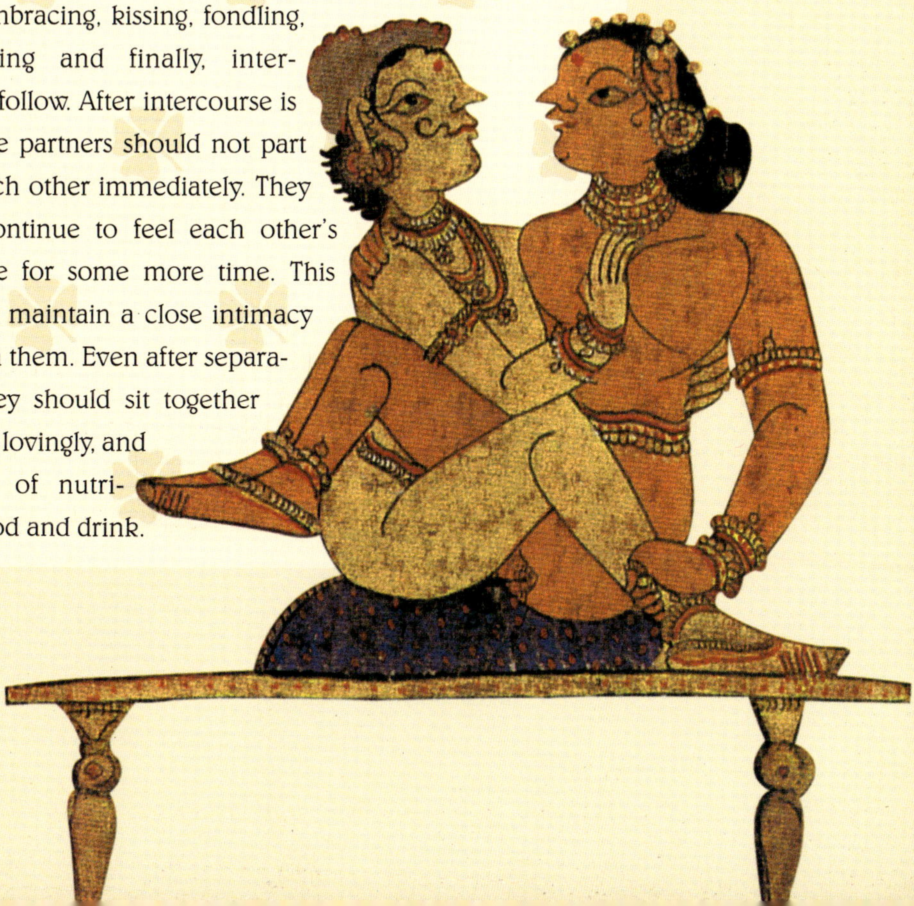

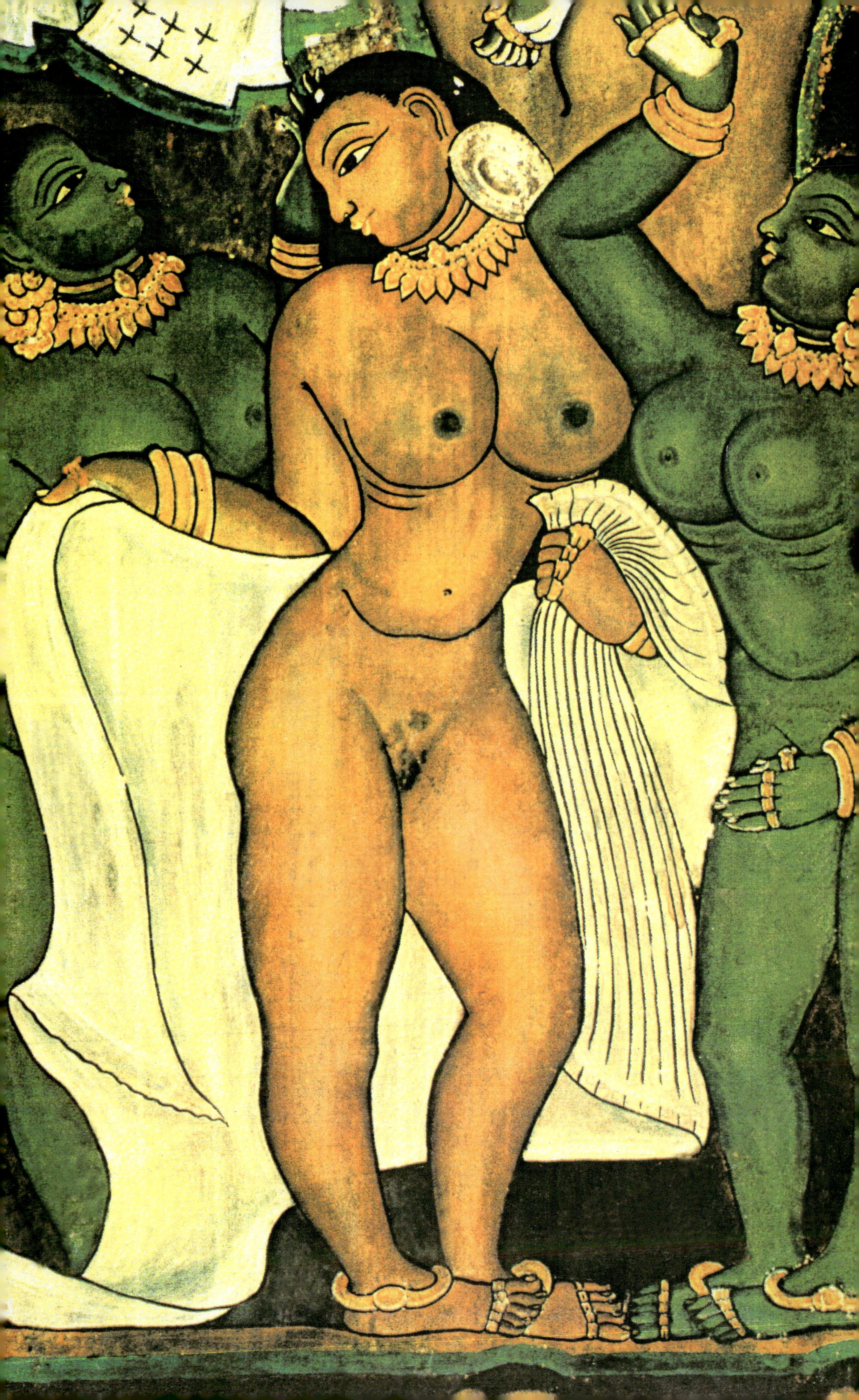

She becomes intimate with her lover, and after that, she gets him to love her

Kama Sutra

women's wiles and WEAPONS

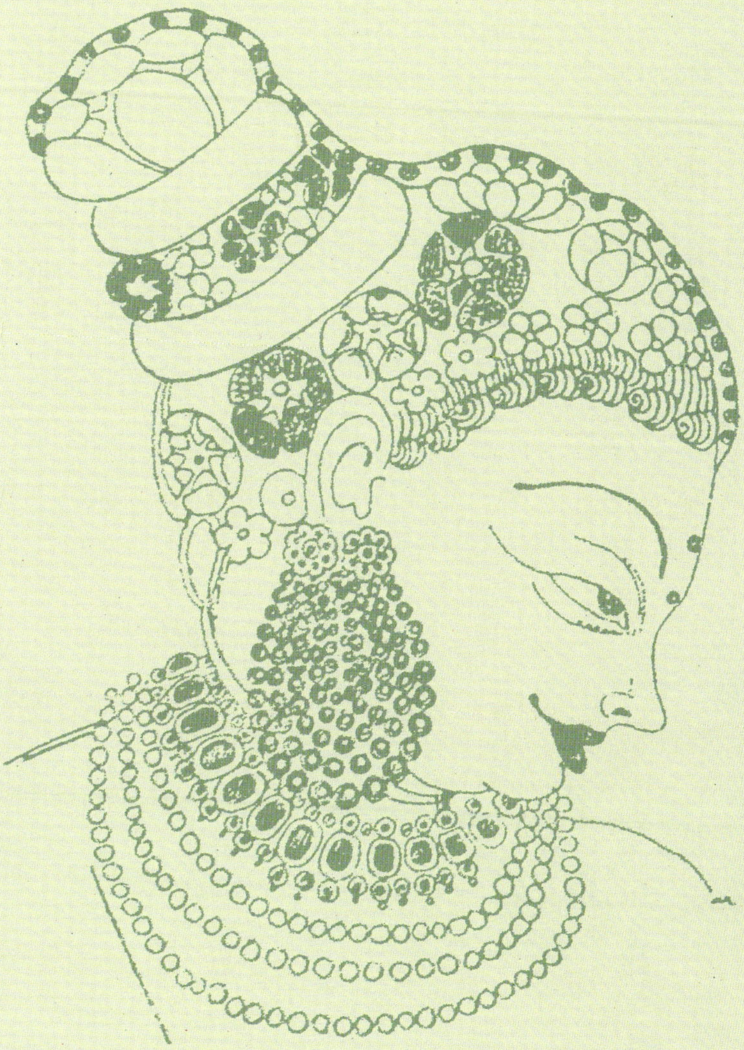

The swing of love: Spring is in the air and joyous times lie ahead, as the young couple closely entwine themselves on the small swing and melt into each other.
Miniature painting, Jodhpur, Rajasthan, 20th century. Private collection.

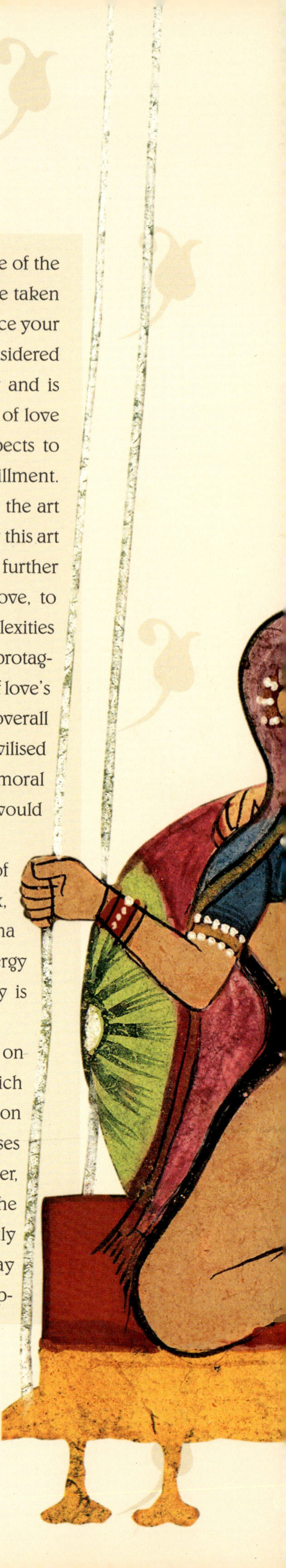

The ancient sage Vatsyayana was aware of the fact that female sexuality could not be taken for granted. He instructed men to 'place your pleasure second to hers'. Rati is considered the embodiment of female sexuality and is meant to initiate women into the art of love making, enhancing both the sensual and sexual aspects to lead them to ascend unknown peaks of desire and fulfillment.

While many sages felt that only men should study the art of love making, Vatsyayana believed that women knew this art instinctively. And it was imperative for them to study it further to hone their skills. Erotic love, to him, comprised the complexities of interactions between the protagonists and dwelt on the enjoyment of love's pleasures as well as an awareness of its sorrows. The overall attitude of erotic love in the *Kama Sutra* is that of a civilised and cultured person who seeks his pleasure within the moral and social order in which he is placed. The same would apply with suitable changes in the modern context.

Men and women also have varying degrees of endurance - those who are quick to reach their climax, and those who carry on for a long time. Vatsyayana avers that a woman loves the man whose sexual energy lasts for a long time and resents one, whose energy is spent quickly.

Book Two of the *Kama Sutra* also contains a verse on the kinds of 'love' or 'erotic desire' such as that which arises out of habit, that which stems from the imagination and not out of the act of love itself, the love which arises out of a comparison between a past and present lover, and that which is born out of the desire for what is presently before one's eyes. Foreplay should all be resorted to keeping in mind the customs of the region a woman belongs to.

Embracing or clasping removes the physical distance between partners. For partners who already know each other, embracing is full of drive. Between partners who are unknown to each other, embracing removes the physical distance and establishes closeness. There are four distinct stages in the process of embracing. These are touching, pulling, rubbing and pressing hard. First the partners touch each other lovingly. Next they are drawn closer. Once their bodies come in close contact, the partners caress and stroke each other. Even their bodies begin to rub against each other. Finally, as the urge grows stronger, the partners begin to press hard against each other in preparation for intercourse. The *Kama Sutra* states that at this stage, the partners should make use of any methods that help to increase the intensity of love.

Kissing may accompany embracing or follow it. While kissing kindles the fire of love, piercing with nails, acts like fuel to keep this fire burning. Nails should be used only when the partners have attained a certain level of excitement. Care should be taken not to inflict

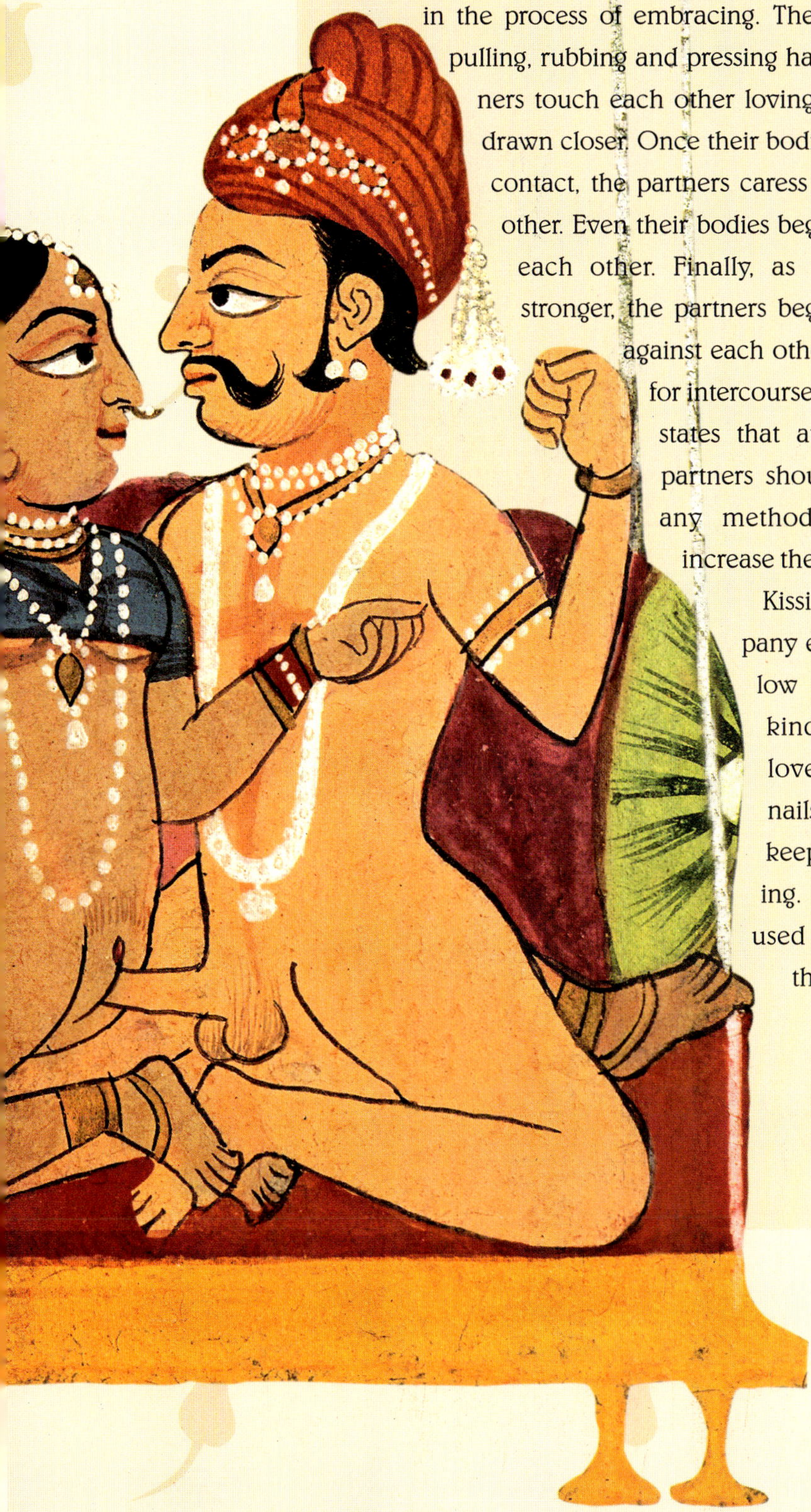

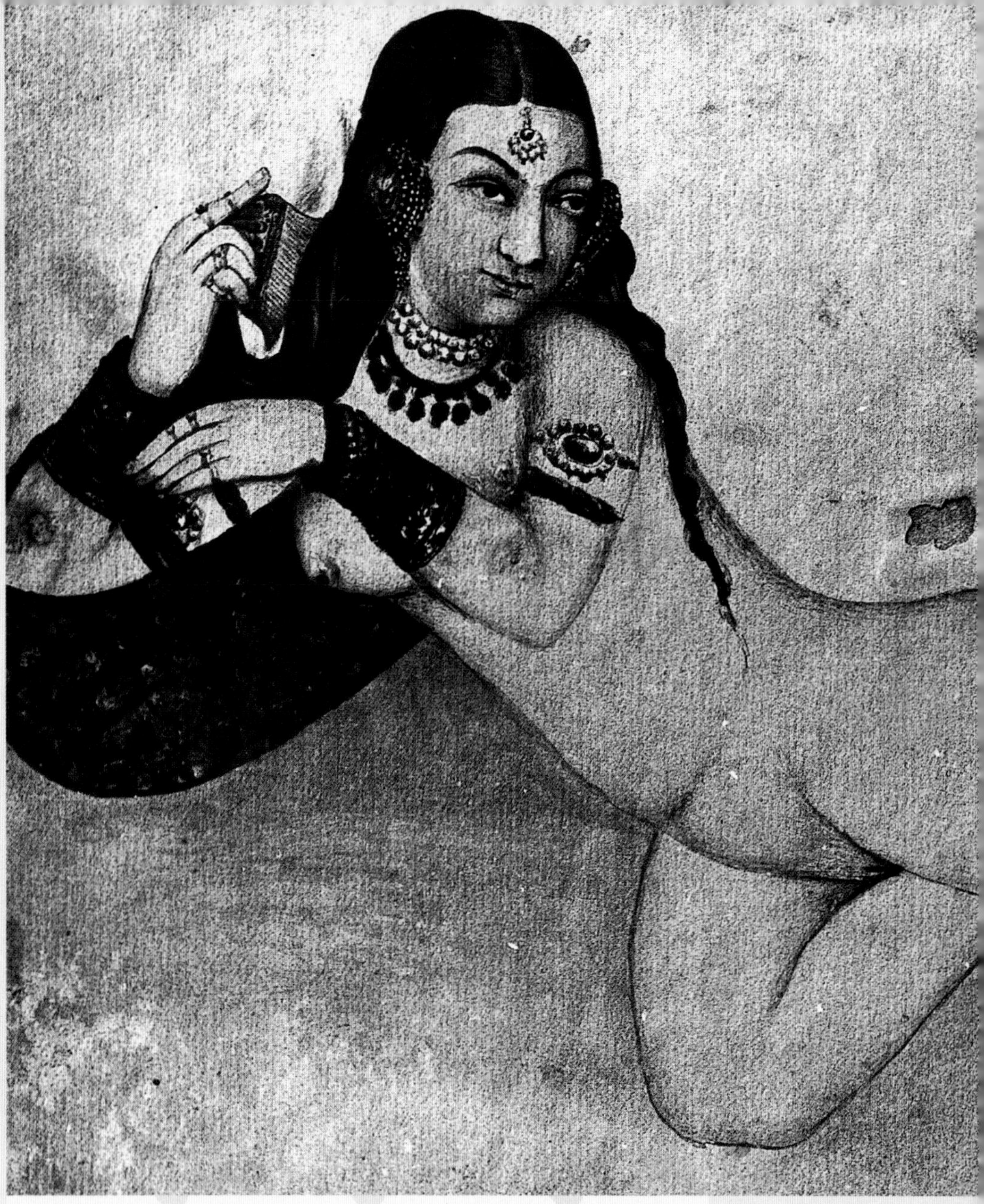

long-lasting marks. Nail marks serve to remind a person of the partner long after the two have parted. Biting, either, accompanies or follows the piercing with nails. It adds to the heat of love but no permanent marks should be left.

WHAT ATTRACTS A WOMAN

Book Seven of the *Kama Sutra* deals with using 'secret recipes' to attain the object of one's desire. The Pali canon states that that man is not dear to a woman who has five personal demerits. They are:

- He is not handsome of form.
- He has no prosperous enjoyments.

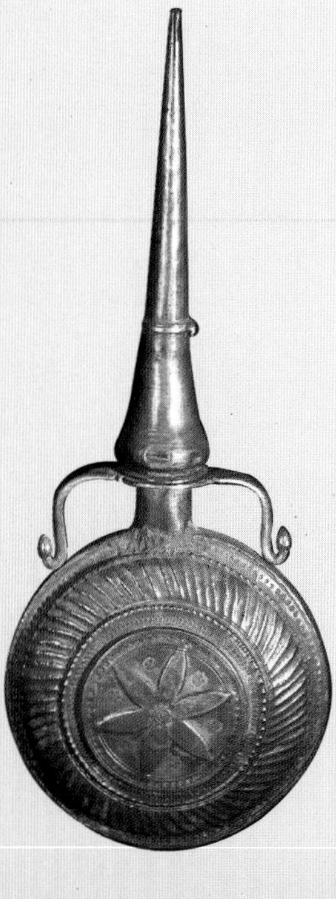

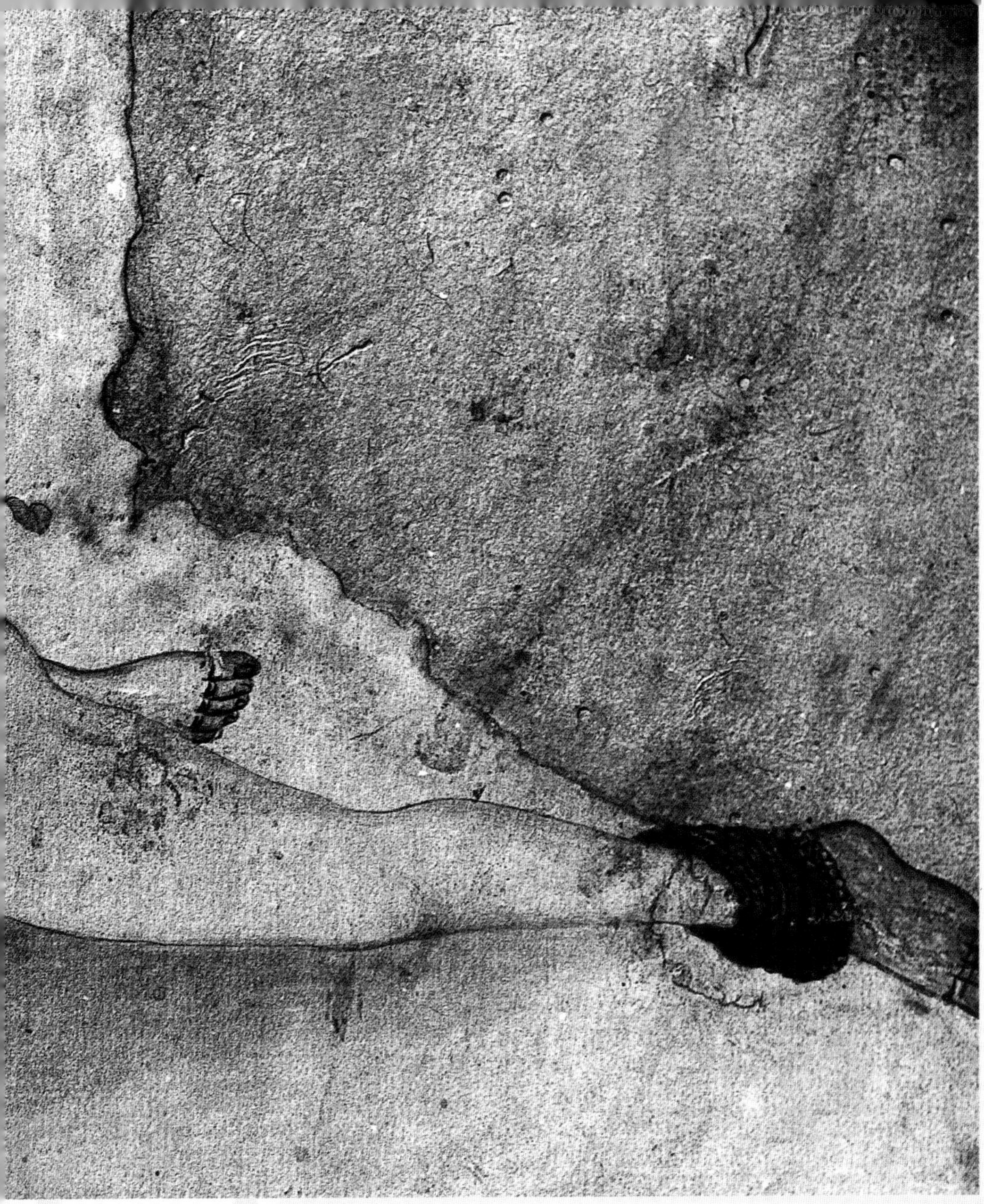

Public woman: Sanskrit presents a nomenclature, abundant in its variety as in its potential for visual imagery. To give expression to the unclothed body of a beautiful woman, it has countless renderings. A good number of them have classical associations and have, therefore, appeared in literary works, since human thoughts have given expression, to the incomparable attraction of the feminine form. A most famous *ganika* in Buddhist legend is the wealthy and intellectual Ambapalli of Vaishali. Even Lord Buddha did not find it inappropriate to sit with her and take refreshments. The courtesans of ancient India, in the great cities of Vaishali, Pataliputra and Rajagriha, were held in the highest regard, and enjoyed a status enviable even to the wives. They were ranked high for their artistic talents, and for their responsible attitude. The *sutras* composed by Dattaka proclaim that *ganikas* should also bear the following feminine features and characteristics - be possessed of beauty with auspicious body marks; should have a taste for good qualities; must have a great desire to attain wealth and position; should take great delight in sexual union; should have a firm implacable mind, and with regard to sexual enjoyment, be in the same class as the man. *Painting, Thanjavur, Tamil Nadu, late 18th century. Private collection.*

- He is ill of conduct.
- He is lazy.
- He is incapable of begetting progeny.

The *Jamini Brahmana* avers that women like chatting with handsome young men. The *Shathapatha Brahmana* maintains: 'He is indeed a blithesome youth who is in the prime of his life; whence one who is in his prime of life is apt to become dear to women.'

The *Kathaka Samhita* feels that 'A woman lusts for a man who sings and not for one who speaks philosophy.' Vyasa states in the *Mahabharata*: 'Women betray a liking for those men who court them, who approach their presence and who respectfully somewhat serve them.'

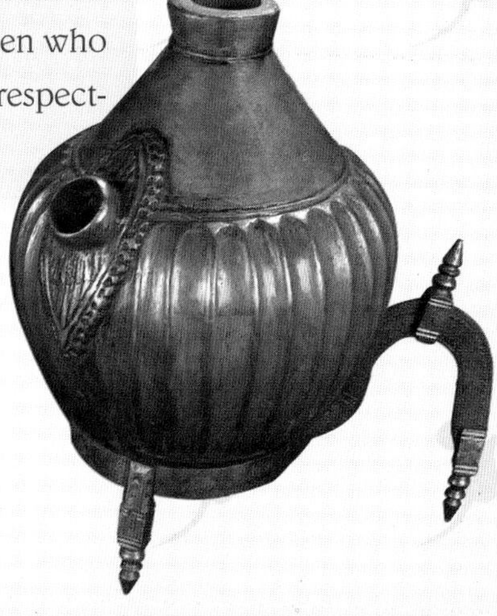

Heroic show of sexual strength: Part of a decorative panel eloquent with erotic encounters: The wooden panel *(facing page)* and also a cut out of a Rajasthan painting *(below)* depict standing sexual encounters. On each side, are standing couples in union from the front and behind. *Miniature painting, Jodhpur , Rajasthan, late 19th century* and a *Decorative wood panel, Chidambaram, Tamil Nadu, 20th century.*

Bharat's *Natyashastra* maintains that there are three kinds of women according to their standing in life:

- *Abhyantara* - Inside Women
- *Bahya* - Outside Women
- *Bahyabhyantara* - Outside-Inside Women

A woman belonging to the household is the Inside Woman. A courtesan is the Outside or Public Woman. A woman who possesses virtue, being a maiden of a high family, is the mixed kind or Outside-Inside Woman. A virtuoso should mark the signs expressive of the love sentiments. A courtesan should be recognised as smitten with love from her external expressions like her impassioned bodily gestures, looks given with askance, touching on the ground with her big toe, displaying her breasts and navel, pricking of the nails and sweeping up her hair.

A woman of high birth, whether married or a maiden, when smitten, looks continuously with glowing eyes, smiles in a secretive manner, speaks with a downcast face, replies with a smile, speaks slowly, covers up her perspiring body, has throbbing lips and appears amazed.

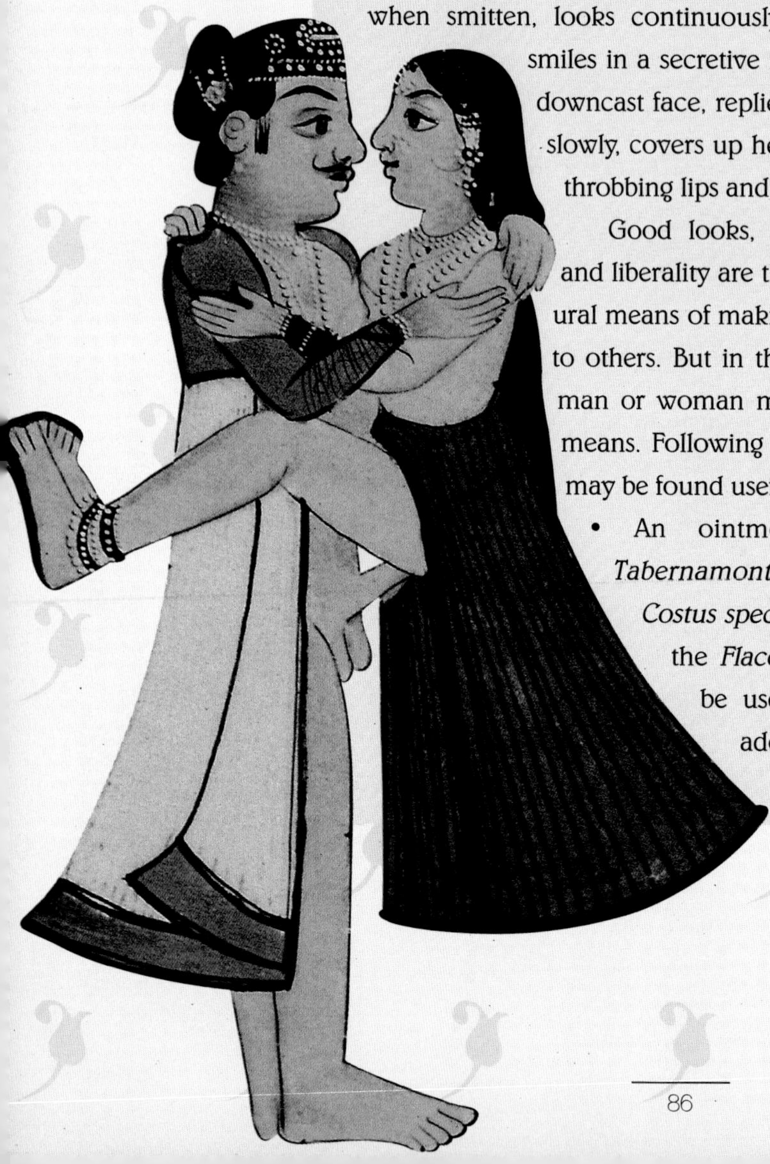

Good looks, good qualities, youth and liberality are the chief and most natural means of making a person agreeable to others. But in the absence of these, a man or woman must resort to artificial means. Following are some recipes that may be found useful:

- An ointment made of the *Tabernamontana coronaria*, the *Costus speciosus* or *arabicus*, and the *Flacourtia cataphrata*, can be used as an unguent of adornment.

If a fine powder is

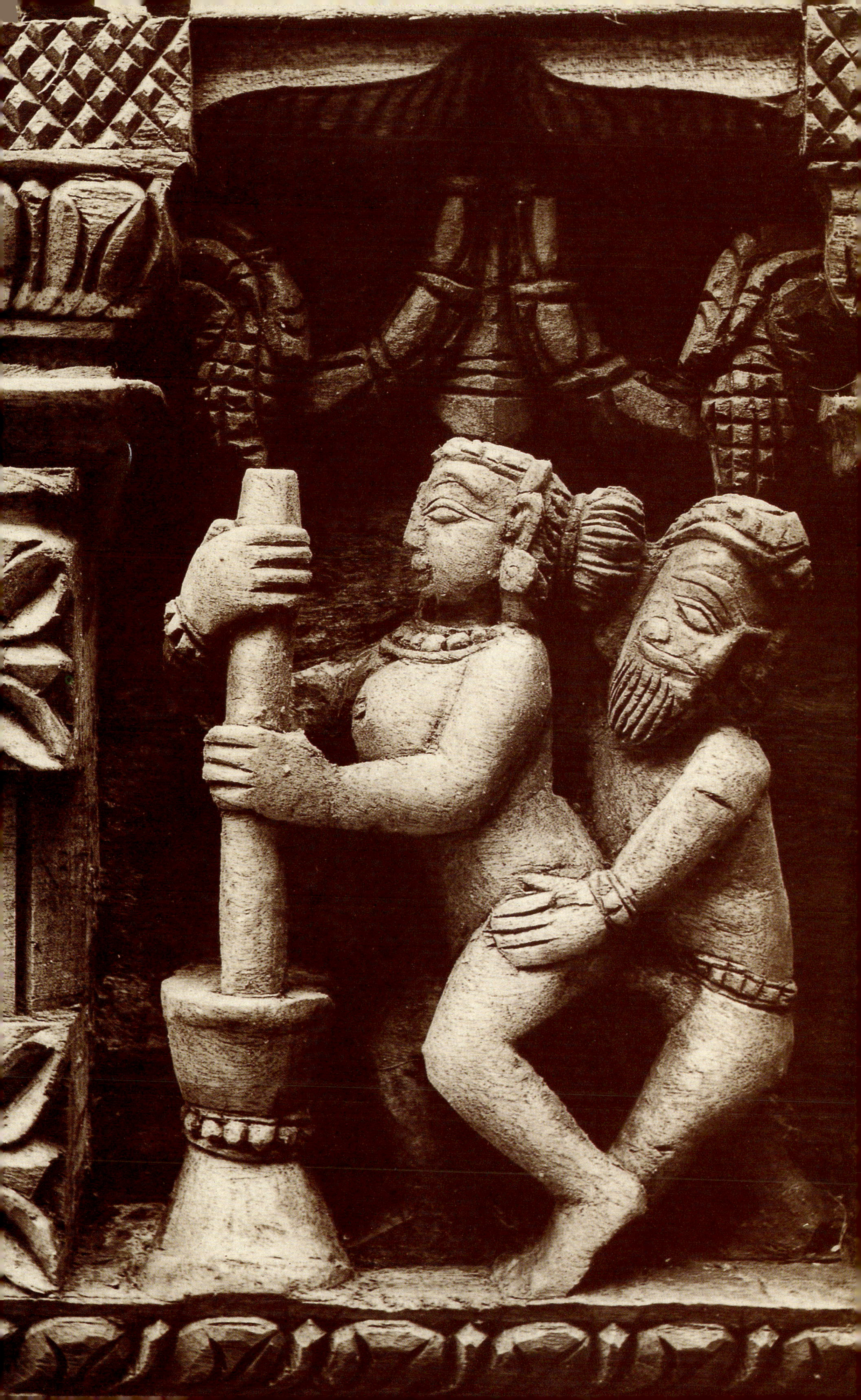

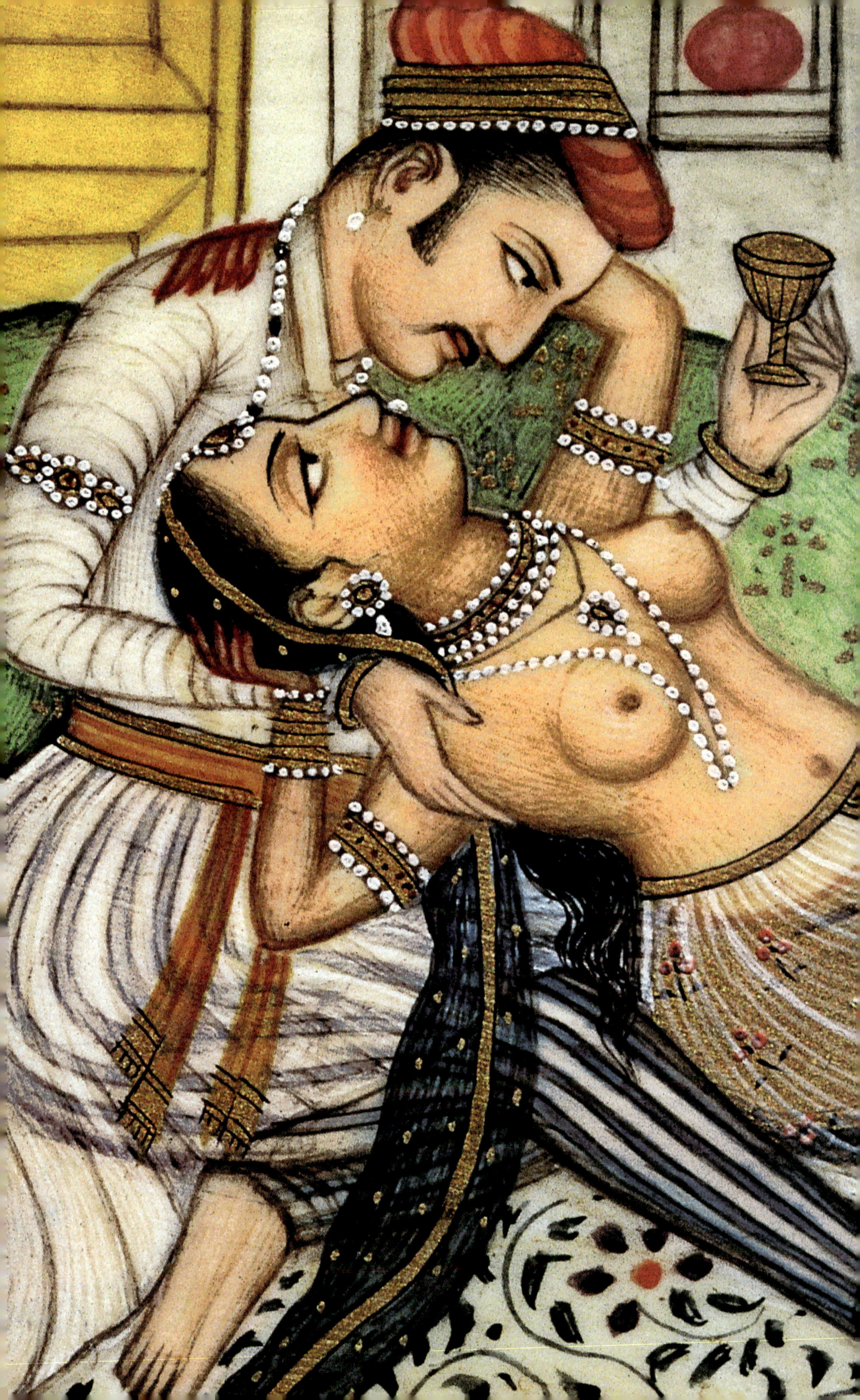

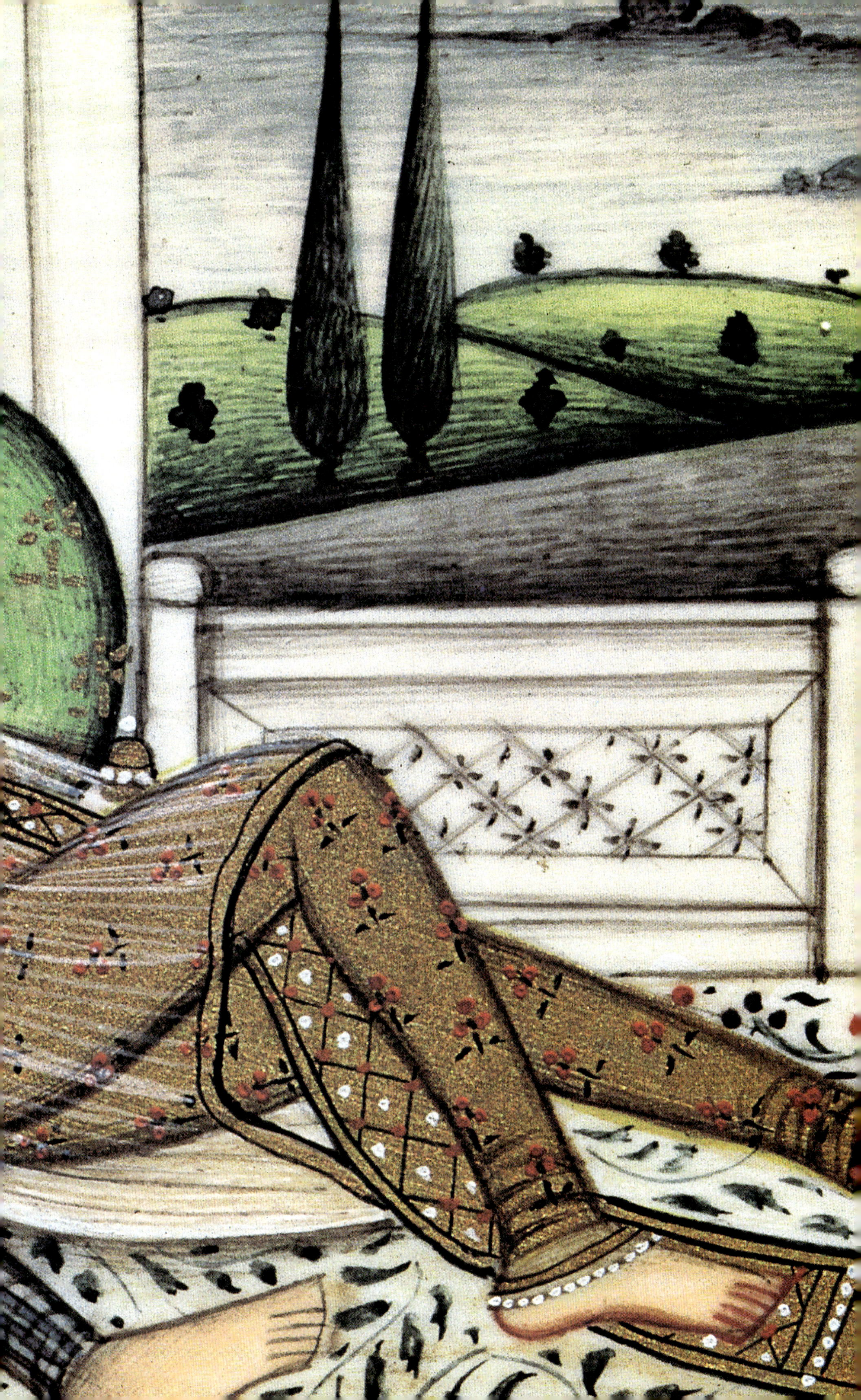

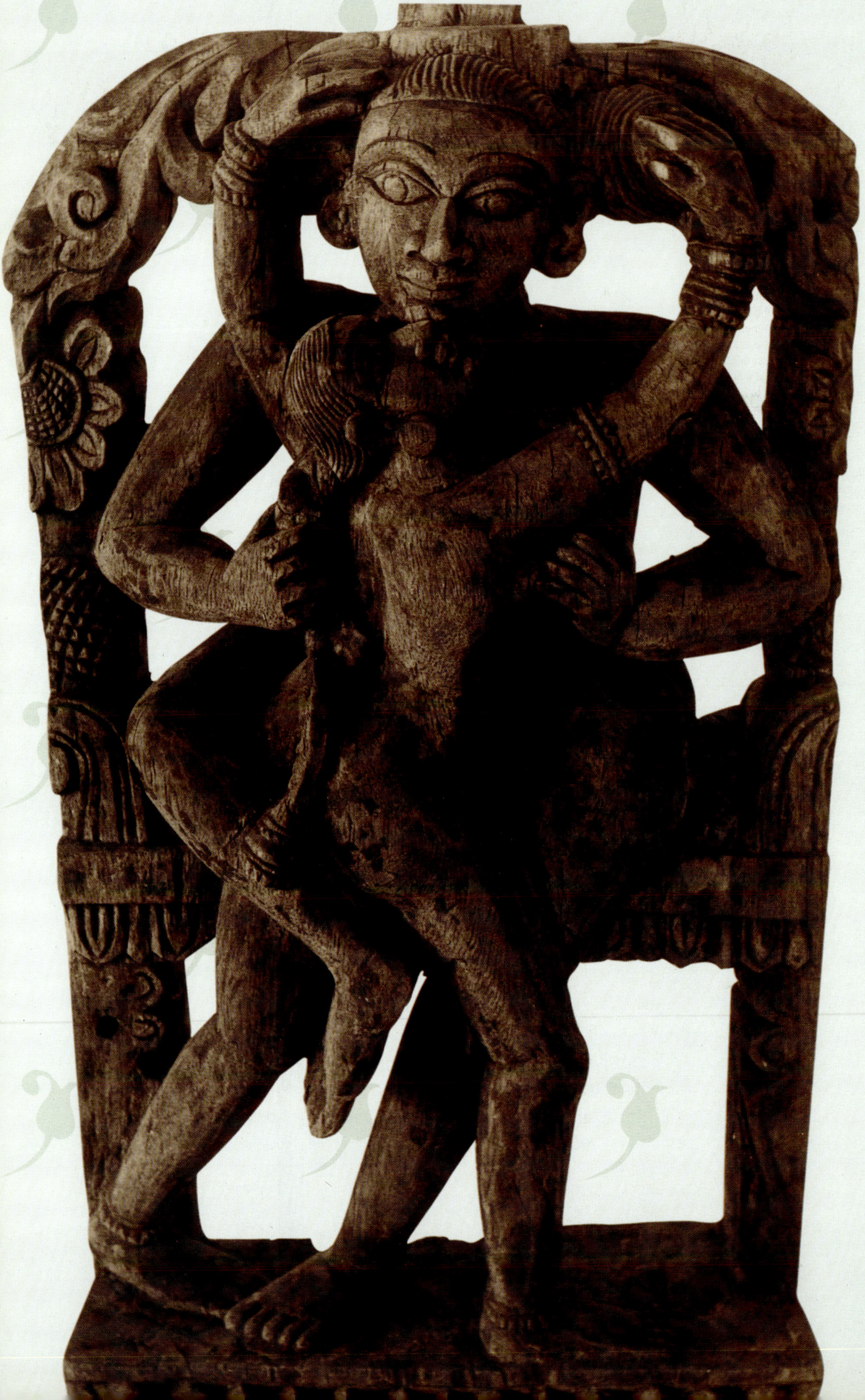

Previous pages: **Wrapped in pleasure:** The *ganika* laps up his attentions and enjoys sips of wine. Dattaka's insight on the inherent skills of manoeuvre of the courtesan is a fascinating study, in subterfuge and strategy. The entourage of these great ladies, runs into considerable numbers. Describing them, Vatsyayana says, "When a courtesan is living as a wife with her lover, she should behave like a chaste woman, and do everything to his satisfaction. Her duty in this respect, in short, is, she should give him pleasure, but should not become attached to him though, behaving as if she were really in love." A courtesan living in this manner, the life of a wife, is not troubled with too many lovers, and yet obtains an abundance of wealth. *Painting on ivory, 20th century, Jaipur or Jodhpur, Rajasthan.*

made of the above plants, and applied to the wick of a lamp, which is made to burn with the oil of blue vitriol, the black pigment or lamp black produced therefrom, when applied to the eyelashes, has the effect of making a woman look lovely.

In today's world, this would translate into the use of kohl or eye make-up to enhance the loveliness of the face.

• The oil of the hogweed, the *Echites putescens,* the sarina plant, the yellow *amaranth,* and the leaf of the nymphae, if applied to the body, has the same effect.

In today's world, aromatherapy becomes a tool for seduction. The essential oils used in aromatherapy are fragrant, and when selected and applied appropriately they may have therapeutic effects. Aromatherapy can be used by either sex.

Essential oils may be applied in a variety of ways, such as evaporated into the air, massaged into the skin, and being dispersed in bath water. However, aromatherapy as a therapy or treatment usually refers to body treatment in which a practitioner applies a blend of essential oils diluted in carrier oil(s) to the client's skin.

Highly concentrated essential oils that are often highly aromatic and are extracted from plants, are often used for healing; incense is employed for religious rituals, used in perfumes and embalming ointments, and for culinary purposes. There are many Biblical references that give an insight into the uses of plant oils and the high value that was attached to them.

In prominent ancient cultures the use of these oils, traditionally known as aphrodisiacs, was very much part and parcel of the lifestyle of the sophisticated. The earliest pictorial references associated with aromatherapy are images on the walls of the Lascaux caves in France, which are thought to date from approximately 18,000 B.C. They were used in ancient Egypt almost 3000 years before Christ for medicinal as well as cosmetic purposes and for embalming their dead.

Ancient civilisations may not necessarily have used scent-

Facing page: **Beginning and end of congress:** "He should then seat her on his left side, and holding her hair, he should gently embrace her with his right arm." The realism portrayed in this remarkable wood sculpture exhibits an artistic handwork, probably a crafts person from Orissa or even Andhra. *Wood carving from a temple chariot, South India, early 19th century.*

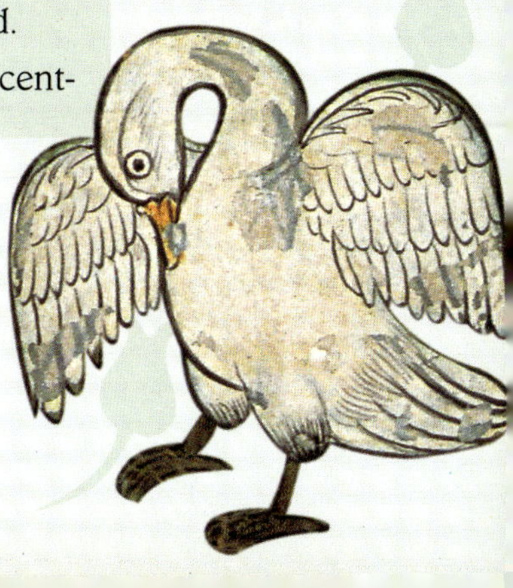

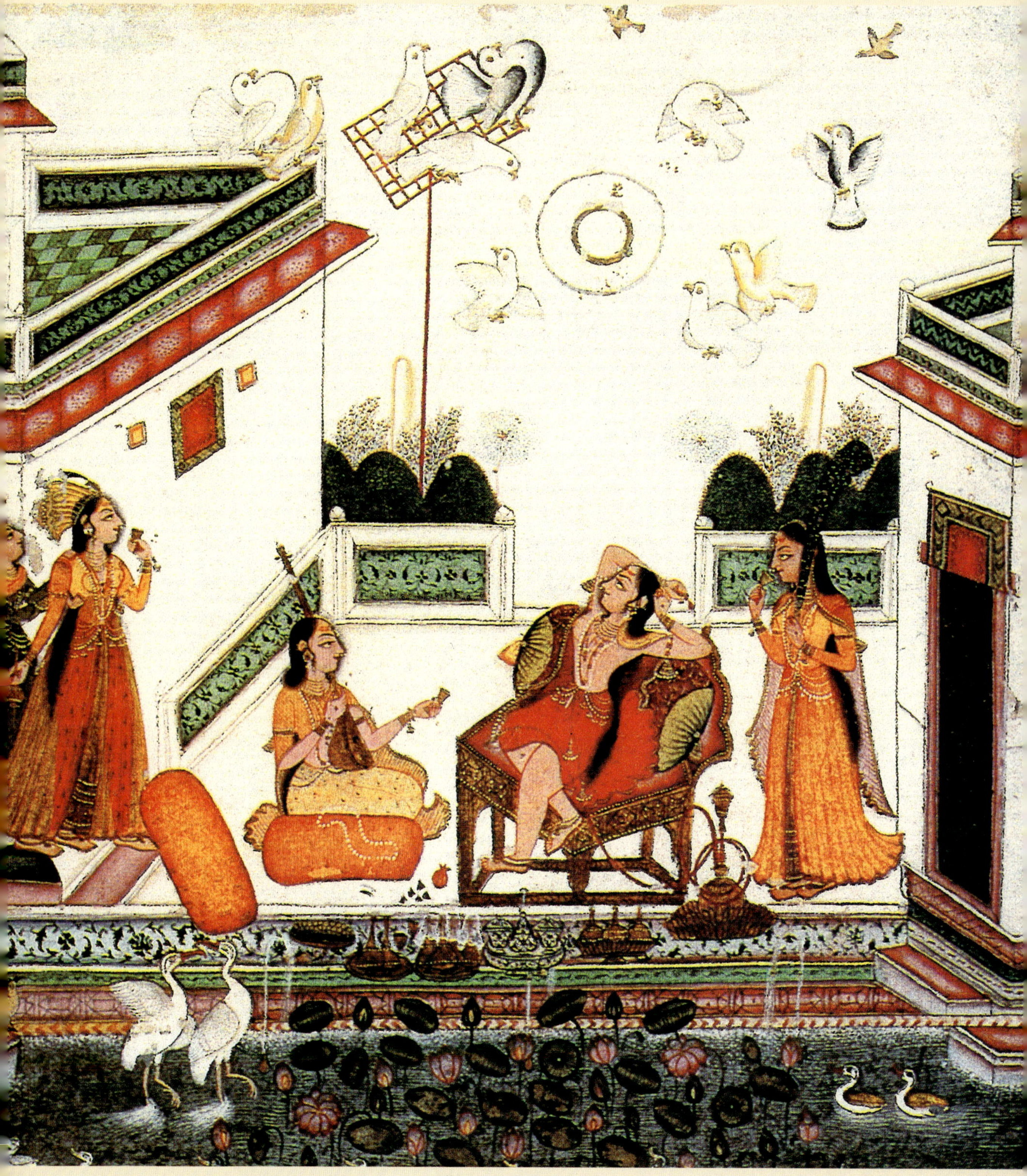

A beautiful courtesan: She bares to the waist, and delights in pleasant memory of her lovers. She revels in an outdoor setting, enjoying the fresh air. The atmosphere is absolutely charming, with the lotus pool in the foreground and pigeons fluttering overhead. *Miniature painting, Bundi, Kota style, Rajasthan, early 18th century. Private collection.*

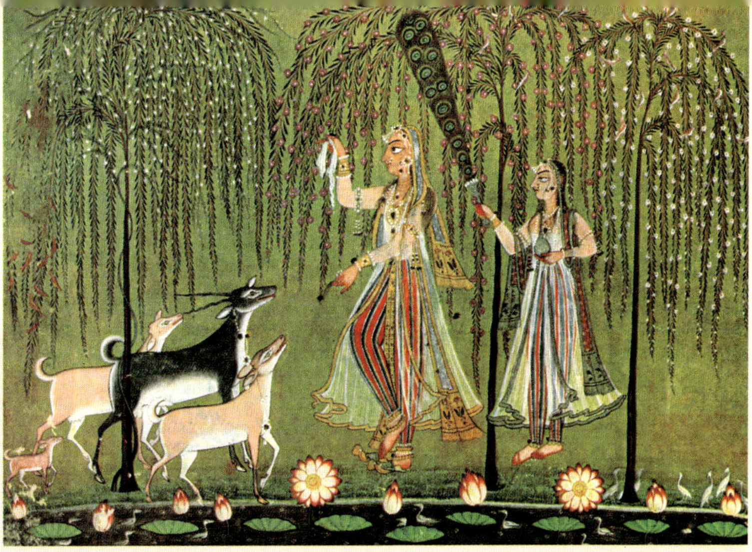

Lost in the forest: The miniature portrays two lonely *nayikas* in the tree laden forest, looking for guidance from a group of deer, who would guide them to safety. The natural ambience is typical of the artistic brush of hilly artisans. *Miniature painting, Kulu Valley, 19th century. Private collection.*

ed oils in the same way as each other, or in the same way as aromatherapy is practised today but there is evidence of use of scented/aromatic oils for the purposes of physical, mental, emotional, and/or spiritual well-being.

During the Renaissance in Europe (c. 1450-1600), explorers and merchants brought exotic herbs and oils back to Europe from the Middle and Far East. Interest in these luxuries grew, especially among the middle and upper classes.

In the later years of the 20th century, massage with aromatherapy oils became extremely popular, and it generally became associated with relaxation and the removal of the effects of stress as well as natural healing and alternative medicine.

When combined with base oils to dilute them, the essential oils are very readily absorbed through the skin, and so they make the ideal massage oil. The person applying the massage oil selects a blend of oils to suit the client and a great deal of skill is required to get this right. The deeper degree of relaxation, the more likely it is that you will be able to get more in touch with yourself.

Aromatic oils of today are based on traditional methods, on the belief that certain odours have alluring and seductive properties. *Sandalwood, ylang ylang, carnation oil, patchouli, damiana, jasmine, ginger, peppermint, ashwagandha* - all these oils are known for its effects in rejuvenating and stimulating the nervous system.

To effectively initiate a mood for romance, the aromatic industry has come out with different mixtures and portions of oil to enhance sexual ability and performance and to create intimacy between partners.

THE ROMANCE BLEND

Patchouli, sandalwood, ylang ylang, jasmine

INTIMACY BLEND

Ylang ylang, patchouli, lavender, rose

TENDERNESS BLEND

Geranium, cedarwood, ylang ylang, lavender

THE SIXTY-FOUR ARTS

The sixty-four arts that should be studied along with the *Kama Sutra* include singing, playing musical instruments, dancing, painting . . .The list includes useful skills like making beds, cooking a variety of foods, even quaint pastimes such as teaching birds to talk! A knowledge of a foreign language, speaking beautifully, calligraphy, flower arranging, ability to distinguish between false and real gems, sewing, saving money, treating birds and animals kindly, ability to judge craftiness and reply accordingly, behaving suitably with others, prudence, personal hygiene - are all general arts that prepare a woman to become a good wife.

As far as the physical aspects of a relationship are concerned, there are 16 arts that a young girl must learn before opening herself up to her husband. These are: reading others' thoughts, expression of love for others, showing acceptance through bodily gestures, allowing slow touching of her private parts, scratching lovingly with nails and biting, undoing the fastener of the lower clothing,

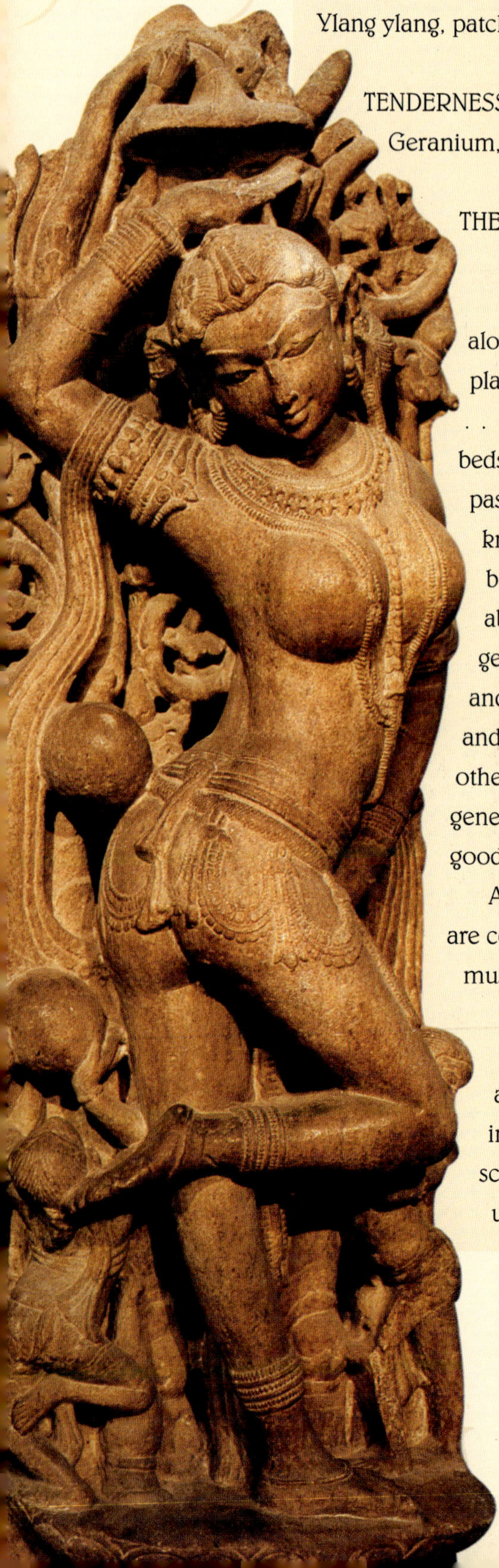

Playful maiden, potential footballer: Young playful girls, adopt voluptuous postures and look most attractive. Inspired artists embellished them as decorative bracket figures. The cutting of stone permits an almost three-dimensional view. On the left, her charming action is so visible as she plays with footballs, several at a time, and a monkey is looking for an opportunity to join in the fun. Sparse or semi clad, her figure is beautiful. *White marble, Rajasthan, 11th century. National Museum.*

straightening and exposing the private parts, artful participation in intercourse, pleasing the partner, experiencing satisfaction and making the partner feel the same, encouraging the partner to have intercourse, posing as if angry, removal of anger in a playful way, pleasing the angry partner, leaving the sleeping partner, going to sleep after coition and concealing the private parts. Apart from these, there are four more additional arts inducing guilt in the partner through tearful eyes for his showing negligence to you, stopping an uninterested partner from leaving, following him if he does not stop, and looking helplessly at the partner who is leaving.

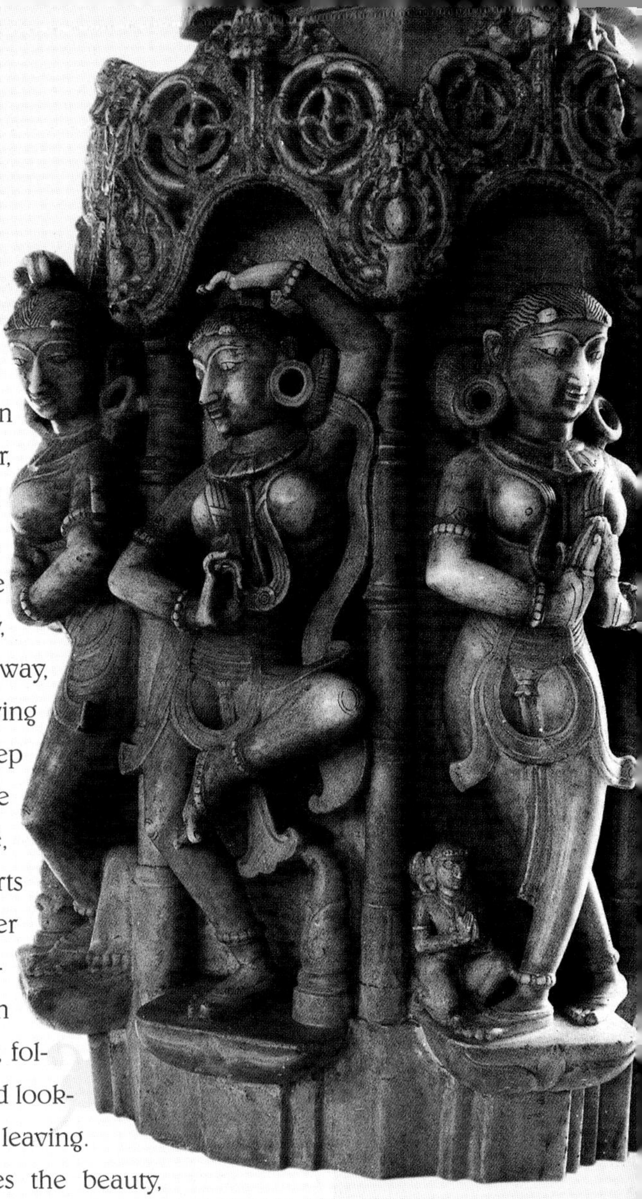

Learning these arts enhances the beauty, character and virtues of a woman. The sixty-four arts, which are auxiliary to the *Kama Sutra* are:

1. Vocal music
2. Instrumental music
3. Dancing
4. Painting
5. Cutting of different designs on the *Bhurga* leaf for adorning the forehead
6. Making various designs with rice grains and flowers
7. Arrangement of flowers
8. Colouring teeth, garments, hair, nails, the body and other toiletries
9. Fixing coloured tiles on the floor
10. Arrangement of the bed, settee, the *divan*
11. Creating musical sounds with the water - *Jaltaranga*

Following page: **A scene of revelry:** The costumes of the court have gone off as amorous women in various stages of undress, dote joyfully on a heroic young nobleman, and delight in the pleasure of his company. *Painting on ivory, Jodhpur, Rajasthan, 20th century. Private collection.*

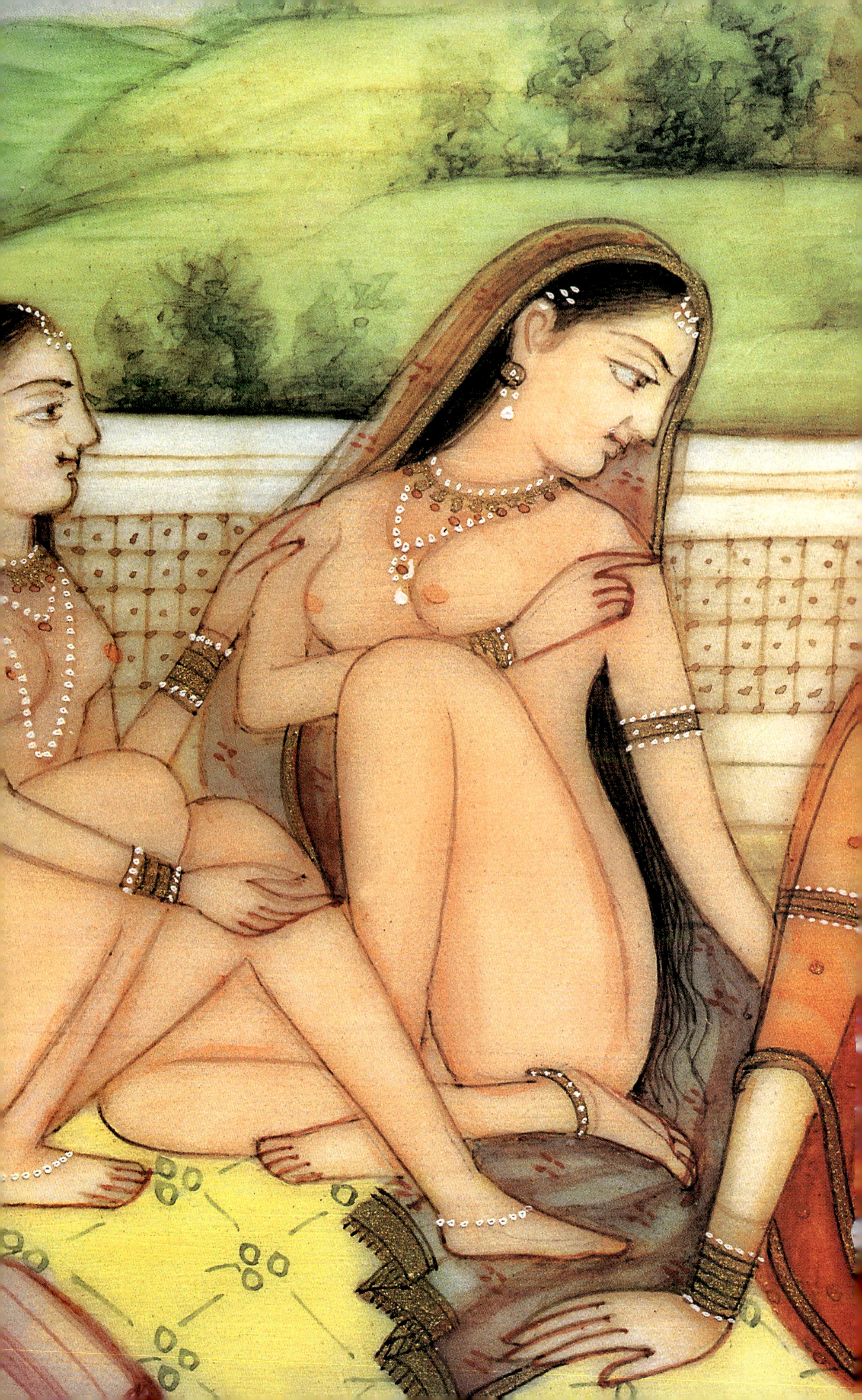

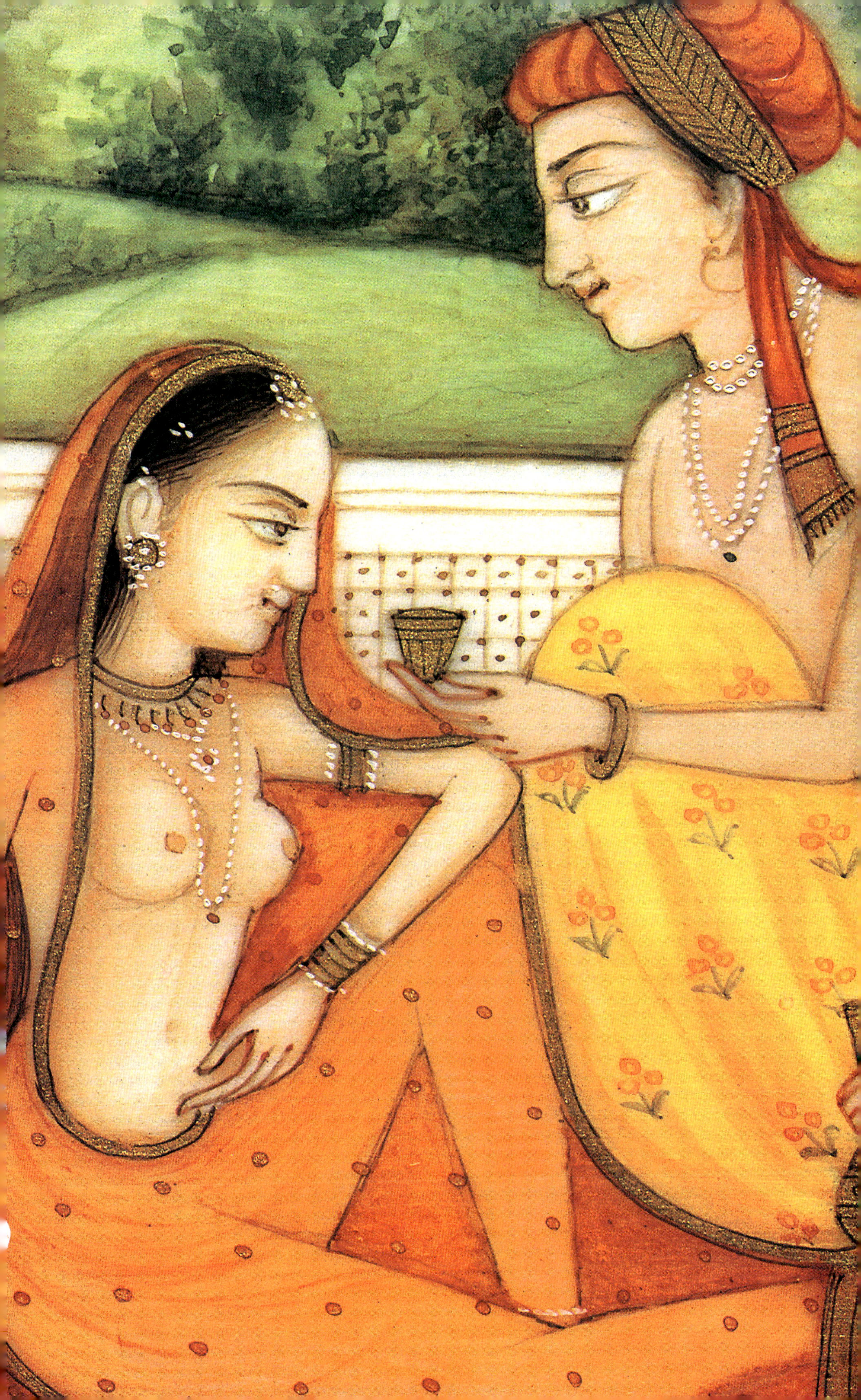

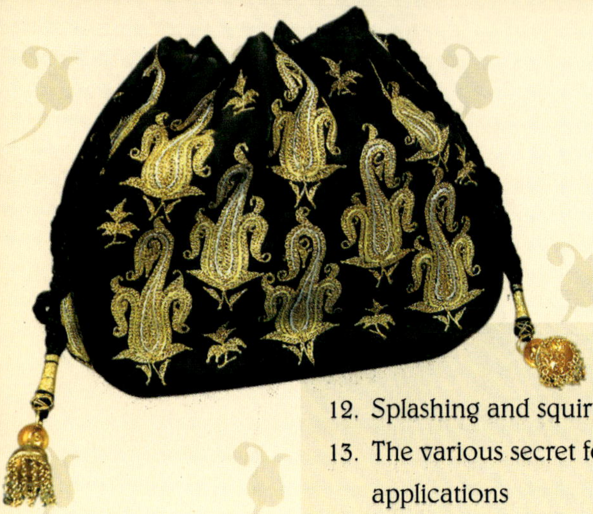

12. Splashing and squirting with water - *Jalkrida*
13. The various secret formulae and *mantras* and their applications
14. Making various types of garlands
15. Making head decorations known as *Shekharaka* and *Apida*
16. Dressing and decorating the body
17. Making designs called *Karnapatra*
18. The preparation and proper use of perfumes
19. Making ornaments
20. Magic and creating illusions
21. Preparation of ointments
22. Deftness in manual work
23. Cooking and similar culinary arts
24. Preparing *sherbets* and drinks
25. Needlework
26. Creating patterns from yarns and threads
27. Playing on the *veena* and the drum called *damaruka*
28. Composing and solving riddles and rhymes
29. *Antakshari*, a conversation or repartee through music
30. Reciting verses difficult to repeat such as tongue-twisters
31. Recitation from books
32. Knowledge of dramas and stories
33. Composing other lines when one is given
34. Caning of wood frames for cots, chairs, and so forth
35. Fabrication of mechanical aids in love making
36. Carpentry
37. Knowledge of architecture and house construction
38. Knowledge of precious stones
39. Knowledge of precious metals
40. Knowledge of jewels
41. Gardening
42. Art of cock fighting and ram fighting

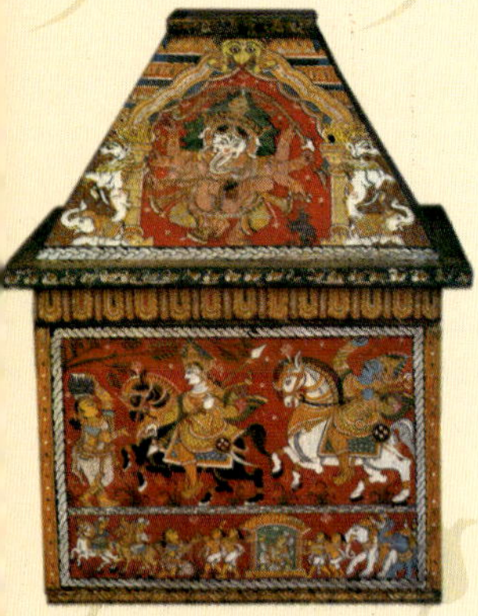

On both sides of the page are handicrafts, relevant to the theme of the sixty-four arts, a good way to make an effort to gain practical knowledge. Young people should take the opportunity to gain familiarity with these practical aspects of daily life.

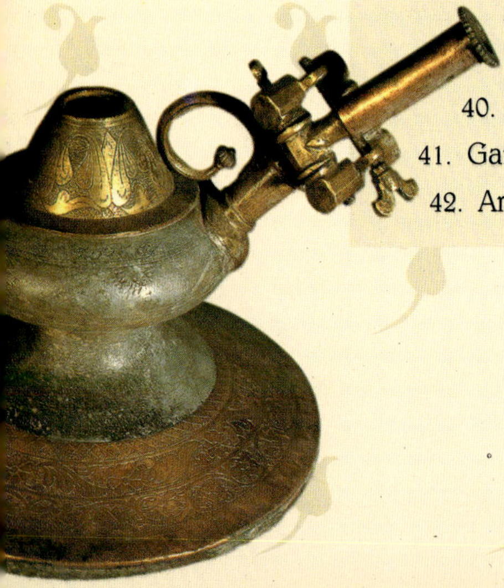

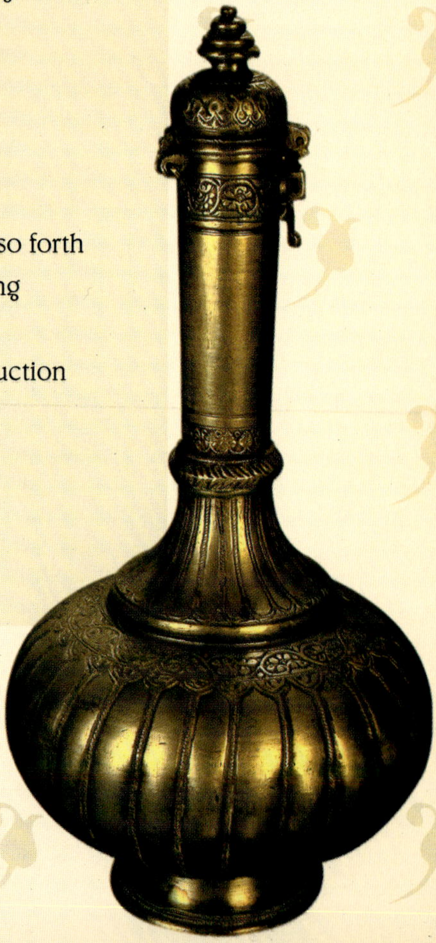

43. Training parrots and mynahs to speak and sing
44. Proficiency in shampooing and dressing hair
45. The art of understanding writing in cipher
46. Talking in a language with deliberate transposition of words or letters
47. Knowledge of the languages of other provinces and of various dialects
48. Art of making flower carriages
49. Art of addressing spells, charms, auspicious & bad omens
50. Constructing mechanical aids
51. Memory training
52. Recitation of verse
53. Deciphering of secret codes
54. Knowledge of etymology
55. Knowledge of lexicography
56. Prosody and rhetoric
57. Art of impersonation
58. Wearing garments artfully
59. Various dice games
60. The game of dice called *Akarsha*
61. Making dolls and play things for children
62. Knowledge of etiquette
63. Knowledge of the science of victory
64. Physical culture

Obviously, these arts were in keeping with the context of the times. Many would be defunct today, what with modern gadgetry and less time available on hand to actually make numerous items listed oneself. However, these sixty-four arts are a good indication of the general talents that a woman needs to cultivate.

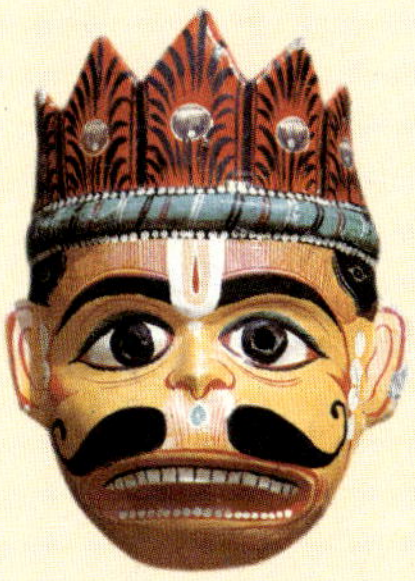

Following page: **Padmini, the lotus woman:** Padmini is really beautiful, swan like, with soft rounded hips and breasts, nose like a sesame flower, face like the Moon, gentle in union with a sweet, lotus smelling pudenda. She is sentimental, soft hearted and easily moves to tears. Physically, she submits and can be pleasing - suitable match for *shasha*, hare or *mriga*, buck type male. *Miniature painting, Mewar, Rajasthan, mid 17th century. Private collection.*

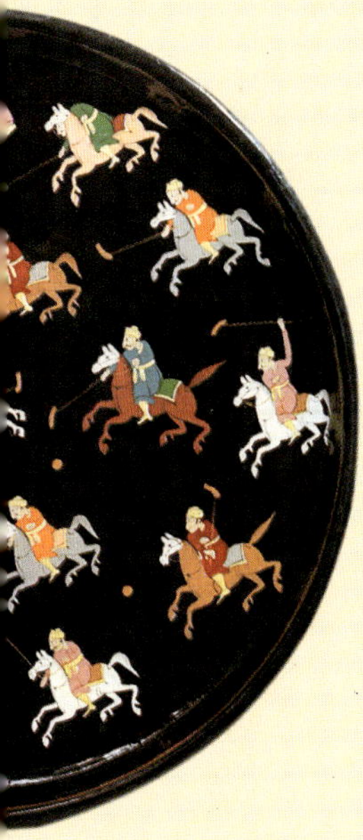

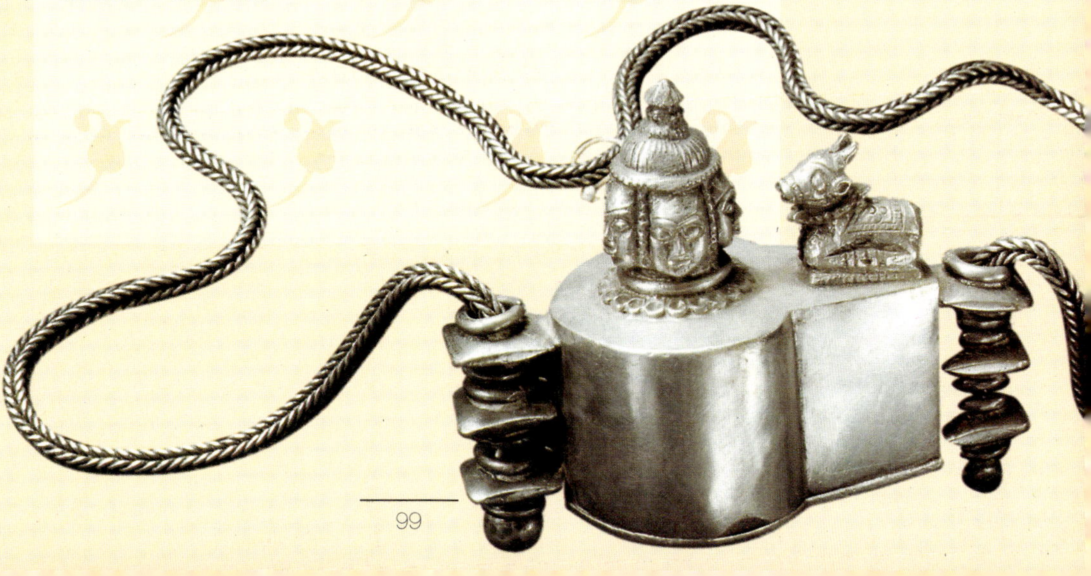

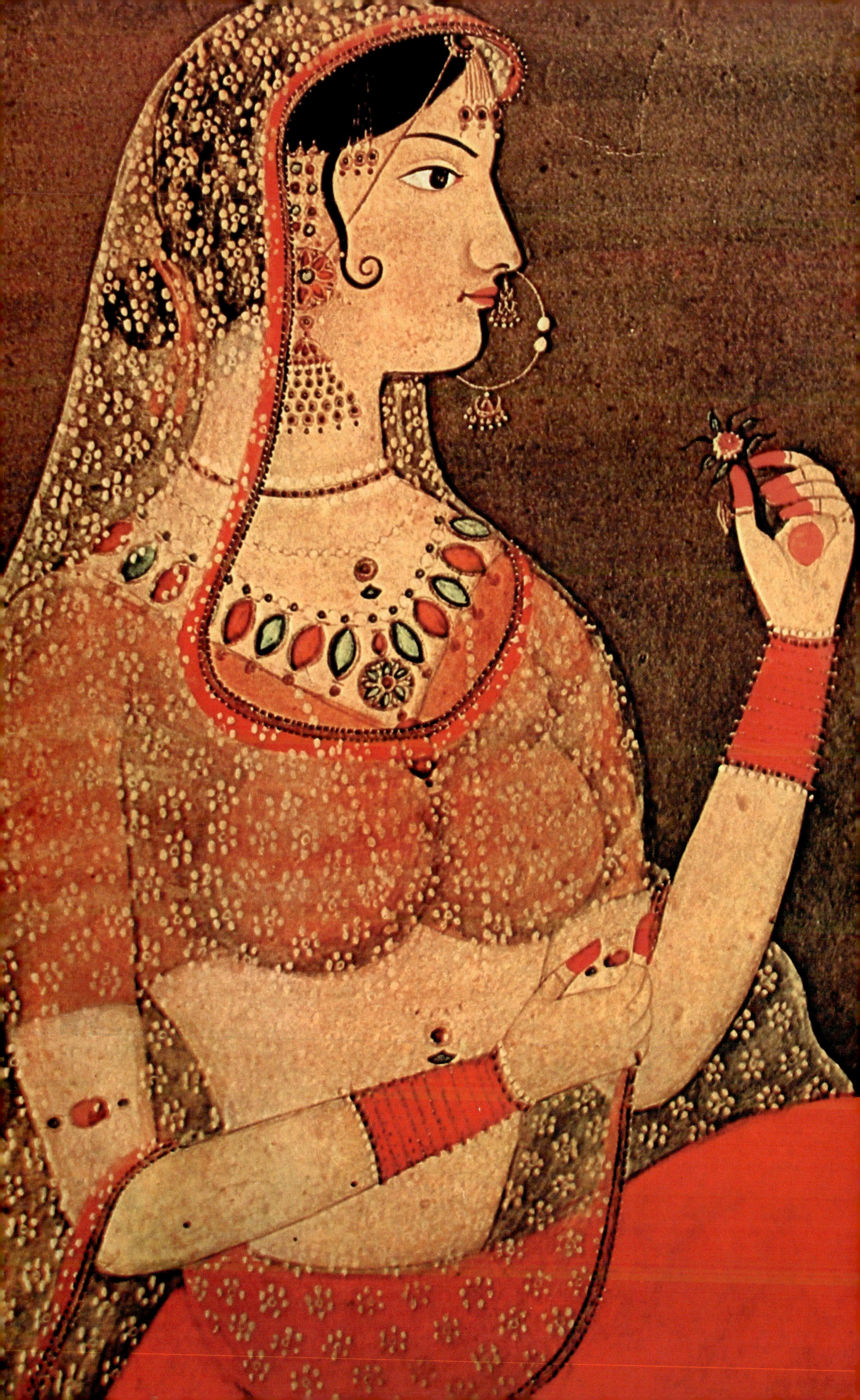

The extent of the love of women is not known, even to those who are the objects of their affection, on account of its subtlety, and on account of the avarice, and natural intelligence of womankind

Women are hardly ever known in their true light, though they may love men, or become indifferent towards them, may give them delight, or abandon them, or may extract from them all the wealth that they may possess

Kama Sutra Book VI

women AT PLAY

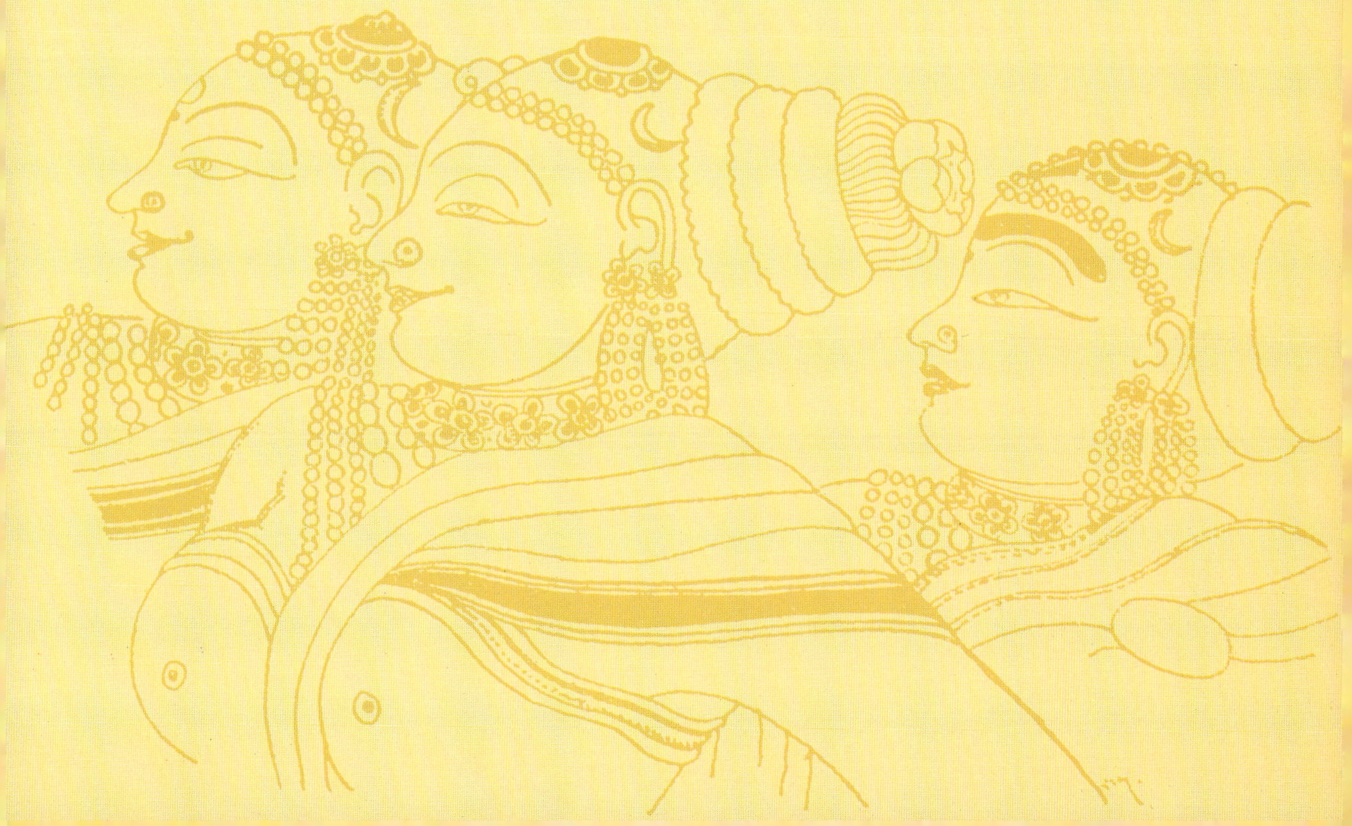

In olden days women were often considered distractions to kings and royal counsellors preferred the monarch to abstain from such temptation since it could distract him from his royal duties. The *Kathsaritasgara* illustrates the example of King Yashodhana. A merchant wanted him to marry his daughter Unmadini, and the king's counsellors were dispatched to inspect the prospective bride. Astounded by her amazing beauty, the counsellors feared that she would distract the king from his *Dharma*. Therefore they informed Yashodhana that she was very ugly. Rather than rejecting the proposal, the king ordered the merchant to get his daughter married to the commander of his forces. Unmadini never forgave the king for rejecting her and wanted to avenge her humiliation. During a spring festival when the king was moving through the streets, she stood naked on the terrace of her house and showed herself to the king. Infatuated by her beauty, Yashodhana sent his spies to learn more about her. When he learnt who she was, he was outraged and banished the counsellors from his kingdom. Learning of the king's desire for his wife, the commander offered to send his wife to him but Yashodhana refused the offer since it was against his *Dharma*. Unable to control his passion though, and realising the malignant effect of *kama*, the king renounced his kingdom and became a hermit.

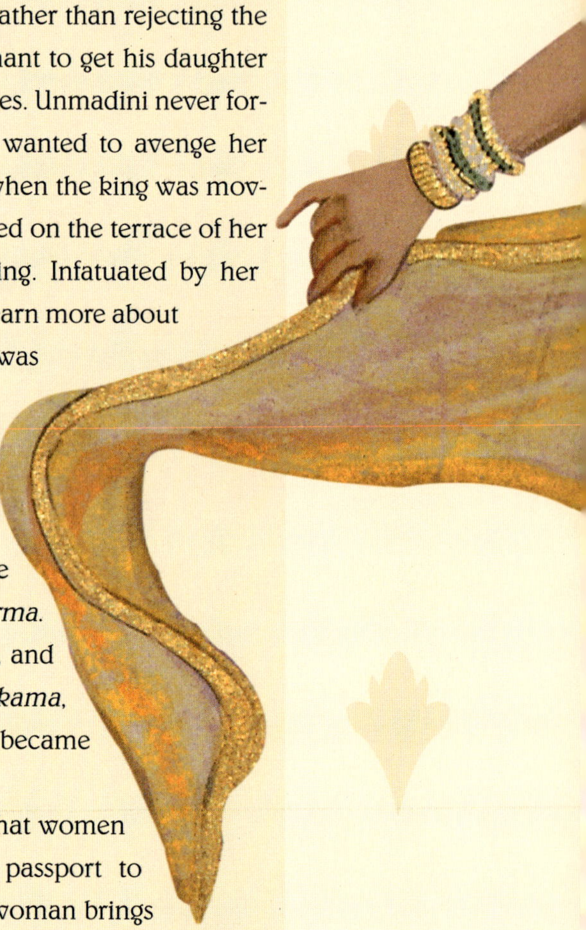

This story is proof of the power that women can invoke. This power is like a passport to unimagined territories. The modern woman brings to mind the subtlety and depths of the *Ganika*, encapsulated in the pages of the sixth book of the *Kama Sutra*, on courtesans:

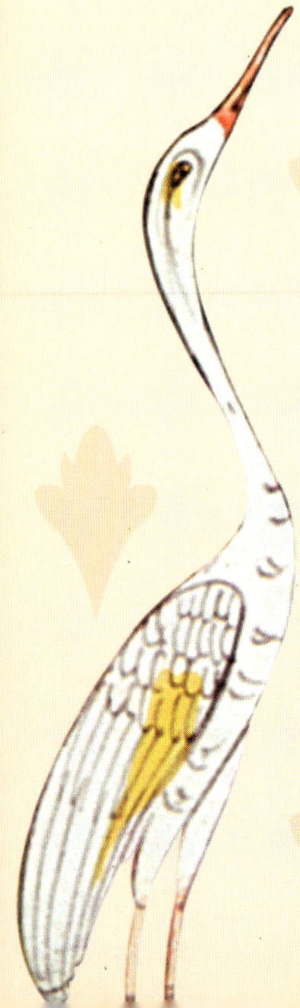

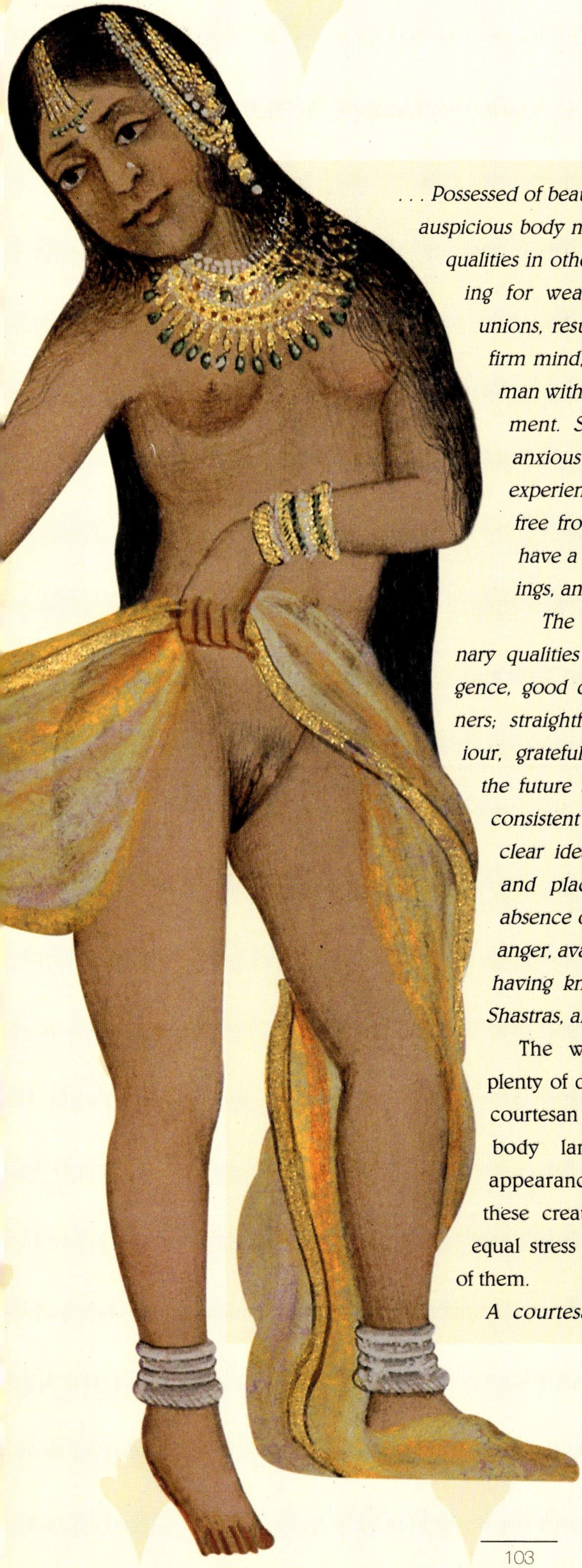

. . . Possessed of beauty and amiability, with auspicious body marks; a liking for good qualities in other people, as also a liking for wealth; delight in sexual unions, resulting from love, and a firm mind, and the same class as man with regard to sexual enjoyment. She should always be anxious to acquire and obtain experience and knowledge, be free from avarice, and always have a liking for social gatherings, and for the arts.

The following are the ordinary qualities of all women: intelligence, good disposition, good manners; straightforwardness in behaviour, gratefulness; considering well the future before doing anything; consistent in behaviour, with a clear idea of the proper times and places for doing things; absence of meanness, malignity, anger, avarice, dull and stupidity; having knowledge of the Kama Shastras, and skilful in all the arts.

The woman of today has plenty of drive and force like the courtesan of yesteryears. Speech, body language, mannerisms, appearance and conduct - all these create an impression and equal stress must be paid to each of them.

A courtesan, well dressed and

Keeping the lover aroused: The style of this extra-ordinary painting and its probable period is made possible by the complete nudity of the full bodied women adorned with spectacular jewellery. This rather blatant direct approach is Dattaka's view, wherein he has described in detail, the state of the mind of the girl, when she protests against an ill arranged marriage and gets an opportunity to make her displeasure public. Vatsyayana says that meetings and separations are questions for the woman, who gives a lot of thought about the nature of her lover. *Miniature painting, Indore, Madhya Pradesh, 20th century. Private collection.*

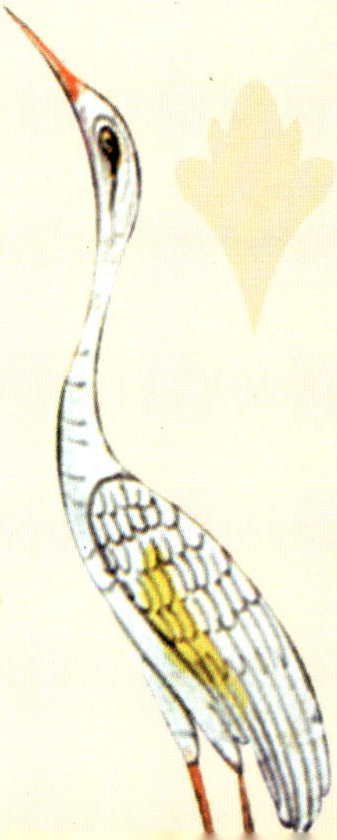

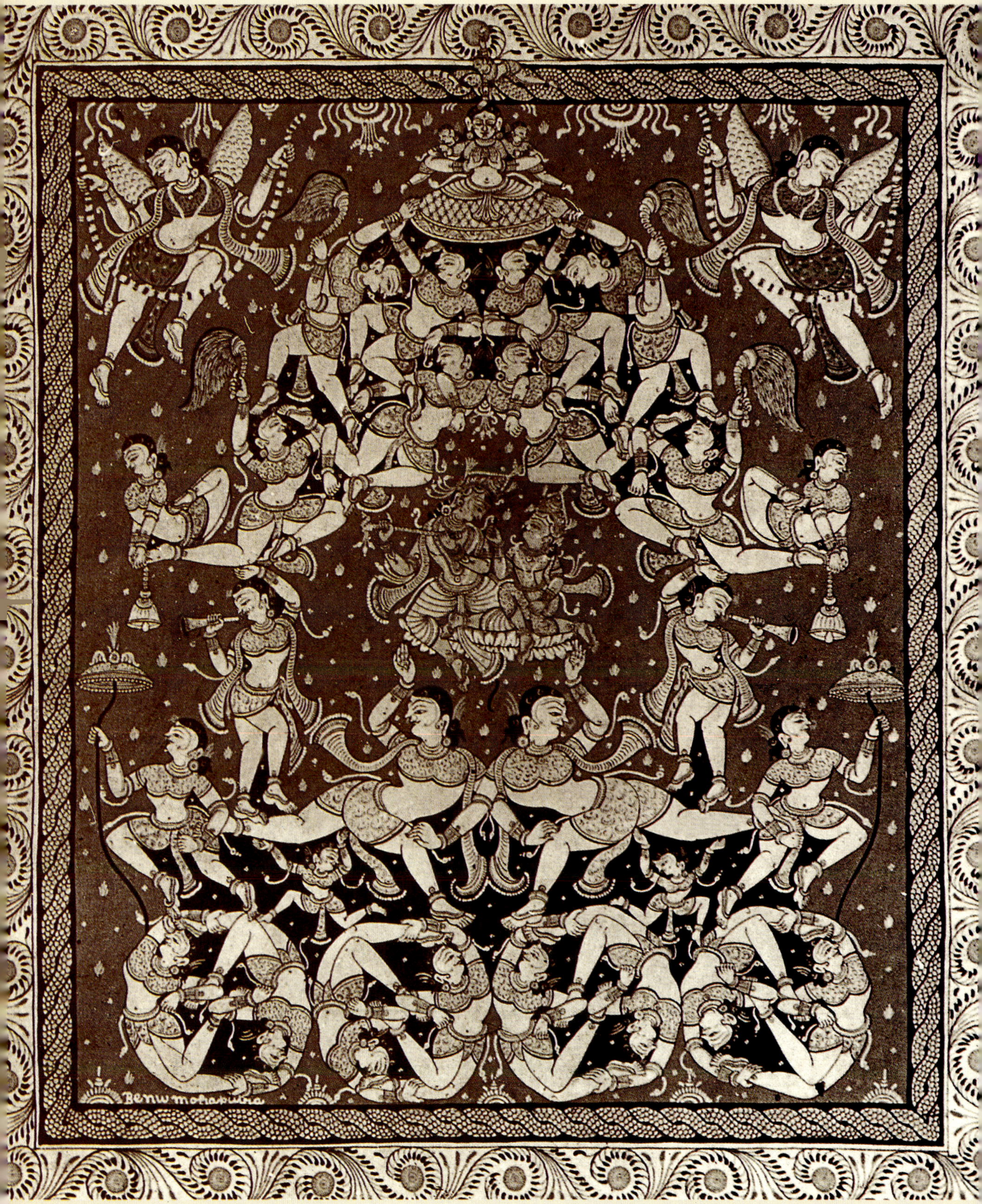

Composite formation of physical beauty: The painting accentuates the physical beauty of maidens, who form an acrobatic representation of a sacred *vahana*, vehicle. It is in such a vehicle that gods are transported in a procession during festivals, to enable large crowds of devotees to obtain *darshan*, blessings. In the central platform are the divine couple - Radha and Krishna, open on all sides for everyone to see. The *gopis* are performing this unusual disposition of their bodies as an act of devotion. *Oil Painting on cloth, Puri, Orissa, 20th century. Lance Dane collection.*

wearing her ornaments, should sit or stand at the door of her house, and without exposing herself too much, should look on the public road so as to be seen by passers-by, she being like an object on sale. She should form friendships with such persons as would enable her to separate men from other women, and attach them to herself, to repair her own misfortunes, to acquire wealth, and to protect her from being bullied, or set upon by persons with whom she may have dealings of some kind or another.

These may have been the mores of a courtesan in times gone by, but the woman of today who is competing in what were predominantly male sectors, requires to use every weapon in her command to provide a befitting combat. Her demeanour is a window to the world. Her outer persona should make it obvious as to who she is and what she aspires to be; her convictions and concerns, her support system from where she gathers motivation, encouragement and applause.

Money is got out of a lover in two ways: By natural or lawful means or by artifices. Ancient sages are of the opinion that when a courtesan can get as much money from her lover, she should not make use of artifice. But Vatsyayana lays down that though she may get some money from him by natural means, yet when she makes use of artifice he gives her doubly more, and therefore artifice should be restored to for the purpose of exhorting money from him at all events.

To achieve her goal, it is necessary for her to mesmerise those around. Achieving her goal requires the same powers of seduction that courtesans of yesterday employed. Well dressed, wearing skilfully done make-up, elegant taste, a sound and stable character, faithfulness to her lover, graceful at social gatherings - she needs to stand out in every which way. In her the two seemingly incompatible modes of love and practicality must function alongside. This is the palette of the modern woman.

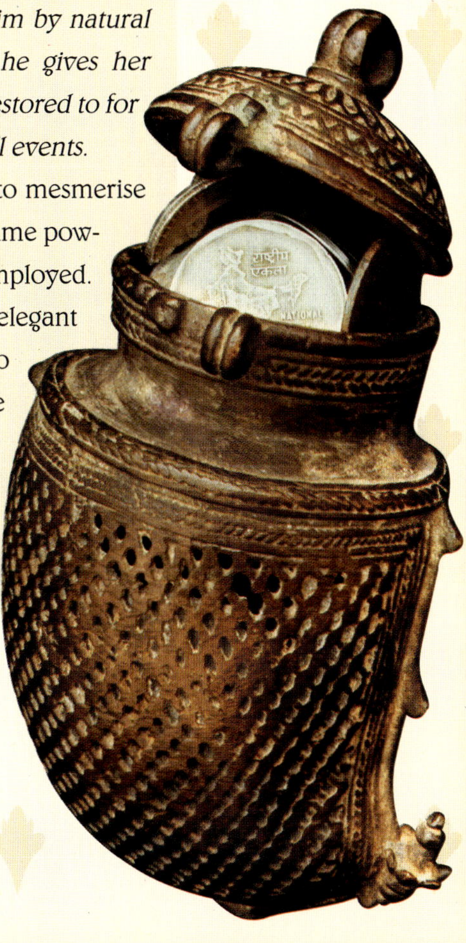

A money pot in the shape of a mango: *Bronze, Bhuvaneshwar, Orissa, 19th century. Lance Dane collection.*

Following page left:
The Kings day-out: This unusual painting features a prominent person who is central to the action. Romance, of course, is the real name of the game, and love is what life is all about. Vatsyayana in his selections commented upon behavioural characteristics of the leader, the king, who in principle upheld the good, and punished or corrected the wrong, and, of course, he was held in respect, and also allowed considerable amplitude in all the good things of life. The story is summarised neatly in this visual segmented painting. It has an element of comic also. The king arrives as expected, and is welcomed by his lady friend. They go out and enjoy nature by doing what comes naturally. She playfully acts like a man, on top of the king, then he reciprocates and acts like the king, which he is! *Miniature painting, Coimbatore, Tamil style, 20th century. Private collection.*

JUDGING A LOVER

A woman should be able to judge the state of mind, the feelings and the disposition of her lover towards her from the changes in his temper, his manner, and the colour of his face. The behaviour of a waning lover is manifest by the following:

- He gives the woman either less than is wanted, or some thing else other than that asked for.
- He keeps giving her hope by making promises repeatedly.
- He pretends to do one thing, but do something else.
- He does not fulfil her desires.
- He forgets his promises or does something other than what he has promised.
- He speaks with his own servants in a mysterious way.
- He sleeps in some other house under the pretence of having to do something for a friend.
- Lastly, he speaks in private with the attendants of a woman with whom he was formerly acquainted. Often a situation arises when a woman wants to reunite with a lover with whom she has broken off earlier. But she should return to him only if he is still attracted to her, and if he is living with another woman at the time, she should examine the situation well before approaching him again. Such a man can only be in one of the six following conditions:
- He may have left the first woman of his own accord, and may even have left another woman since then.
- He may have been driven away by both women.
- He may have left the first woman of his own accord, and been driven away by the other.
- He may have left the first woman of his own accord and be living with another woman.
- He may have been driven away by the first woman, and left the other of his own accord.

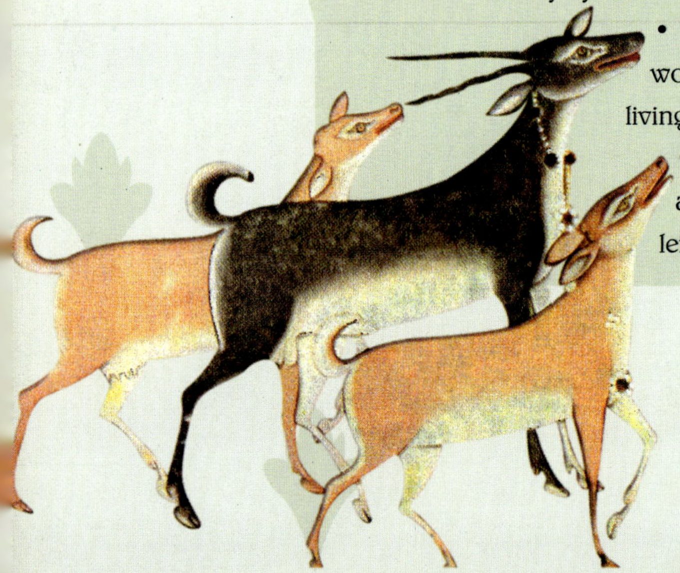

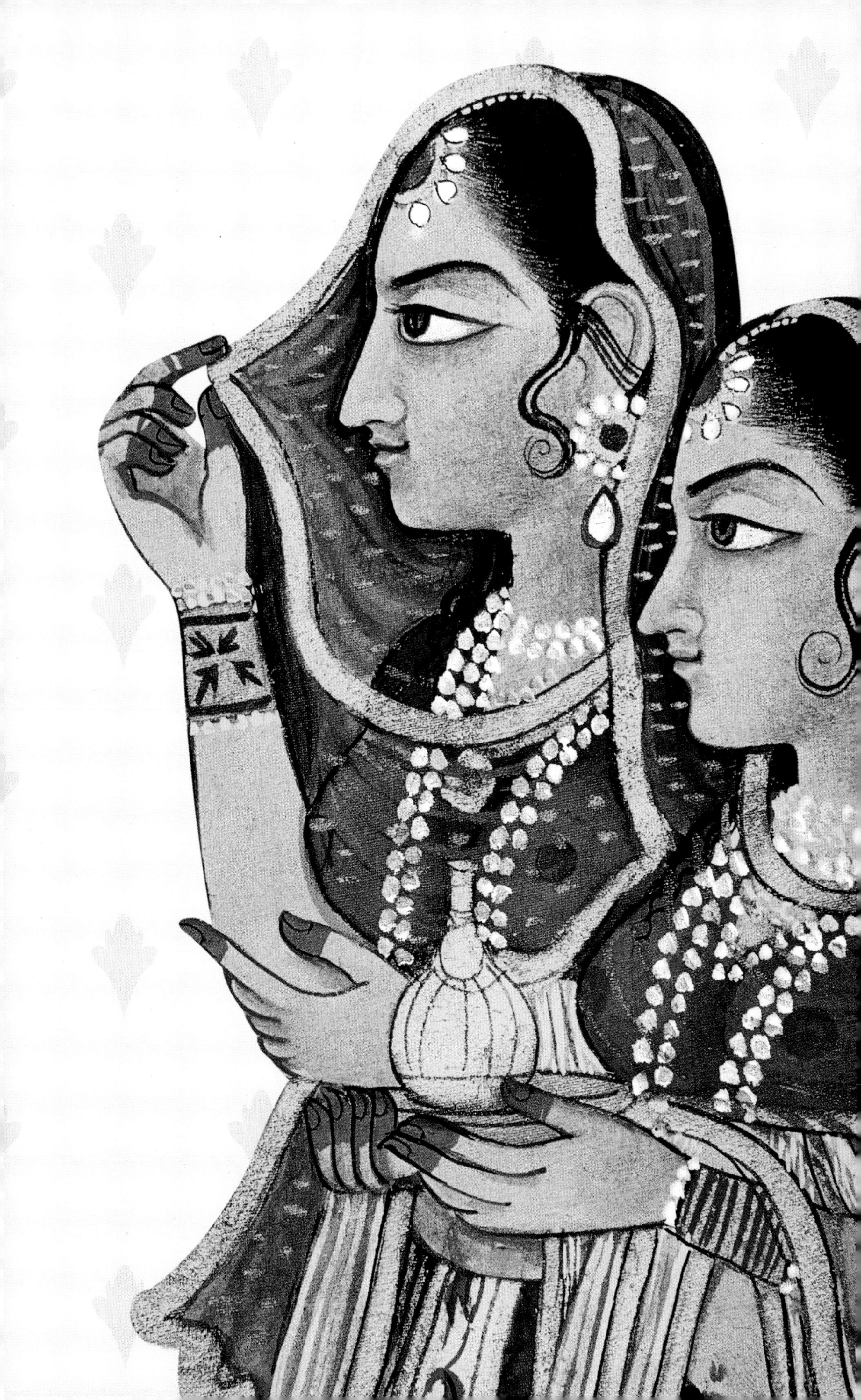

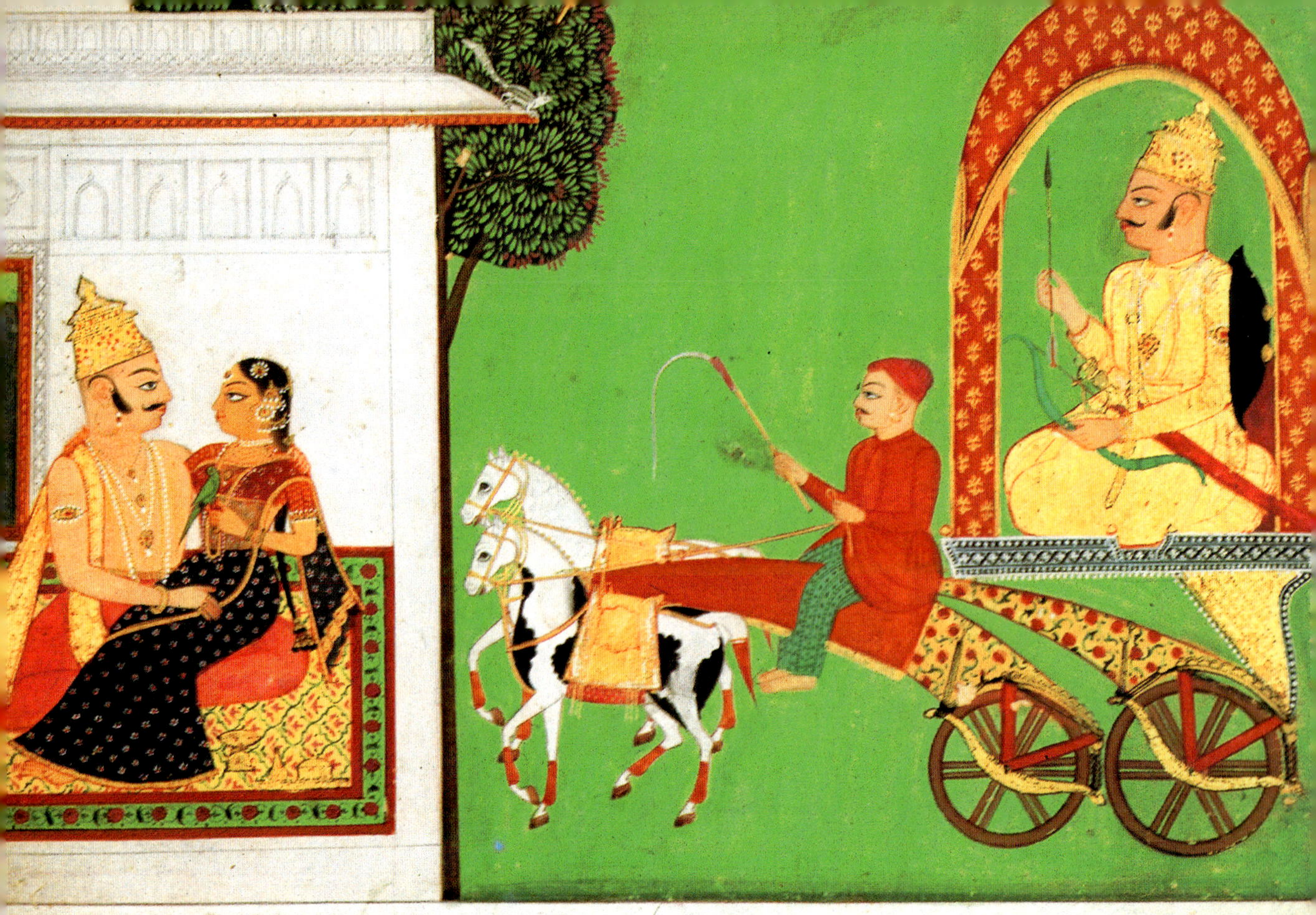

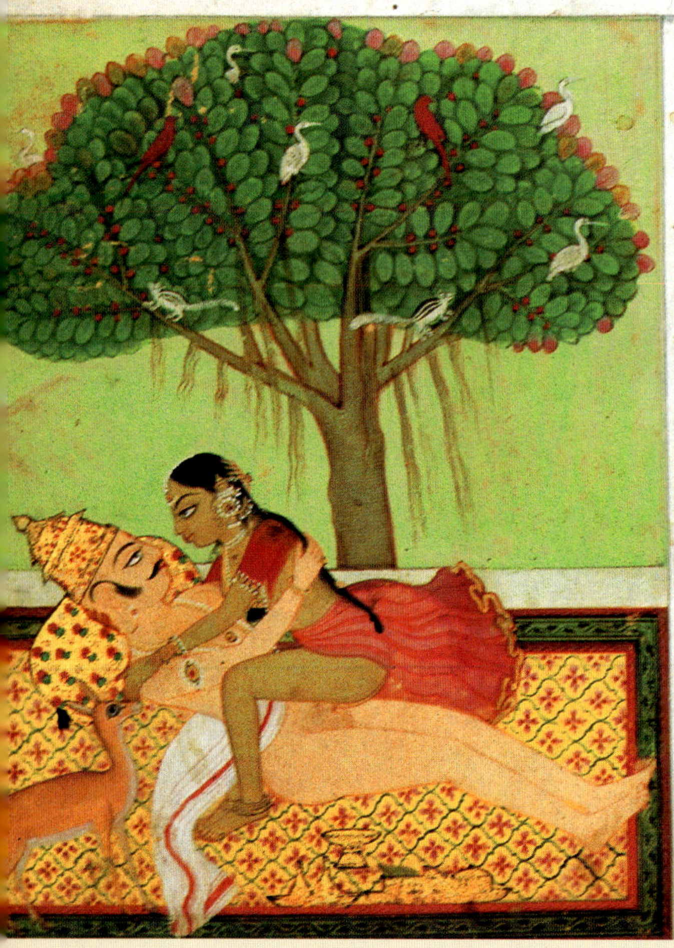

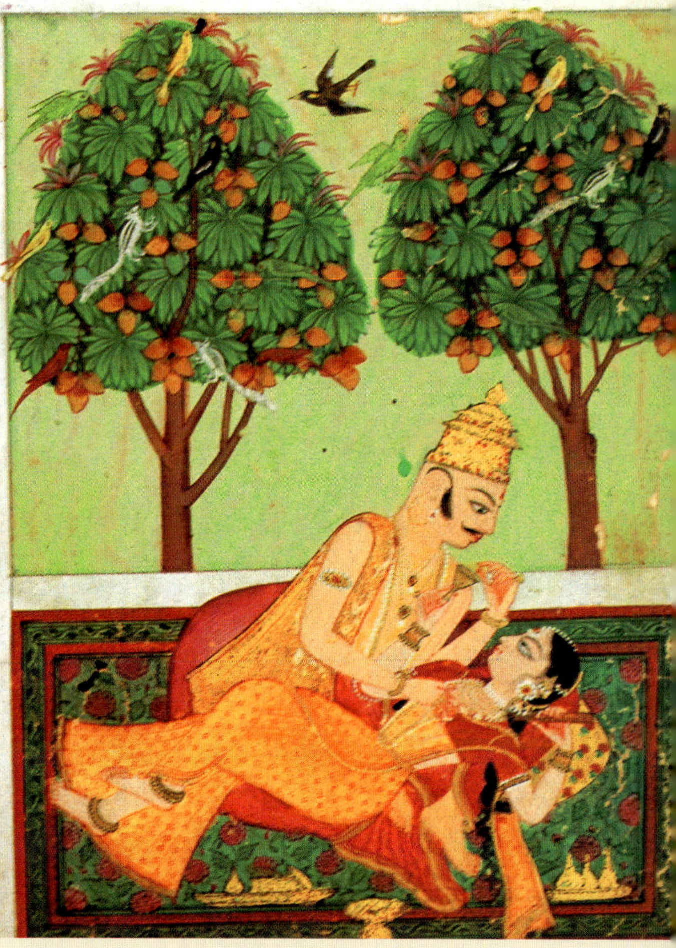

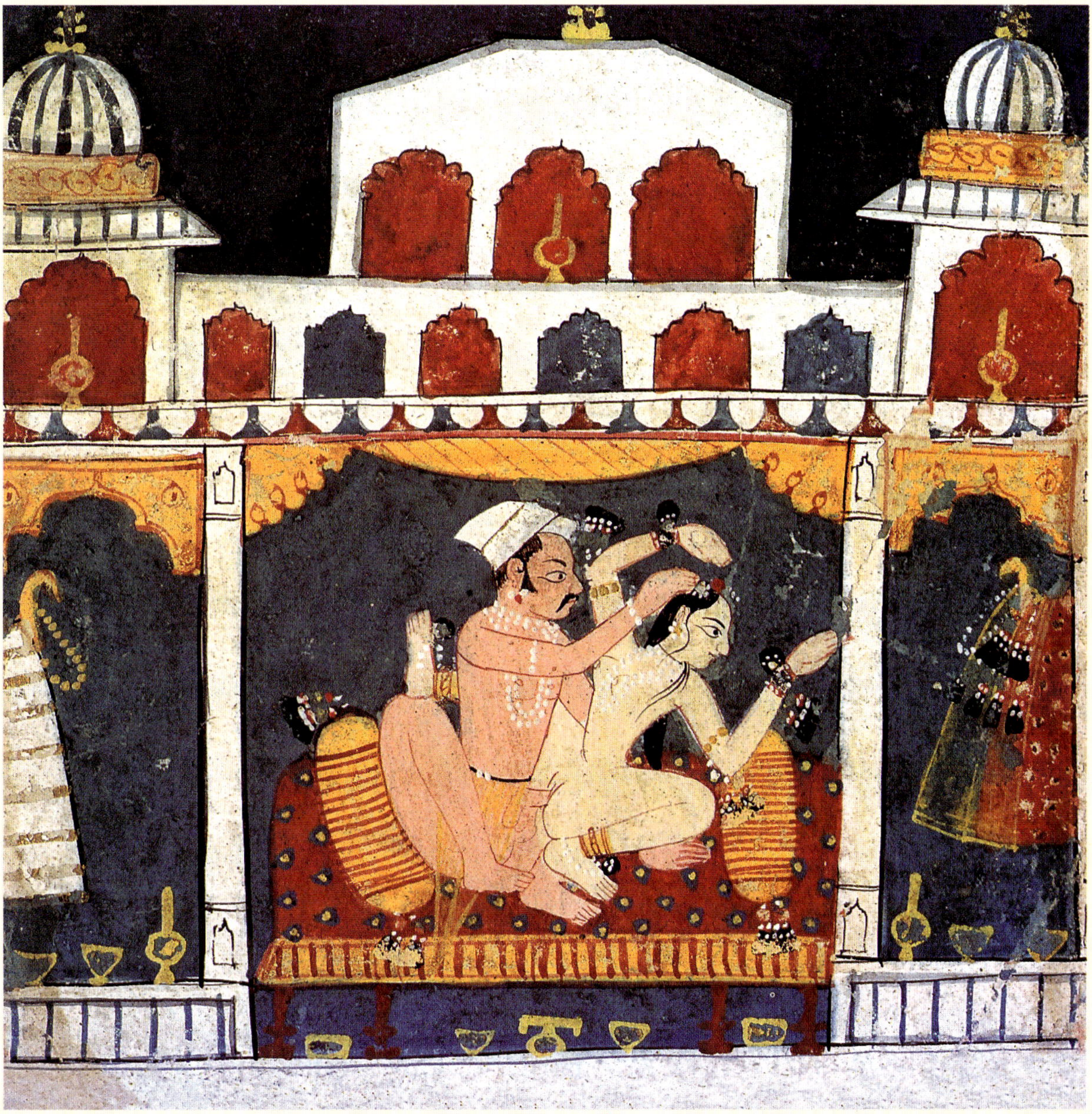

A play in the love game. Striking with open palm: This and another example to follow are dramatic, in forceful imagery, dominated by solid strong colours, a regional device most particular to this series. They visualise *prahanana*, 'a mode of striking' with the open palm of the hand. They represent the view expressed by Vatsyayana when he says, "Sexual intercourse can be compared to a combat, on account of the contrarieties of love and its tendency to dispute." It is accepted that the experience of pain, during the culmination of the thrust and push, adds greater excitement to this - the most pleasurable of all love acts, and even after the explosion of the final thrust, a brief pause, and the couple can revert to tickling and kissing. So, the game can go on, for as long as the lovers can pursue their mutual enjoyment. *Miniature painting, Malwa, Rajasthan, early 17th century.*

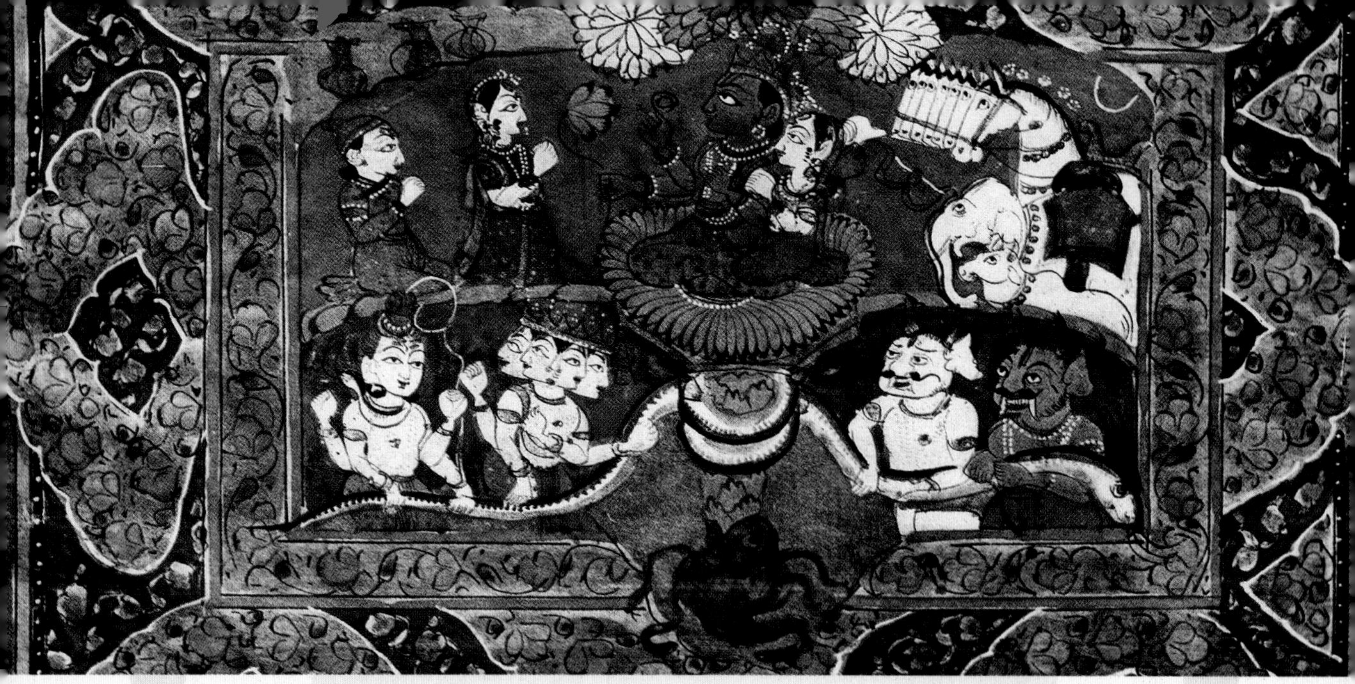

- He may have been driven away by the first woman, and may be living with another.

Now if the man has left both the women of his own accord, he should not be pursued on account of the fickleness of his mind.

As regards the man, who may have been driven away by both women, if he has been driven away from the second one because she could get more material gain from another, then he should be resorted to. But if he has been driven away due to his own bad qualities, he should not then be resorted to.

In the case of a man, who may have left the first woman of his own accord, and been driven away by the other, if he agrees to return to the former and give her enough to sustain herself materially, then he should be resorted to.

If a man has left the first woman himself, and is living with another woman, the first woman (if she wishes to get him back), should first ascertain if he left her because he felt that the second woman had better qualities, and that not having found such excellence, he was willing to return to her, on account of his affection for her. Or, whether, having discovered more faults in the second woman, he was now able to appreciate the first woman's qualities, and wished to return to her.

Or, lastly, to consider whether he was a weak man or a man fond of enjoying several women, or one who never did anything for the woman he was with. Only after considering these things maturely, should a woman decide whether to resort to him or not. In short, she should ascertain whether he

***Samudra Manthan* or churning the ocean for *amrita*, the nectar of immortality :** Lord Vishnu had made his *avatar* as *kurma*, the giant tortoise, and had stationed himself at the ocean bed. On his back, the great mountain Mandara was placed to serve as the churning stick. The great serpent Vasuki, became the rope by wrapping himself round the mountain. The *devas*, 'gods', and the *asuras*, 'demons' took hold of either end and with great effort, proceeded to churn the ocean. As they churned, first the deadly poison came out which contaminated the atmosphere. Shiva swallowed it down. Then slowly, emerged from the depths, a number of matchless treasures known as the *chaturidasa-ratnam* 'fourteen jewels'. Most of these became the prototypes of similar things in heaven and earth. Then Dhanvantri stepped out, in flowing white and golden robes. The 'immortal physician of the gods', held aloft in his hands the most precious gift of all, *amrita*, the nectar of immortality in a great golden *kumbha*, 'a glittering chalice.' The wily *asuras*, under the masterful guidance and skilful manoeuvres of their king, seized the golden *kumbha* and fled with all speed. The *asuras* would have consumed the nectar, had not the equally astute gods persuaded Vishnu, to assume the guise of a sensuous beauty Mohini, a beautiful and charming woman, who lured the demons to give her the nectar and handed it over to the gods. The gods, without any delay, consumed the nectar and regained their powers. *Amrita* is also called *nirajar* 'not aging' and *piyusha*, 'immortal juice'. It is to Vatsyayana's credit that while compiling his *Kama Sutra*, he included the work of Kuchumara, who had taken note of those aspects of sexual life, which depend on the value of nature's remedies. *Miniature painting, Kashmir, 20th century. Private collection.*

is still fond of her; or whether, knowing her good qualities, he was not satisfied with the second woman; or whether he merely wanted to get back with her to wreak revenge; or, whether this was a means to rid himself of the second woman and then do the same to her too. If he is willing to return due to any negative plans, he must certainly not be resorted to.

The sages even advised courtesans that if two men were courting her, she should take up with the man who would look after her interests better. If both men are willingly to look after her, she should select the one with the better qualities.

UNACCEPTABLE PROPOSALS

When a man pursues a woman and she does not return his affection, it could be due to a number of causes:

- Affection for her own husband, if married
- Desire of lawful progeny
- Want of opportunity
- Anger at being addressed by the man in an over-familiar manner
- Difference in status in life
- Doubt of reliability due to excessive travelling by the man
- Thinking that the man may be attached to some other person
- Fear of the man's not keeping his intentions private
- Thinking that the man is too devoted to his friends and would give them greater preference than her
- The apprehension that he is not in earnest

In fact it is always advised that instead of yielding to a man immediately, the woman ought to delay and feign unawareness to ensure that the man's feelings get keener. Delay is a useful tool to assess his sincerity and intentions.

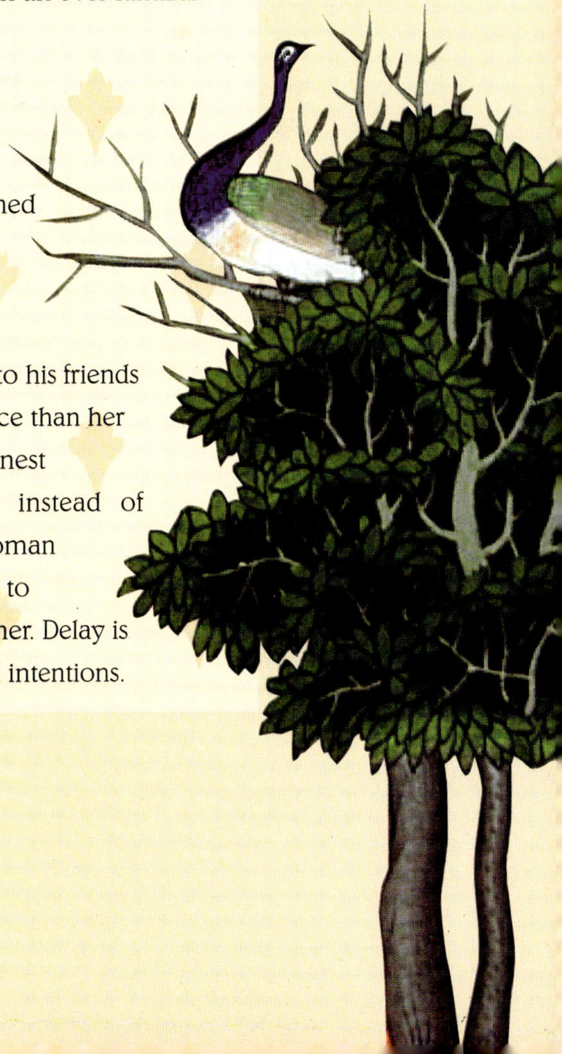

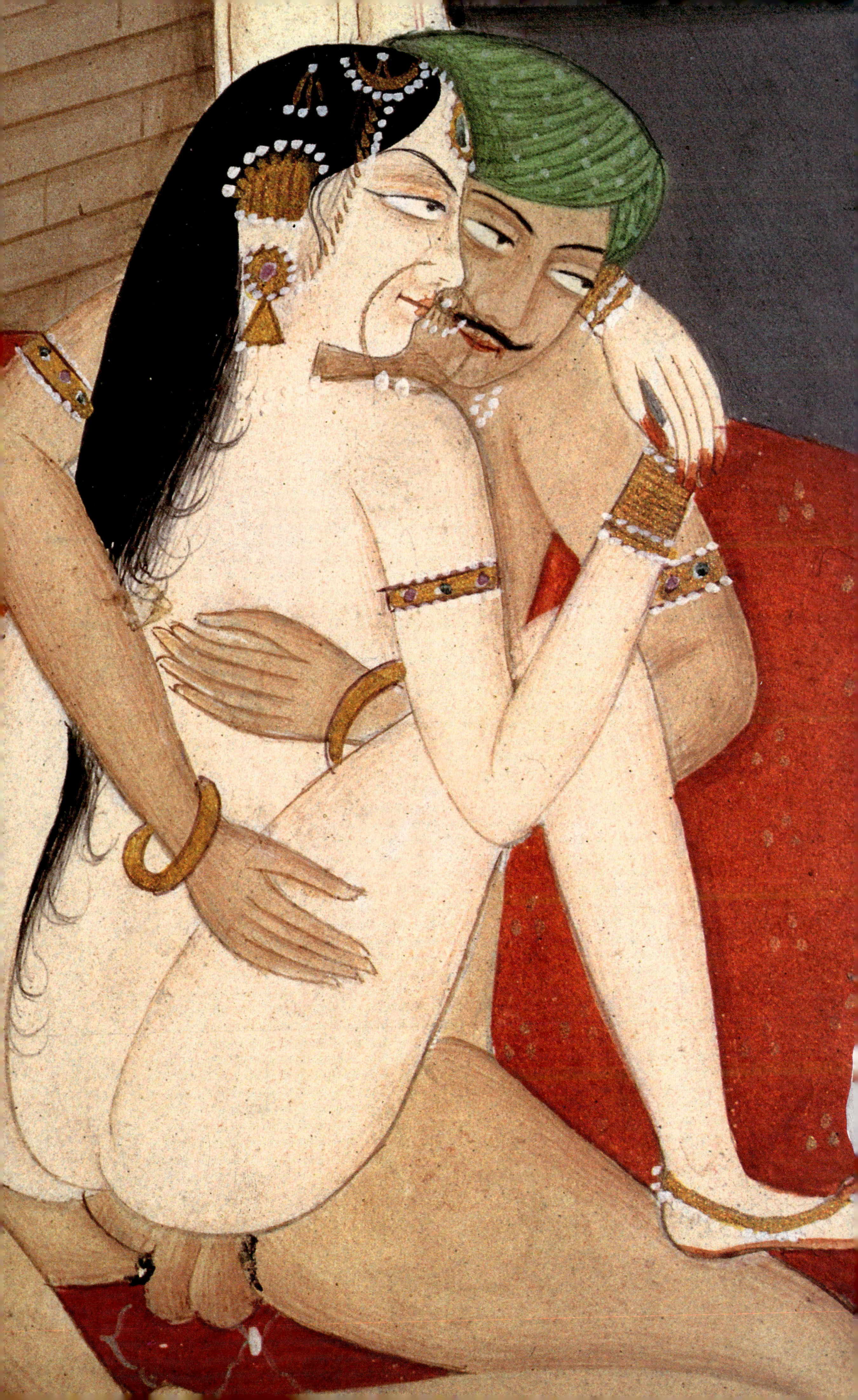

Though a woman is reserved, and keeps her feelings concealed,
yet when she gets on the top of a man, she then shows all her love and affection.

Kama Sutra, Book II

women ON TOP

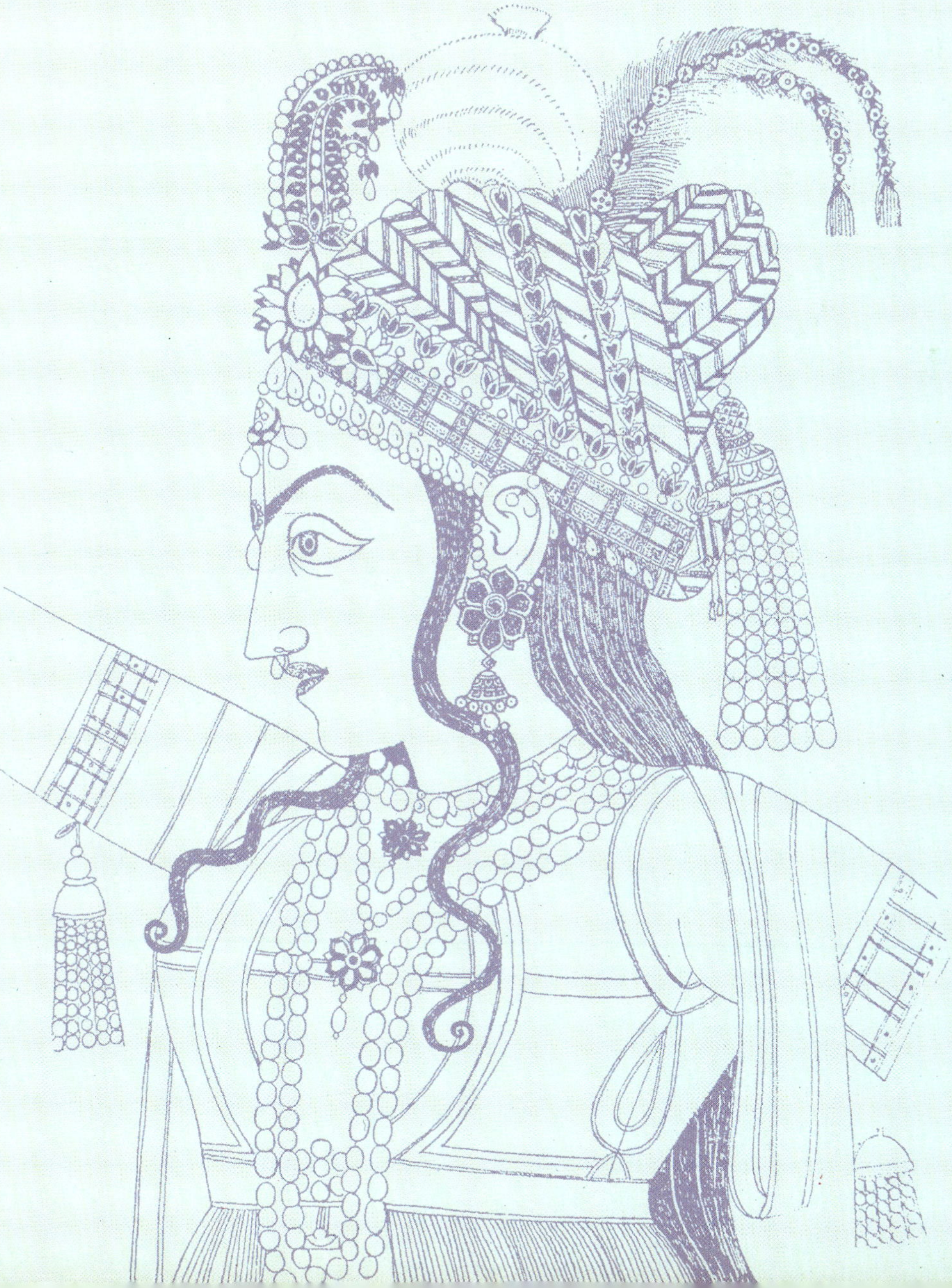

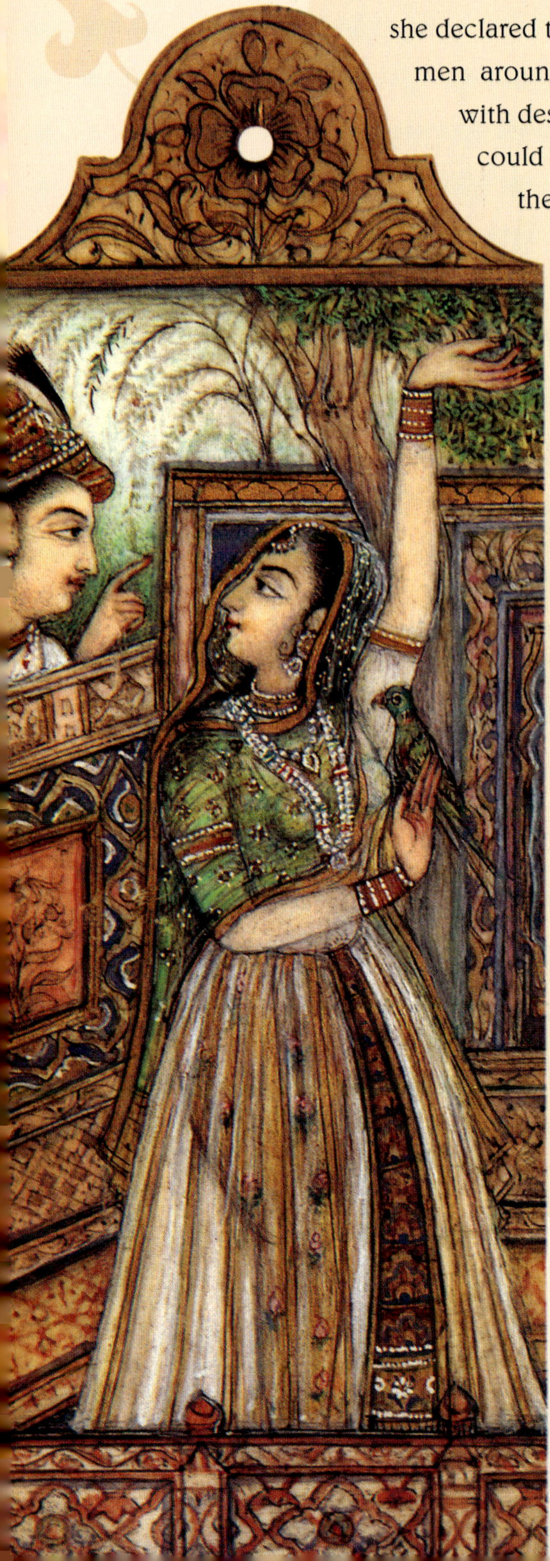

The erotic manual, the *Kokashastra* was written for the sole purpose of enabling husbands to satisfy their wives adequately so that they would not want to be with other men. A folk tale states that a woman once entered a king's court completely naked and on being asked to explain her state of undress, she declared that it did not matter since there were no men around her. Her body, she declared, burned with desire and not a single man in the kingdom could satisfy her. She alleged that it was due to the inadequacy of the king that she had to walk around naked. She proceeded to challenge him to provide her with a lover who would satisfy her. Hearing this a Brahmin, Koka Shastri, with the king's permission, took the oversexed woman home and spent the night making love to her so persuasively that before dawn, the woman was almost fainting from fatigue and orgasms. Koka dragged the woman to the king's court and informed them of her sexual subjugation. The woman then covered her body in the presence of the entire court and the king ordered Pandit Koka to write a treatise that would teach all men how to satisfy their wives.

In ancient Hindu society the beauty and sexuality of a woman was considered a dangerous stimulant to primal, indisciplined urges. All women who were aware of their beauty were considered crafty and a threat to the

Lover on the prowl: As an artistic and attractive scene is conceived, the artist had, using his powers of observation coupled with inspiration, imbibed a touch of drama combined with a picturesque and luxurious ambience. It unfolds with the sudden presence of the hero, who wondering around a lotus pool, spotted the heroine in a fabulous marble pavilion. He takes the opportunity to wish her. Her response is favourable and her gestures encourages him to go ahead. *Miniature on ivory, Jaipur, Rajasthan, 20th century.*

Previous page left: **Woman on top:** Vatsyayana expresses two views occasioning this pose. When in the event, the couple has been enjoying continuously all night long. To keep the flagging lover going, she sits on top of him. The other occasion is, when the lover of a young woman likes her to behave in an assertive bossy manner. This is an occasion, when the heroine is in full charge and command. *Miniature painting, Pahari Hills, Kangra, 19th century.*

Following page: **Birth of the princes of Ayodhya**: This is an important scene from the *Ramayana*, depicting King Dashratha's queens giving birth. Queen Kaikeyi, his favourite, is adorned with golden paint. *Mural painting on the interior walls of the Dutch Palace at Mattancherri, Kerala, 17th century.*

social order. Kaikeyi, the wife of King Dashratha of Ayodhya in the epic Ramayana, is one such example. She was beautiful and courageous, and accompanied her husband to the battlefield as well. Once, in the thick of battle, Dashratha's chariot was maneuvered across enemy lines and the bolt of the chariot came loose. Kaikeyi noticed this and inserted her thumb into the hole of the bolt to keep the wheel in place and the chariot steady. On learning this Dashratha offered her two boons, which she reserved for the future. When the throne was being passed on to Lord Rama, Kaikeyi made use of the boons granted to her and forced her husband to banish his favourite son and heir to the throne, to the forest for fourteen years, so as to crown her own son, Bharat, as king of Ayodhya. Dashratha deeply regretted losing his heart to the wiles of a beautiful woman.

Moreover, when a woman was extremely beautiful, it was taken for granted that she could not be faithful. In ancient India such women were ordered to become courtesans and serve as public wives. Unfaithful women caught by husbands and rejected by society also sought refuge in brothels. They were not treated with dishonour, but were seen as safety valves for the unbridled sexual urges of men, which could otherwise subvert social order. The courtesans were renowned for their capriciousness. The *Katha-sarit-sagar* illustrates one such instance. The king of Pratishthana, Vikram Singh, was driven out of his

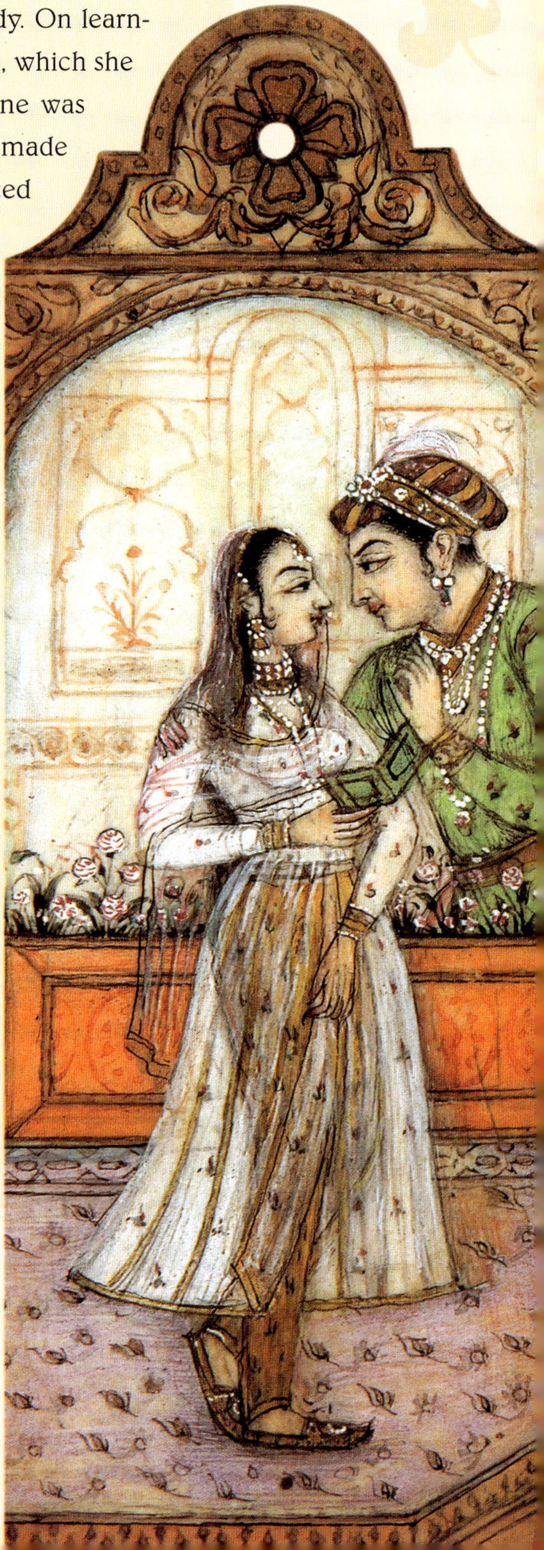

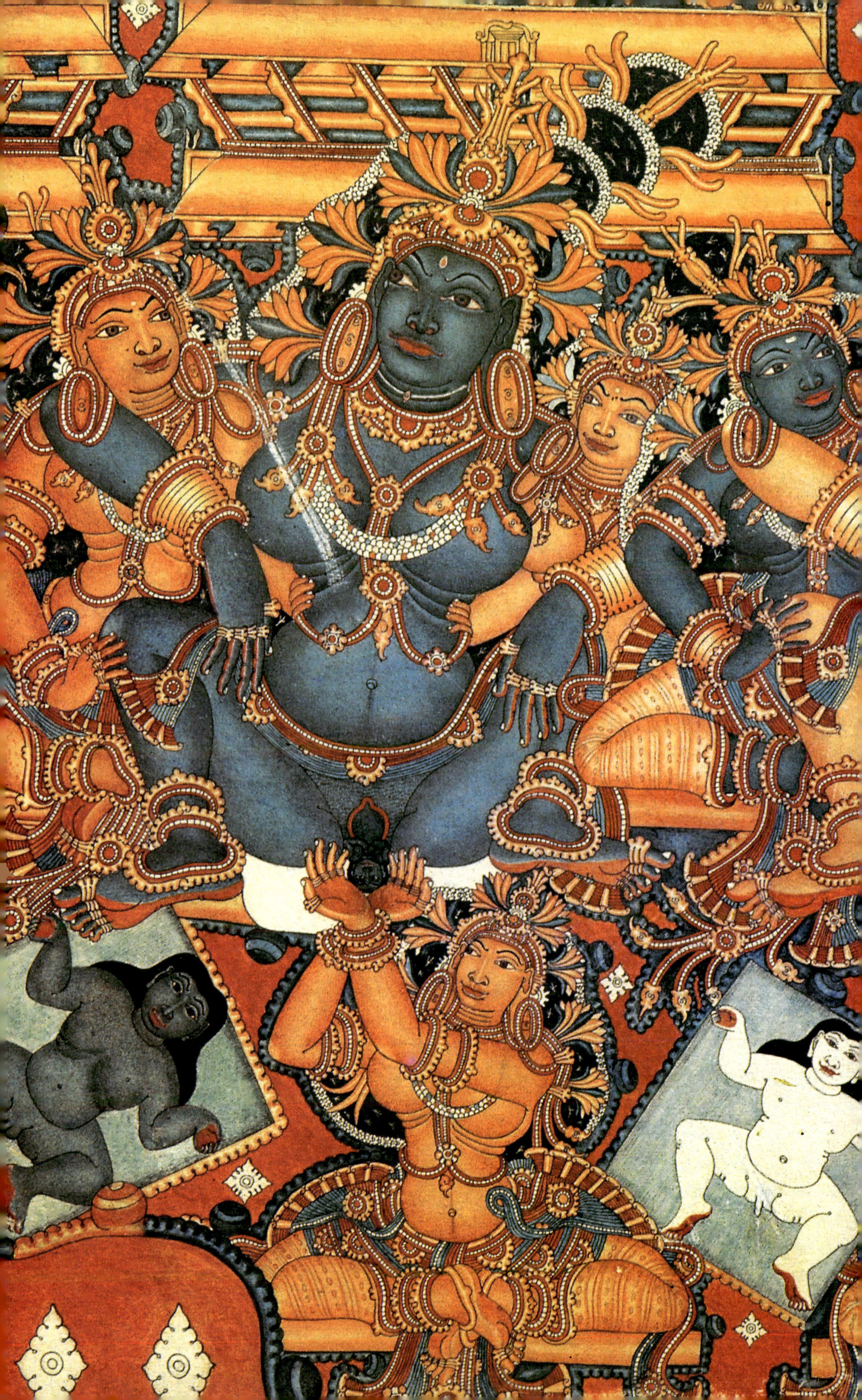

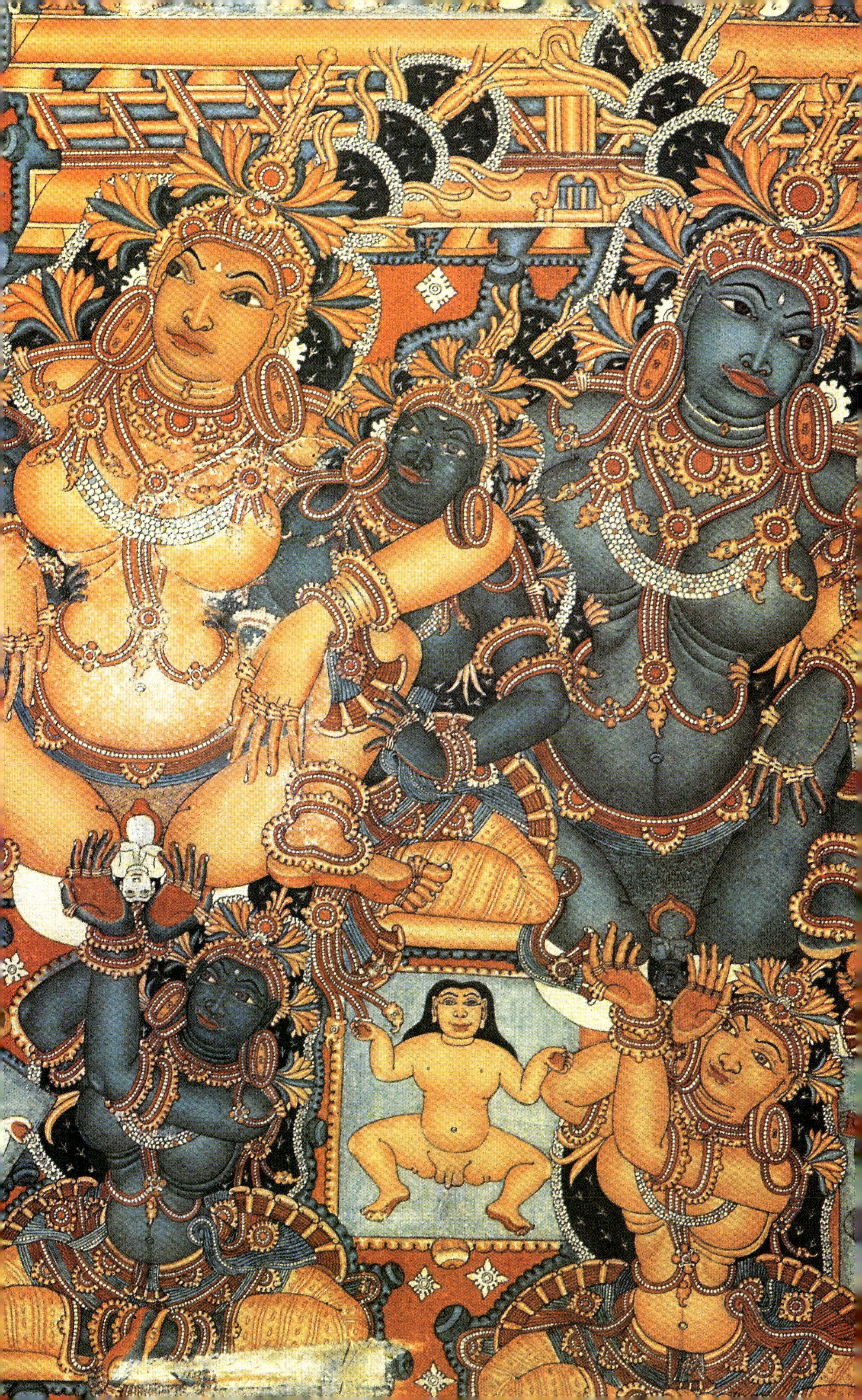

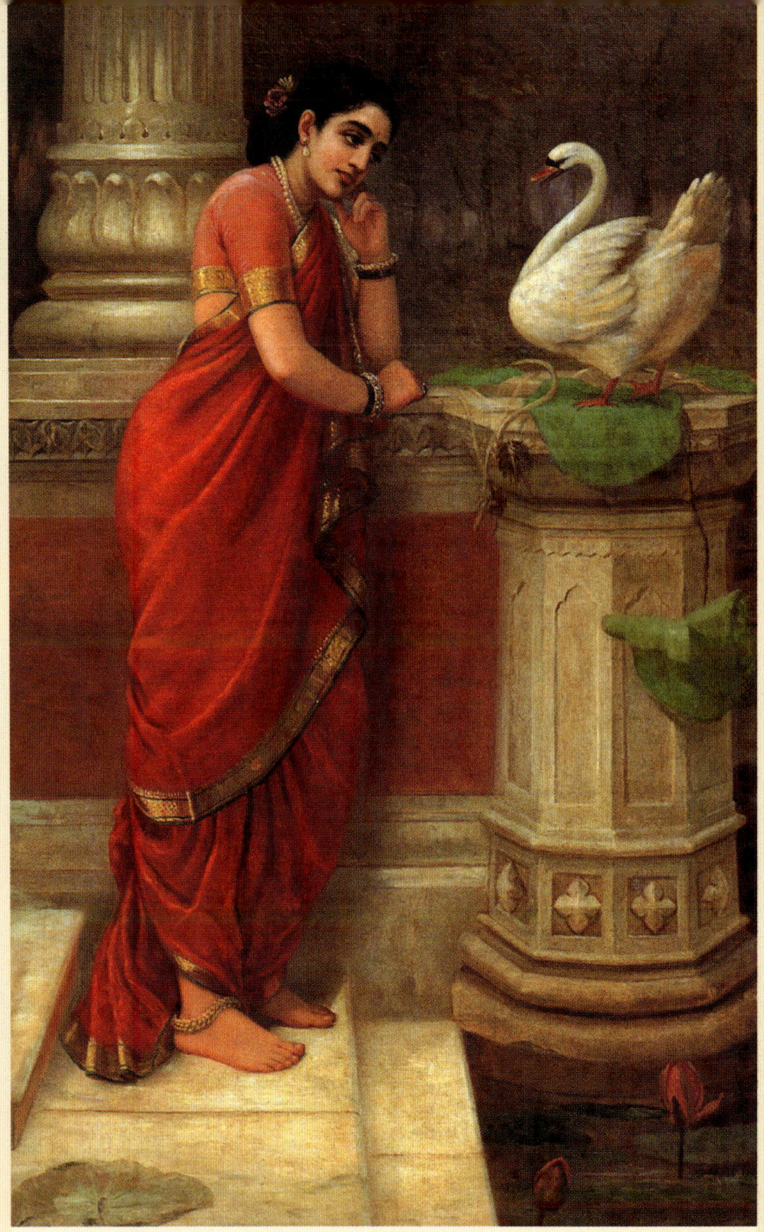

Hamsa Damayanti: Damayanti, her poise and graceful stance has a lyrical naturalism. Nala's go between, the swan, communicates to Damayanti, the love Nala feels for her, even though they had never met physically. When the *swayamvara* was held, the gods invited themselves to the competition. They tried a deceit, by disguising themselves as Nala. But not being human, their eyes did not blink. Damayanti faultlessly chose Nala. For twelve years, joy and happiness filled their lives. But mishaps as well as grave mis-judgements made a sorrowful tale! The *Mahabharata* tells the full story of Nala's downfall. *Painting oil on canvas by Raja Ravi Varma, 1899. Art Gallery Tiruvanathapuram Museum, Kerala.*

city by intruders. He disguised himself and took refuge in the house of the courtesan Kumudika in Ujjain. The king was impressed by her service but his companions warned him to be wary of a beautiful woman's affections. To test her, the king feigned death and as they were about to light the funeral pyre, Kumudika expressed her desire to die with the king; her decision convinced the king of the depth of her love for him. When he revealed his true identity, she offered her entire wealth to him to raise his army and win his lost kingdom back. When asked why she was doing this, she replied it was in the hope that he could also attack and conquer Ujjain and save her lover who was locked in a prison there! The king then realised that it was impossible to gauge a courtesan's heart.

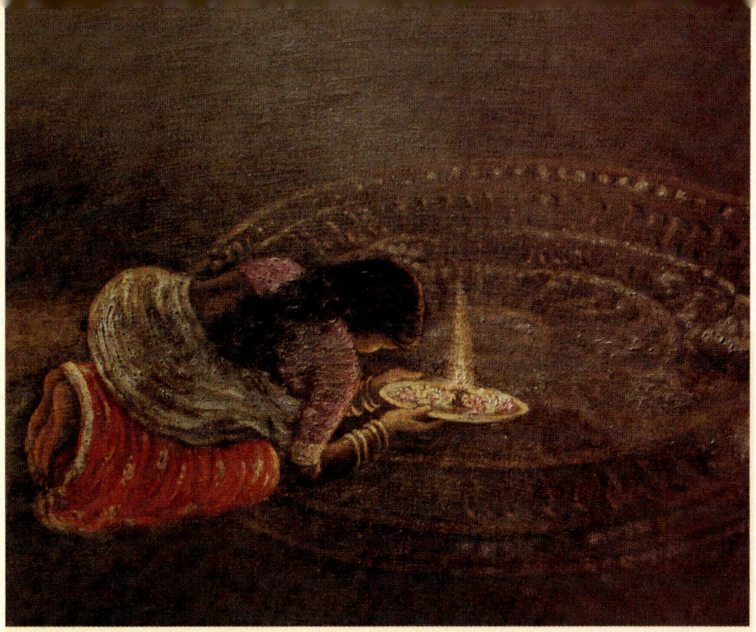

The most famous polyandrous woman of sacred Hindu lore was Draupadi, heroine of the epic *Mahabharata*, and common wife to the five Pandava brothers. According to the *Devi Bhagvattam*, Draupadi in her previous life, had pleased Lord Shiva with her devotion and was granted a boon. She asked for a husband who was noble, strong, brave, handsome and wise, and Shiva in his innocence, granted her five husbands instead. Draupadi was an extremely beautiful, intelligent and virtuous woman, with a body that smelled like a fresh lotus flower. There are few women in Hindu mythology who were aggressive and who spoke their mind in a world of men. Draupadi was one of them. She is considered by many as the first feminist of Indian mythology. At the time of her birth, a celestial voice had proclaimed: 'This unparalleled beauty has taken birth to uproot the Kauravas and establish the rule of religion'.

The agenda of the *apsara*, nymph, in the *Vedas* and *Puranas* was to seduce and enamour the sage, to test his resolve for liberation and to obstruct his quest for occult powers. A tale from *Jataka* of the *Mahabharata* states that Sage Rishyashringa had been kept in seclusion, away from women all his life. He lived a life devoid of sexual desire. Once, while carrying a pitcher of water, rain fell in such torrents that his pitcher broke. Enraged, he prevented Indra from releasing water from the clouds for twelve years, which caused a drought. The only solution to this was to make Rishyashringa lose his spiritual prowess. On the advice of the *devas*; Shanta, the daughter of a local

***Puja*, worship:** Seen here, is a skilful rendition of devotion, when the devotee kneeling before the diety, eases her body forward to lie prostrate on the ground. The gesture requires physical skill but it is a gesture of abjuration, an act of complete faith. *Contemporary painting, Tamil Nadu, 20th century. Private collection.*

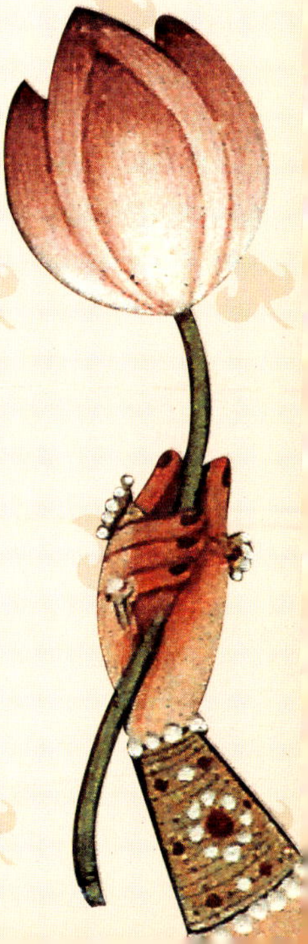

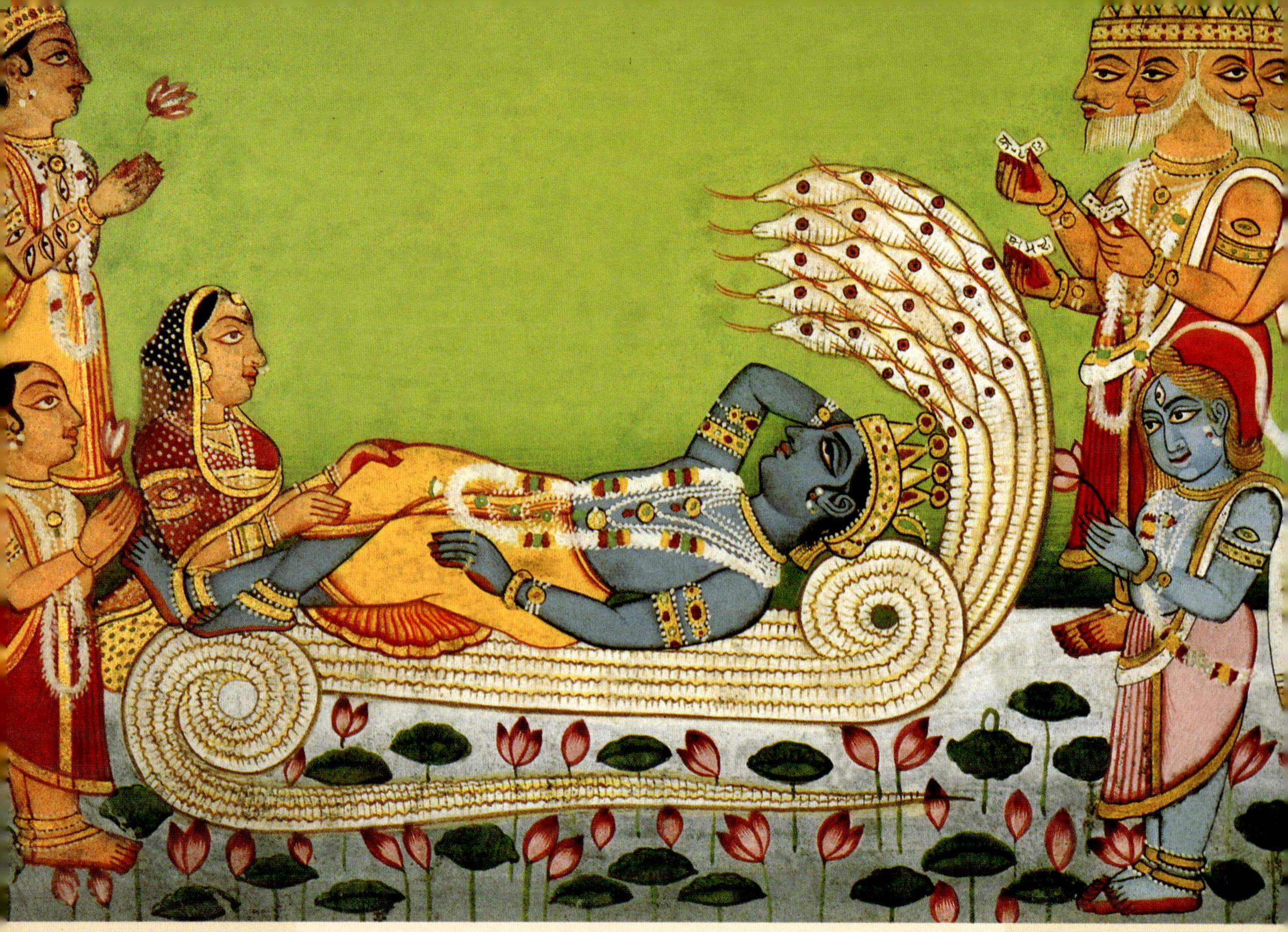

king, was sent to seduce the sage. The sage was by turns aroused, curious and attracted to her alluring beauty. They made love and as a consequence, he lost his control over the forces of nature and it began to rain.

The famous real-life courtesan, Umrao Jaan, as an old woman, narrated her life story to Ruswa. The girl Amiran, later named Umrao Jaan, had been kidnapped and brought to Lucknow in childhood by two criminals, who sold her to the grand madame Khanum. Khanum's house was frequented by all the aristocrats and nawabs of Lucknow, who often threw their entire fortunes away on the sophisticated and talented courtesans. Umrao was taught to sing and dance in the classical Indian style called *Kathak* and soon showed talent as a poetess of *ghazals*. Her artistry won her the favour of some of the richest *nawabs* in Lucknow.

Mohini was regarded as coexisting with Vishnu; she was not, strictly speaking, an incarnation but a form that Vishnu assumed at will. This was a vital difference but then that assumed form did everything the *avatar* would have done anyway, so the distinction is moot. Mohini was not

Reclining on the cosmic serpant: Lord Vishnu, reposes on the soft coils of the serpant Sesha. It occasioned the presence of Lord Rama and Lord Shiva as well as Sridevi, his devoted consort, who is gently massaging his leg. *Miniature painting, Pahari Hills, Guler, 19th century.*

exactly Vishnu's *maya* either, though she certainly made the fullest use of it. Mohini was called the Enchantress, but she did not enchant the mind so much as drove it bereft of reason by infusing every particle of it with desire - for her! Mohini was supernaturally beautiful, beautiful in a manner a woman could never be, for the latter would be real, but she was a facsimile of the Creative Feminine and could be starkly, cruelly flawless. (In the dramatic tradition of Japan, for a long time the hero was played by a female actor as only she could convey the abstract essence of male heroism, any male attempt being invariably and inevitably flawed by the common clay of being a man.) Mohini was the reverse of that principle, a fantastic version of femininity, her attraction being precisely that she was not a woman; she seemed to be, and in reality was, a woman like no other. Trying to possess this impossibly beguiling 'woman' is what drove men mad.

The first appearance of Mohini was during the great myth of the Churning of the Cosmic Ocean. The demon horde got hold of the Nectar of Immortality in cooperative effort with the gods, but then refused to share it. A fight would have meant serious casualties, and an explosive stalemate was broken only by the appearance of this ravishing creature. She offered to arbitrate, and in the grand tradition of all tricksters, proceeded to rob the lustful demons blind. She doled out the nectar to the gods first, making sure that not a drop was left by the time she came to the demons. They were held in thrall by her personality as well as the hope

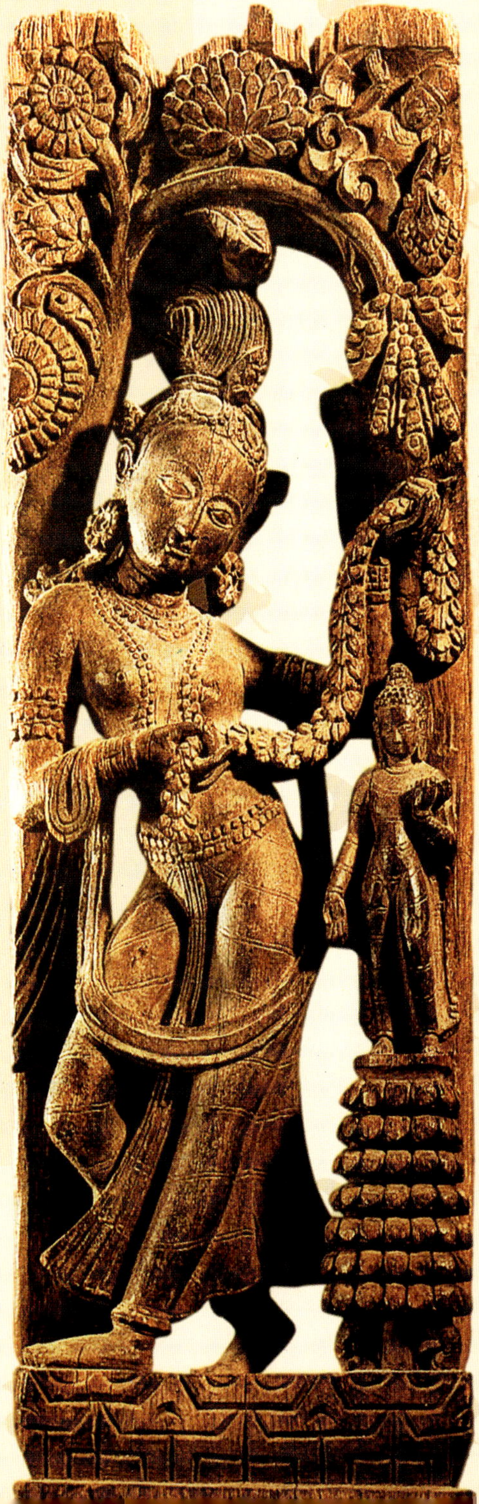

The garland bearer: This sculpture carved in wood, represents an auspicious occasion as the offering of flowers conveys respect and blessings.

Wood, Architectural architrave, Lumbini, Kathmandu Valley, Nepal, 17th-18th century. Private collection.

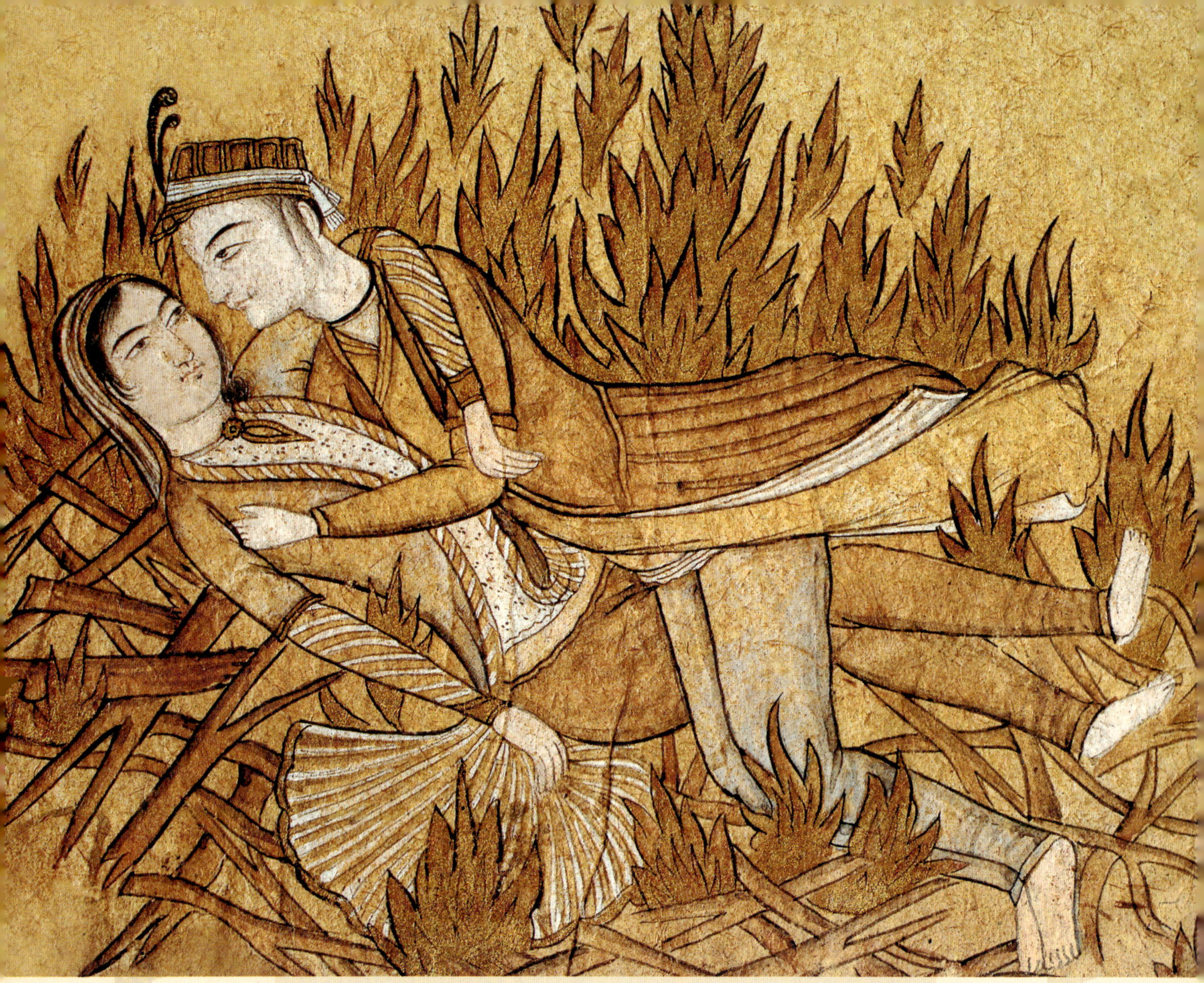

that if they behaved, she would share her favours with one of them at least. The demons were massacred because they abdicated their reason.

Mohini next appeared to save the great god Shiva. Named the Simpleton God by his frustrated admirers, Shiva had just granted a demon who was coming out of horrendous penances to please him, the ability to turn anything he touched into ashes. This earned the demon the epithet of *Bhasmasura*, the Ash-demon, and matters would have gone well if the demon had not decided to test the efficacy of his world-conquering boon on Shiva himself first. Shiva had to take to his heels, and was chased by the demon through all quarters of the universe. This impossible situation could not be resolved by anybody, for nobody dared to come near the Ash-demon. Nobody except Mohini. Upon seeing her, Bhasmasura forgot his conflagration experiments and instantly wanted to marry her. She

An inspiration to light up hidden fires: A fanciful visualisation, where the artist has portrayed inflamed passions of love of the amorous couple on a fiery bed. *Miniature painting, Pahari Hills, Guler, 19th century. Private collection.*

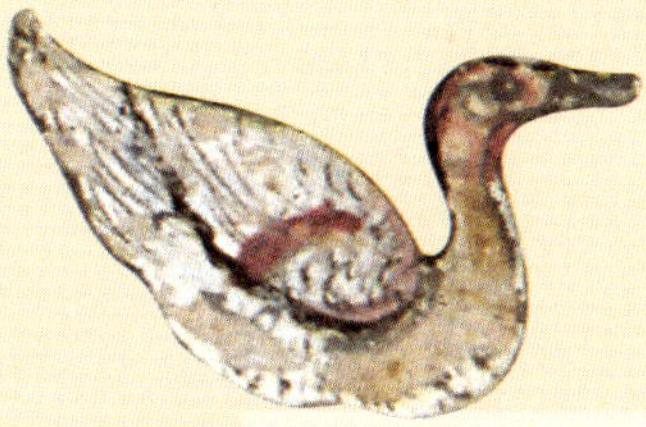

answered that she was under a vow that she would only marry the man who could match her in a dance competition. It says much for the general levels of culture prevalent that the demon was a great dancer too, as befitted a devotee of Shiva Nataraja, the Lord of the Dance. Bhasmasura felt confident of holding his own. The great competition began and the infatuated demon gave a very credible account of himself until the ruthless humour of the trickster came into play. Mohini began to dance, using various *mudras*, positions of the hands, which required her to frequently touch her head. The poor demon, enraptured by her, did not realise what he was doing and reduced himself to an ash heap!

Apsaras, divine courtesans, who adorned the court of Indra, Lord of the firmament, entertained the gods by dancing merrily to the accompaniment of music by *gandharvas*. Urvashi, an *apsara*, is said to have been born on earth as a *devadasi* and imparted the divine knowledge of dance and music to human beings. The *devadasi* institution was established all over India. The Chinese pilgrim Hiuen Tsang who visited India in the seventh century, testified to the existence of a well-established institution of temple dancers. After the advent of Muslim rule, the *devadasis* disappeared from the scene in north India but the practice continued in the south until the beginning of the twentieth century. In their heyday, under the generous patronage of the Pallava, Chola, Pandya and Nayaka kings, *devadasis* were honoured with titles and gifts, and their names are even mentioned in temple chronicles and inscriptions. They were trained from childhood in the arts of dance and music and were also taught classical literature in Sanskrit, Tamil and Telugu. The *devadasis* commanded respect in society and were treated as symbols of good luck. The exchange of *devadasis* between the temple and the court was an accepted practice. Though married

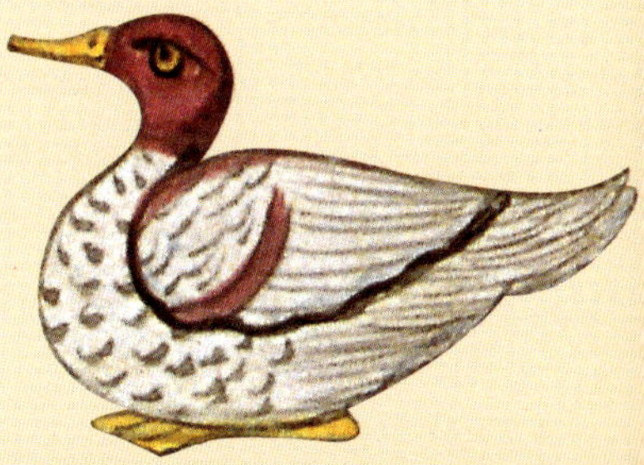

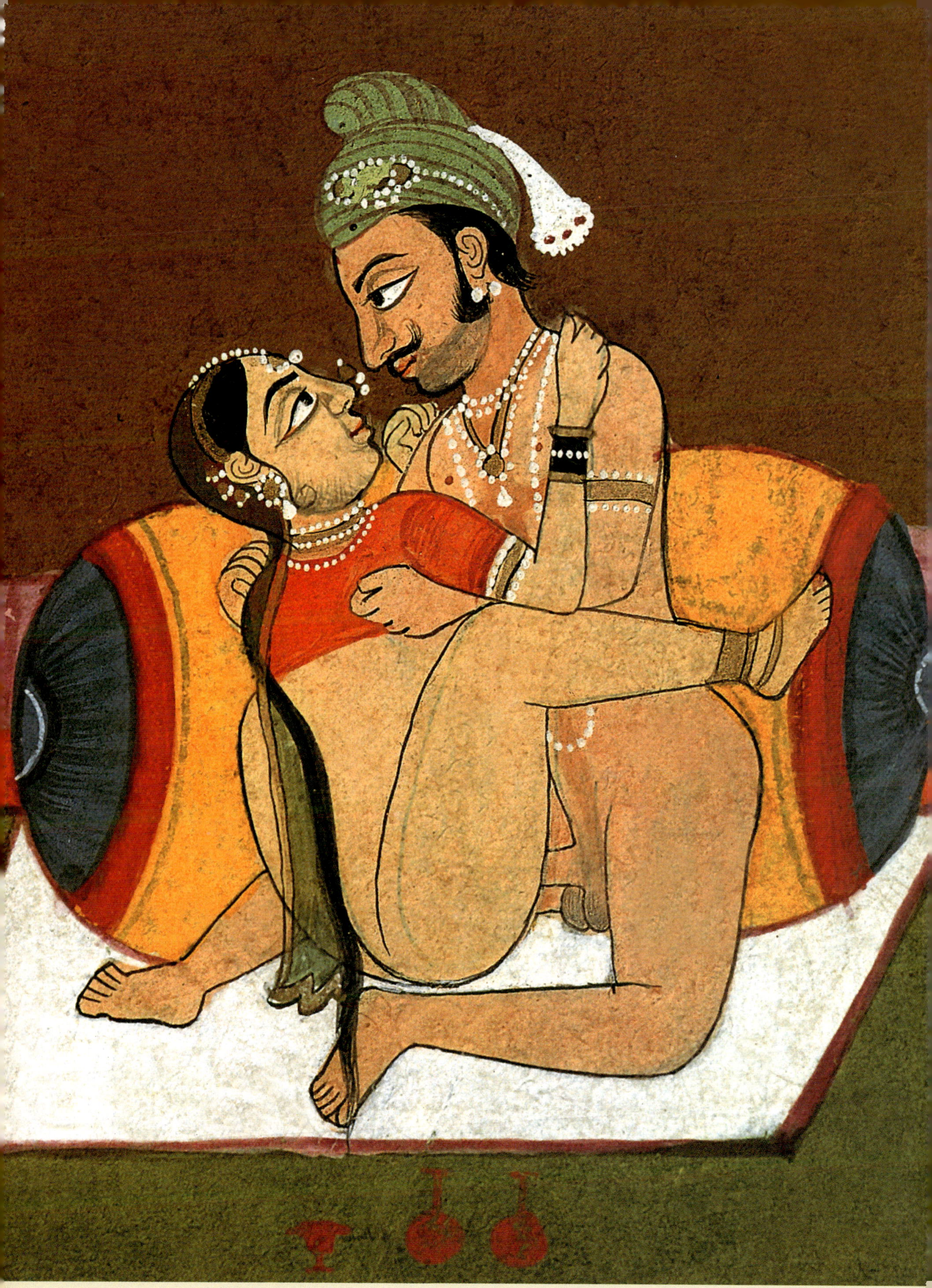

Equal union: The two paintings represent two dramatically different *asanas*, both showing equal union. These are both half-pressed postures, where the sweep of the attenuated lines of the bodies brilliantly portrays the wiles of the conjugal lovers, whose physicality is remarkable. *Miniature paintings, Jodhpur, Rajasthan, late 20th century.*

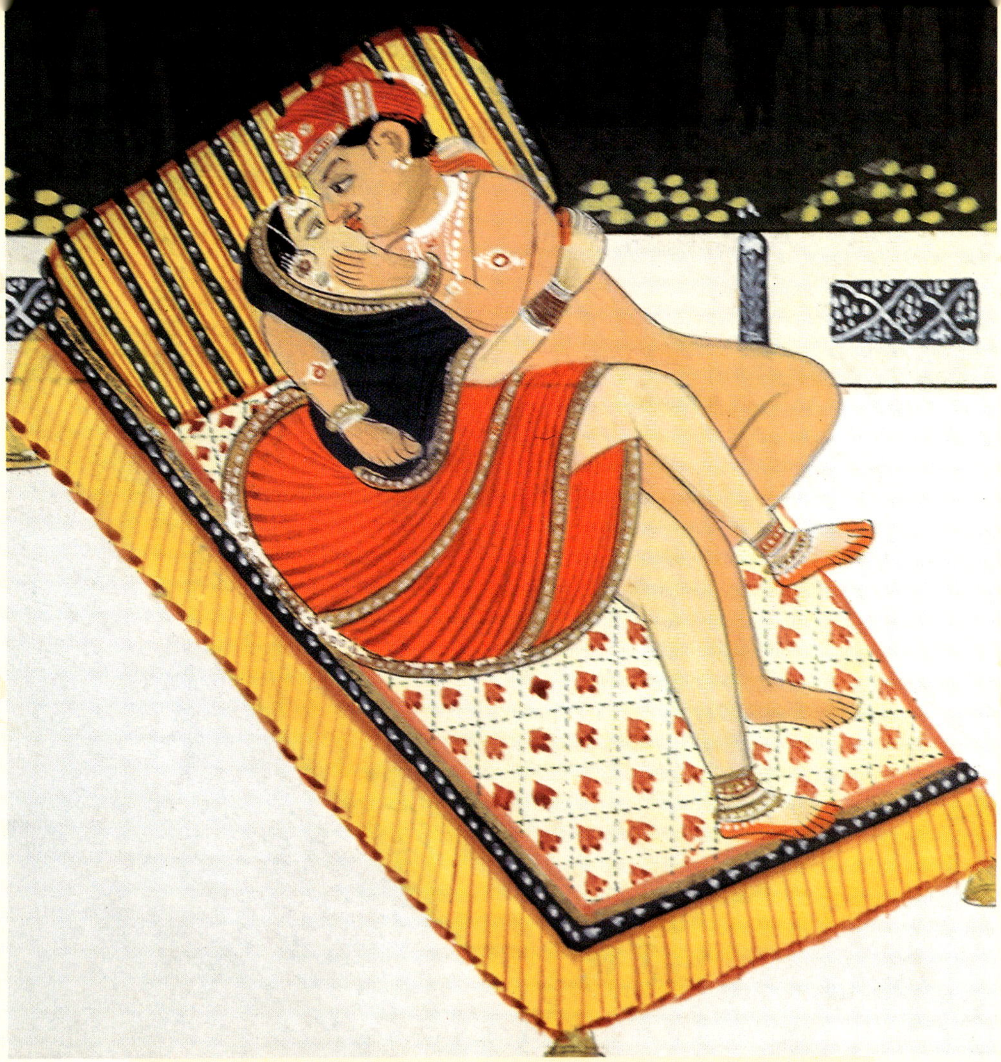

to the temple deities, some of them, gifted with rare beauty and accomplishments, became royal courtesans and consorts of kings.

Some royal or aristocratic women did enjoy greater freedom and indulged in male-dominated activities. During the Gupta period (4th-6th centuries), women held prominent positions in the administration of the state. Women were also involved in political affairs in later times. During the rule of the Mughals (16th-18th centuries), none could surpass Noor Jahan, whose strong personality supplanted even the ablest of politicians and soldiers. This trend continued up to the Vijayanagar period (14th-16th centuries), with women contributing to political, social and literary activities. They were trained in wrestling and handled swords and shields. In 19th century colonial India, there were queens such as Lakshmi Bai of Jhansi (1835-1858) and Ahalya Bai Holkar of Indore (1735-1795), who participated in wars. However, such women were

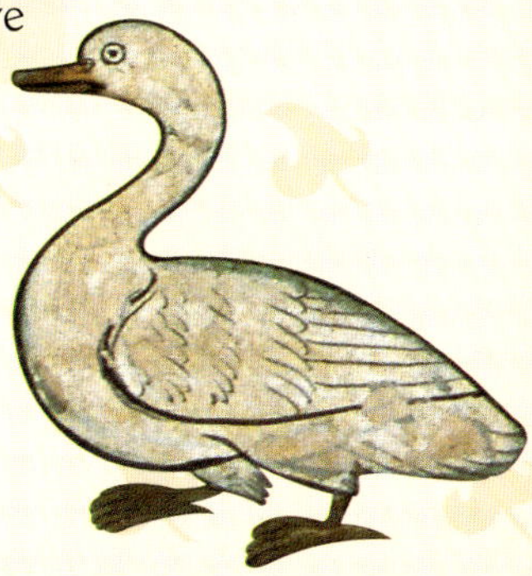

exceptions in Indian history as the average women played a more passive role in society.

A few women had the privilege of education too. Before the rise of the Muslim empires, education was restricted to the Brahmin caste. The Muslim rulers however encouraged education, making it available both to Muslims and Hindus. Girls usually attended the same schools as boys until puberty. Older girls were often taught privately or sent to special schools called *makhtäbs*. Daughters from wealthy households were taught in their homes by learned women or men.

Kathleen Erndl's investigation of how the concept of *Shakti* has empowered Hindu women and been adopted in Indian feminism supplements these thoughts. Feminism was not a Western import but has its roots in the *Shakti* cults of old; it was not a negative reaction of rebellion, but a rediscovery of a positive creative force empowering men and women alike. *Shakta* female saints have a higher status than their Vaishnava counterparts. Unlike in the west, speaking of God as female is not shocking to the Hindu tradition. However, the challenge facing Indian feminists is how to generate a sense of commonalty among women cutting across caste,

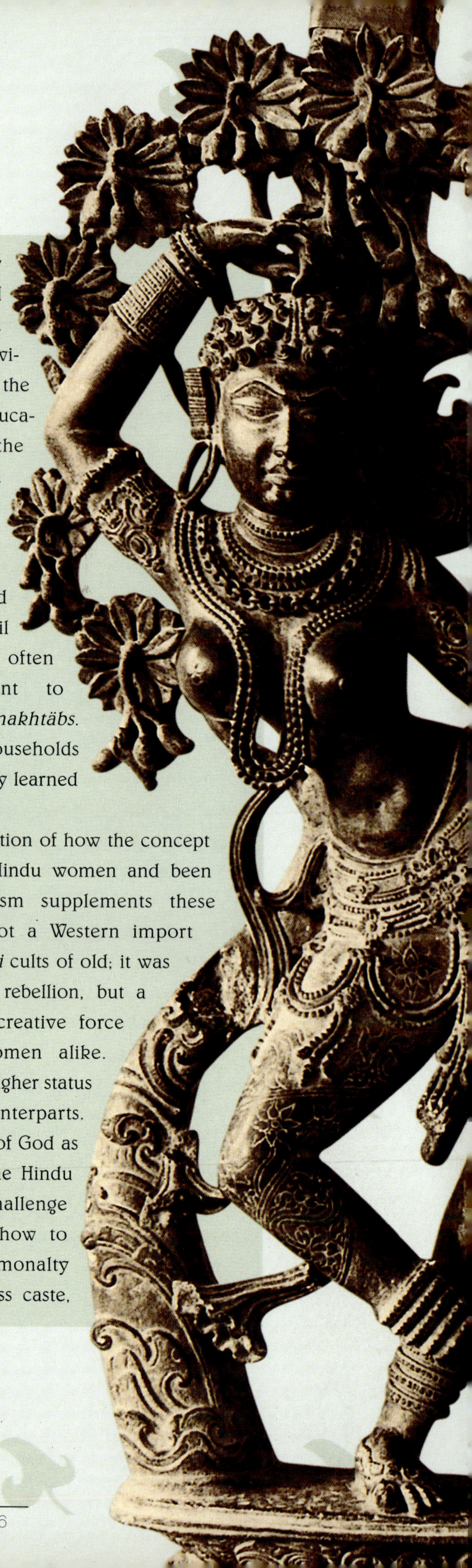

class, language and kinship barriers.

Tracy Pintchman asks a basic question: whether powerful, independent goddesses are conducive to female empowerment in society. This is in the context of the theory that in goddess-less traditions the Hindu goddesses provide a resource for rediscovering the goddess. Durga is represented as a golden-faced woman of great beauty with ten arms that hold a formidable array of weapons. She holds a spear piercing the demon *Mahishasur* and her mount is a lion. According to the *Devi Mahatmayam*, the goddess was created by the light of the three gods, Brahma, Vishnu and Shiva. She slayed the king of the *asuras*, demons, *Mahishasur* the buffalo demon, and was thus called *Mahishasura Mardini*.

No other form of divinity worshipped by the Hindu is so difficult of acceptance as Kali - the dark and terrible naked Mother, named after the night black complexion of her skin. Kali is easily amongst the six most popular forms of god worshipped amongst Hindus today. There is a concentration in Bengal, Assam and parts of South India however, for historical reasons. In the *Devi Mahatmayam*, Kali is finally brought into the ambit of the formal faith. In this version, Kali is an emanation of the great goddess Durga, or more specifically, she is a personification of emergent wrath on the part of the older goddess when she goes to battle. She is red eyed from quaffing wine as well as wrath, has a garland of human heads, wears tiger-skin clothes and has a lolling tongue that she occasionally employs to emit frightful roars that fill up all quarters. Her preferred mode of destroying demons is to either chew them up or cut off their heads. Kali is a symbol of all that man fears most in woman. The large number of male heads lying around in the myths of the goddess is seen as symbolic castration.

Razia Sultan (1236-1240) is a much-romanticised figure

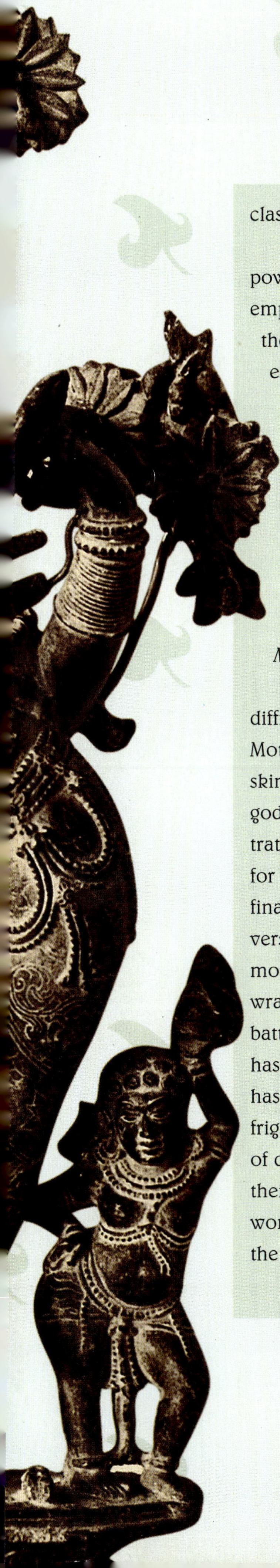

Mohini - the temptress: The Gods in desperation called upon Vishnu to save for them the vital *amrita*, the elixir of life, which was to emerge from the churning of the ocean. Vishnu entered upon the scene, visible to the *asuras* as a beautiful, naked, sensous woman. Besotted by her, the *asuras* were totally out of control and could not retain the *amrita* kept in a golden chalice. With one elegant sweep, Mohini took up the vessel and gave it to the gods, who drank it immediately. *Black stone, Chalukyan style, Gadag, Dharava, Karnataka, 10th century. National Museum.*

in Indian history. As late as three centuries later, the legal aspect of her accession was still a matter of heated theological debate. Of course, what makes her more interesting was that she had an affair with her Assyrian slave, Yakut. By all accounts, Razia vindicated her father's faith in her. She was a very shrewd ruler, and for all her feminine beauty, an autocrat who kept the nobility in its place.

THE *KAMA SUTRA* ON WOMEN

Despite popular opinion, the *Kama Sutra* is more than an illustrated guide to good sex. It is a guide to living a well-balanced, satisfied life. Although the text is widely known and often talked about, only a small minority of people has actually read it. No doubt several of the passages in the *Kama Sutra* were specific to the time and place in which it was written, making it difficult, if not impossible, to relate them to modern society. For instance, rape, though not encouraged, was an accepted form of love making in the third and fourth centuries. However, many of the passages are in fact relevant to today's society. For example, when the author, Vatsyayana, writes about 'how to get rid of a man without literally kicking him out', and tells women to use techniques such as not paying attention to his needs, not laughing at his jokes, and nagging, the same actions would produce the same results even today.

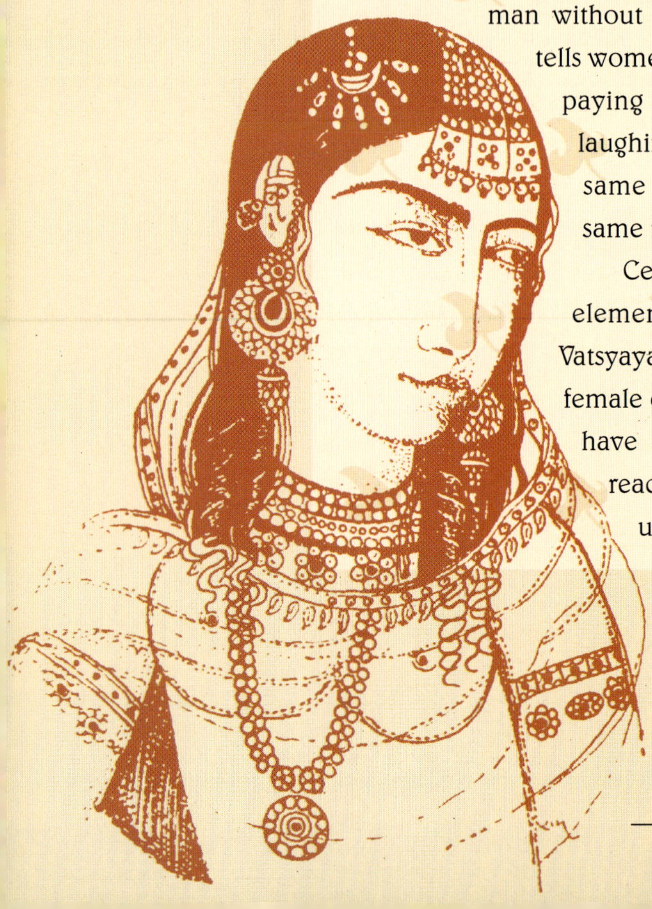

Certainly there seems to be an element of feminism in the text: Vatsyayana, who was male, talks about female orgasms and a woman's right to have them, a concept that did not reach Western mainstream thought until very recently. More surpris-

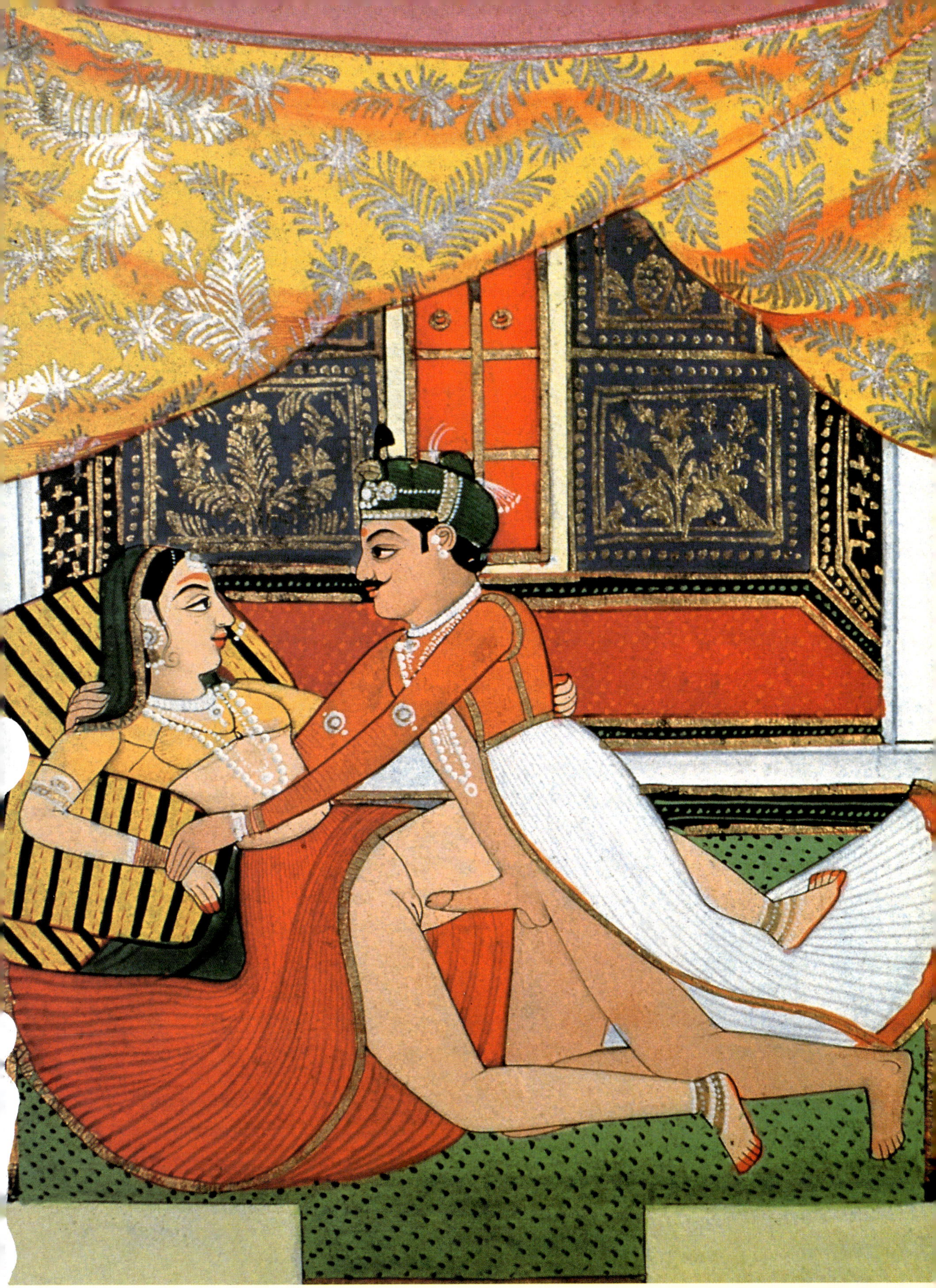

The bow shape posture: The artist has chosen to show the ardent lover, poised and ready, to implant his beloved, who has adopted the bow shape posture to receive his entry in a widely open stance. The venue is a richly designed alcove in the typical Rajasthan style with gold leaf foliage on the walls. *Miniature painting, Jodhpur, Rajasthan, late 20th century.*

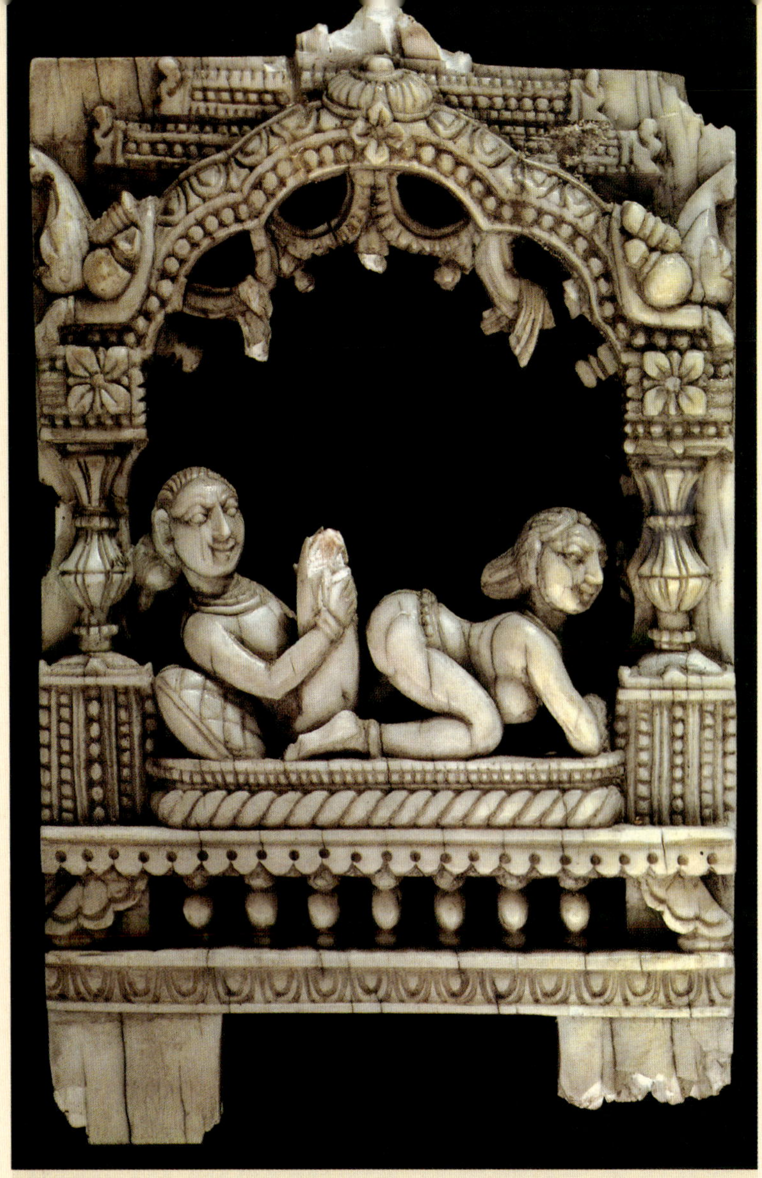

Woman on top: This miniature ivory gem is part of a large set dismantled from an ivory *palana*, love couch. Potentially an invaluable aid, it encouraged 'real life' implication to match all the sixty-four *asanas*, love postures. Possibly a trusted duenna, elderly chaperone, conversant with sexual arts, acted as an instructress and guide. Such an elderly companion, would for instance, be able to outline in detail, the idea of 'role reversal' when the active, young and sexually fertile heroine, takes over from her exhausted hero, who in a turn down state and incapable is willing to accede to, and lies comfortably on his back to enjoy the novelty offered. These ivory plaques and decorated love couches were almost certainly used to invite the girl to implement the variations that the artists invented. *Carving from an ivory bed, Orissa, early 20th century.*

ingly, there is even advice for women on how to fake it! Courtesans, who were women working as prostitutes for the upper class, actually used the *Kama Sutra* for their work and also affected its content.

However, despite its liberal nature towards women, there are definite stereotypes used throughout the text, namely man's 'active nature' versus woman's 'passive nature'. Although the roles are occasionally reversed, the text conveys the idea that these roles are exhibited consistently in all aspects of life, not just sex. Richard Burton's late 19th century formal and euphemistic translations reflect the patriarchal, societal values of the time.

The *Kama Sutra*, which is actually a compilation of seven books from the third and fourth centuries, was read mainly by upper class Indians of the time, yet its

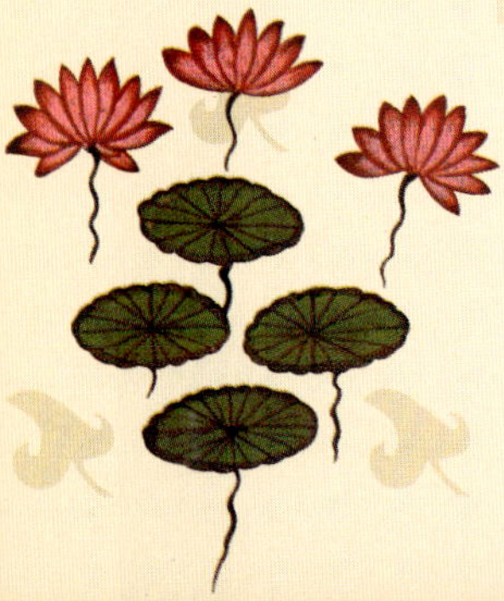

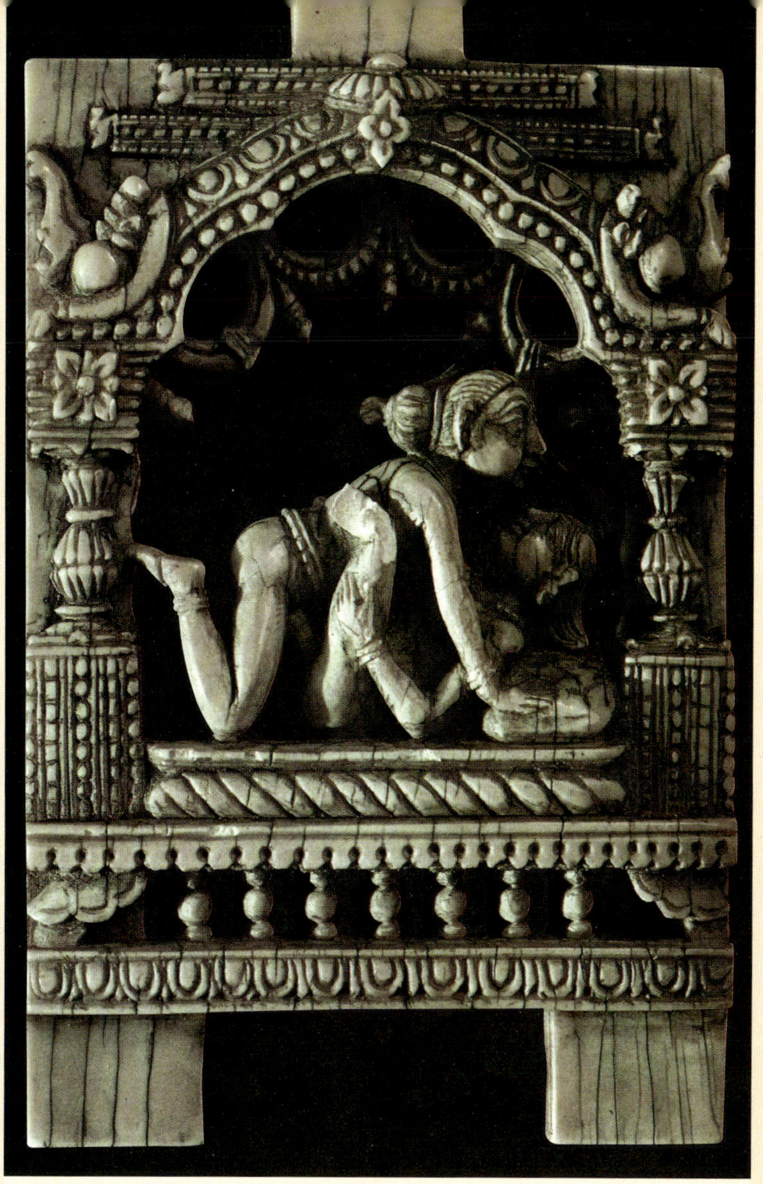

teachings spread to virtually every class level. Indians seemed to realise, as the *Kama Sutra* suggests, that sex is an essential part of human well-being. It is akin to our need for food; we cannot live without it, yet each person's tastes are unique.

In the most basic sense, feminism is exactly what the dictionary says it is the movement for social, political, and economic equality of men and women. Breaking down that one very basic definition, feminism has three components. It is a movement, meaning a group working to accomplish specific goals. Those goals are social and political change - implying that one must be engaged with the government and law, as well as social practices and beliefs. And implicit to these goals is access to sufficient information to enable women to make responsible choices.

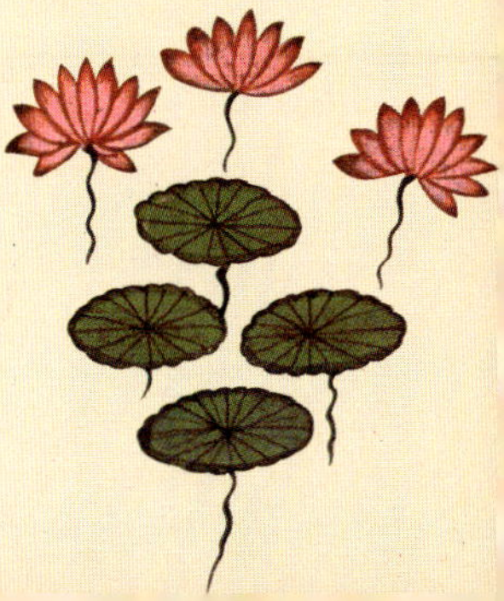

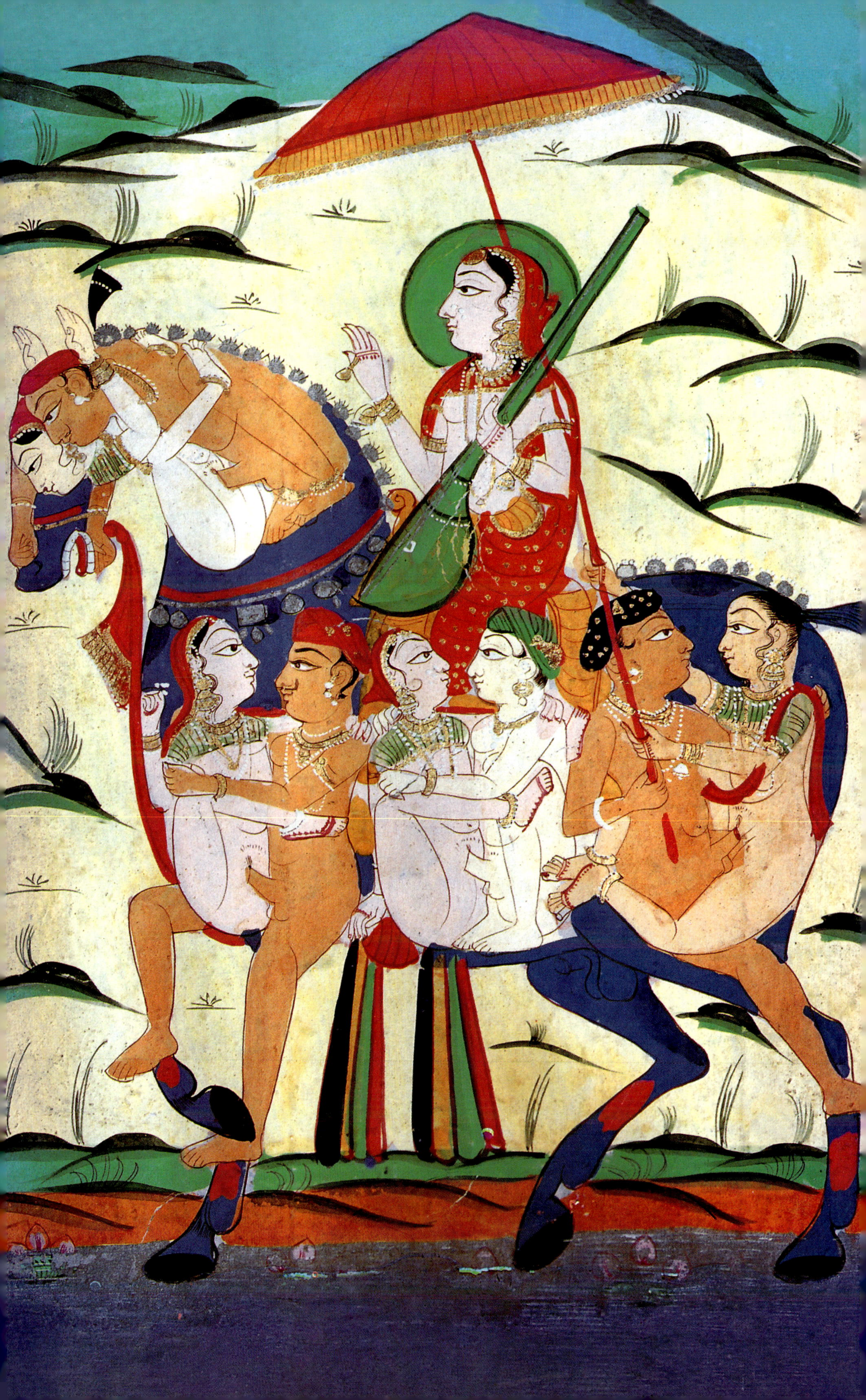

Through love - gifts, hints,
And courtesies with just one meaning,
She becomes intimate with her lover, and after that, she gets him to love her

Kama Sutra

every woman's PERSONAL KAMA SUTRA

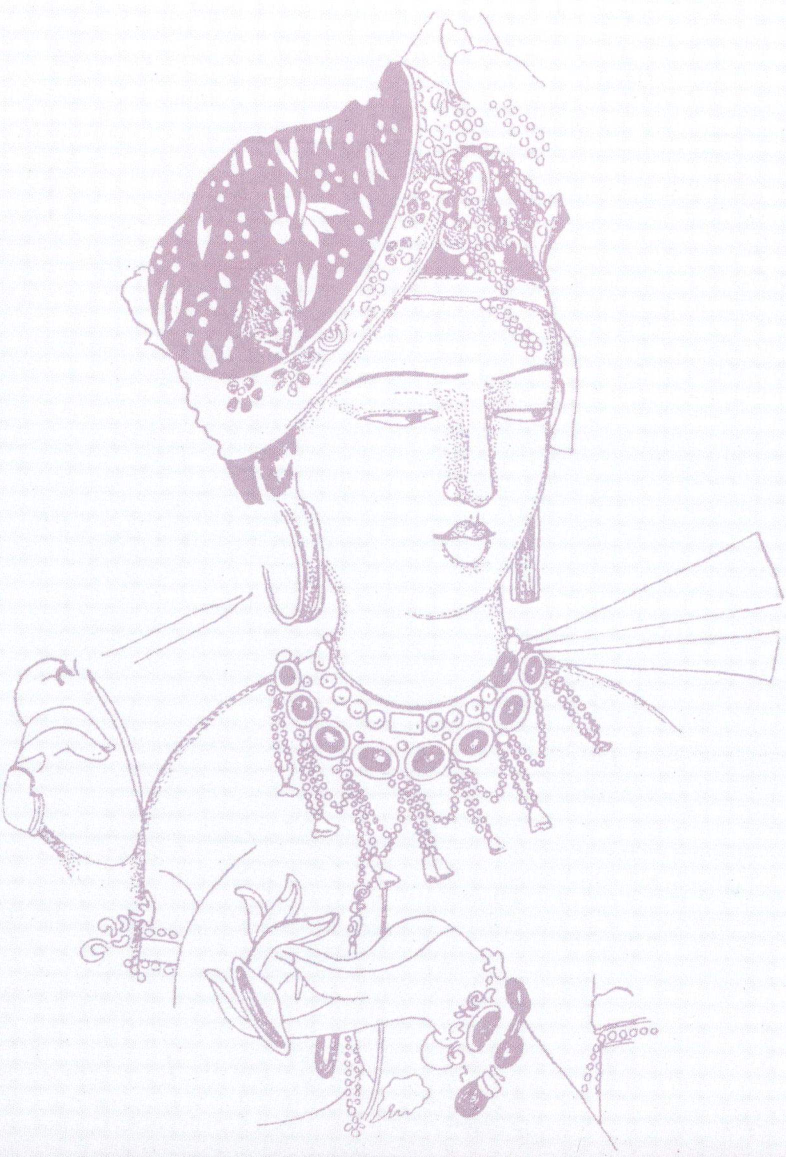

Previous page: **Composite sexual postures:** Lovers are embodied in the shape of a horse. Sitting on the saddle is the heroine, playing a melody to accompany the pace and the prancing of the animal. And in her attitude, importance is given to the figures, who are serving as *chattri*, umbrella bearers. The leading lovers advance the pace of the horse to suit their own body movements. *Miniature painting, Jodhpur, Rajasthan, 18th century.*

Releasing herself from the feminine mystique of domesticity, the New Age woman has simultaneously entered the labelised market of consumer titillation and commercialised sexuality, trapped by popular sociology, magazines, and popular fiction, in the 'be sexy and smart competition' mode.

Stated simply, illustrations and photographs of scantily clad and nude women, once considered disreputable, now grace billboards, calendars, television, movies and magazines. The exposed female body appears ubiquitously as our primary public symbol of 'eroticism'. Mother India, *Devi Maa* and *Dharti Maa* have been replaced with Superwoman!

No longer a homemaker redefining beauty myths, the New Age woman is more than being a power woman, a soccer mom, a trophy wife, homemaker and child bearer. From decision-making in every field of national endeavour to managing stress and conflict, within the home and the workplace, the 'new' woman in spite of gender crossings at work and in her public domain, is essentially a woman. In her private domain she is at once the perennial Eve, where she is the one seduced and the seductress. The modern Eve is a bundle of paradoxes. The power of femininity lies in the celebration of being a woman.

From the mythic past have emerged the repositories of great wisdom and energy. Ancient thinkers understood the importance of the difference between men and women, and instead of

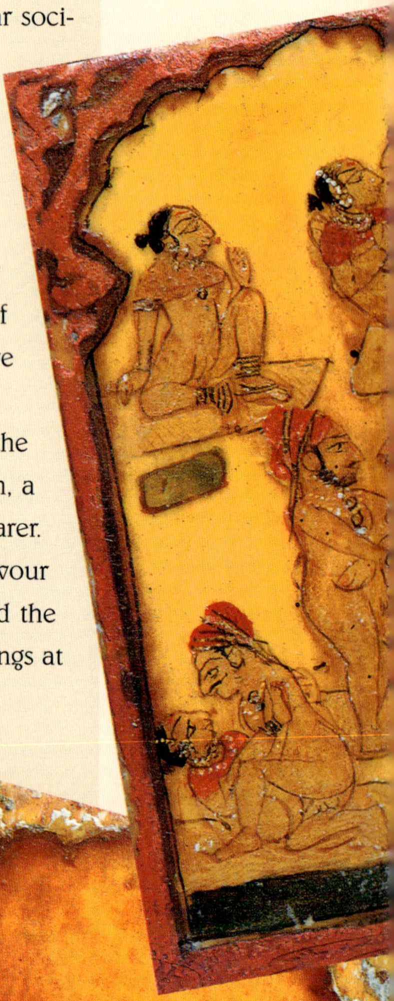

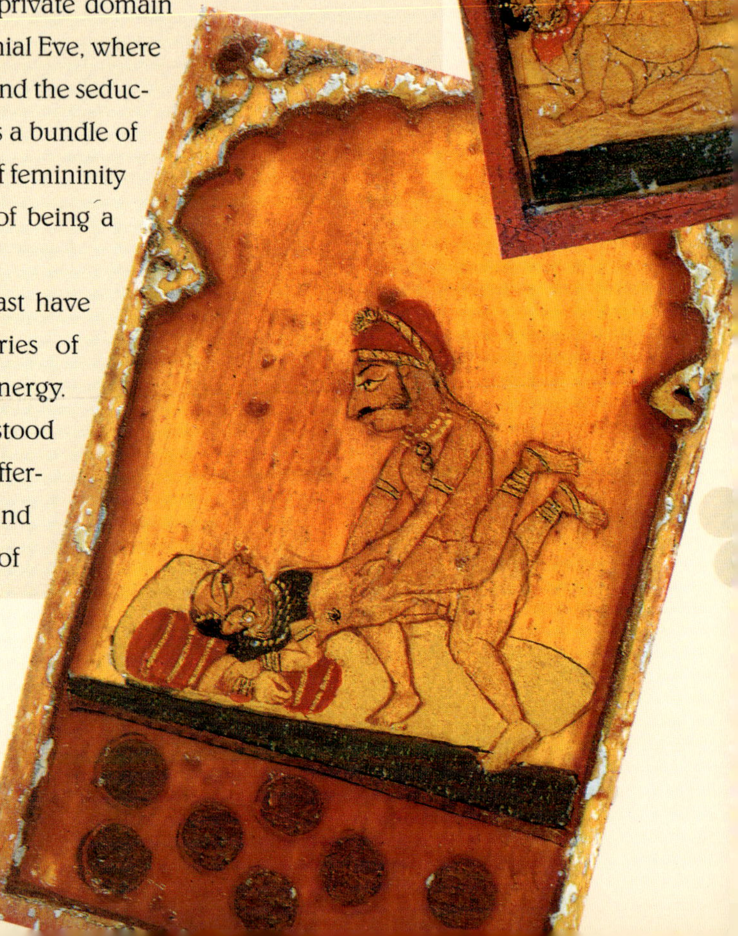

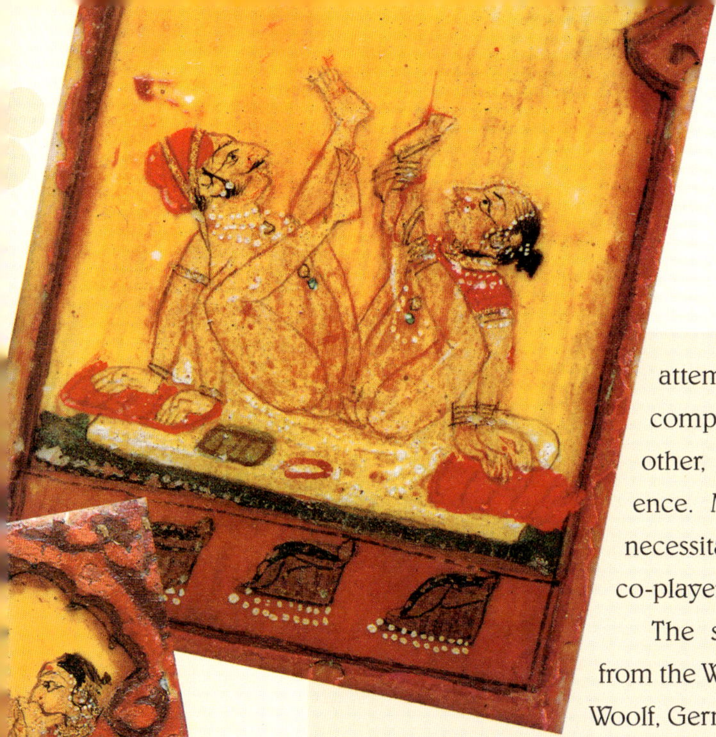

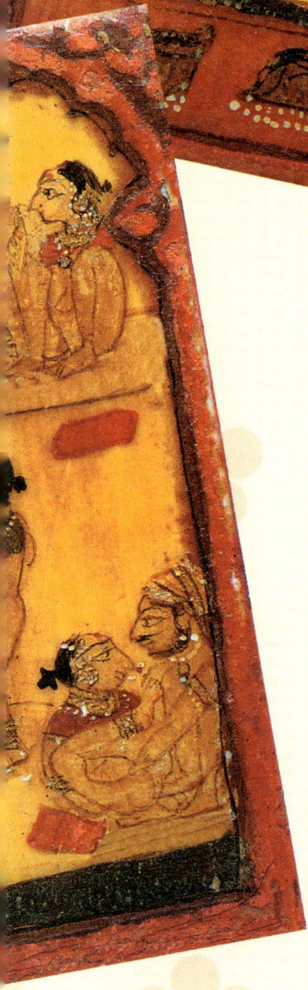

attempting to equate the two or compromise one in favour of the other, they celebrated the difference. Modern life has, however, necessitated that women become co-players professionally with men.

The strident feminist discourse from the West, associated with Virginia Woolf, Germaine Greer and Simone de Beauvoir in the 1960s, matched the vigour of the American suffragettes in the 1920s in using gender as a tool to craft a new identity. The body became the central metaphor, foregrounding sexuality. Feminists redefined themselves and were credited with having effectively displaced norms of male domination.

Contemporary women theorists like Julia Christeva, Luce Irigaray and Helen Cixous, basing their work on psychoanalysis, have been influenced by Freud's account of sexual identity. Gender equality has been processed as a demand within diverse fields: defence, politics, education. But the distinction between male and female, which is essential, endowed and sustained by nature, cannot be negated or in any way undermined.

In India, where the *feminine* force or *shakti* becomes, at times, even more potent than the worship of the male *linga*, the woman has always been central in art, thought, philosophy and literature. As the *Adya Shakti*, Supreme Energy, to the beautiful Parvati, the consort of the primordial Lord Shiva, she is the site of sexual celebration which copes with the erotic energy of her spouse Shiva. As Radha, she becomes the muse for the representation of the romantic heroines of the numerous *bhakti* poets. But where, on the one hand, she is celebrated as a goddess, on another level, she is a commodity as is evident from advertising and cinema.

The Indian woman has always been associated with fertil-

Playful love games: Ivory playing things, decoratively painted with sexual activities indicate the insatiable interest in the more positive actual sexual manoeuvres. The high level of artistic merit these cards exhibit, lend us to believe that they were commissioned from an artist, by a high personage, who enjoyed pleasures of a sexual nature with groups of women, and who desired to participate in such rampageous behaviour. They were used to encourage sexual sport. This view is lent support by the ivory card with explicit sexual behaviour, involving one man with two women and an observer, and another, which shows the male holding the woman by her hips, in the turned position, like a wheelbarrow, which is a fanciful posture. *Painting on ivory playing plaques, Udaipur, Rajasthan, late 19th century.*

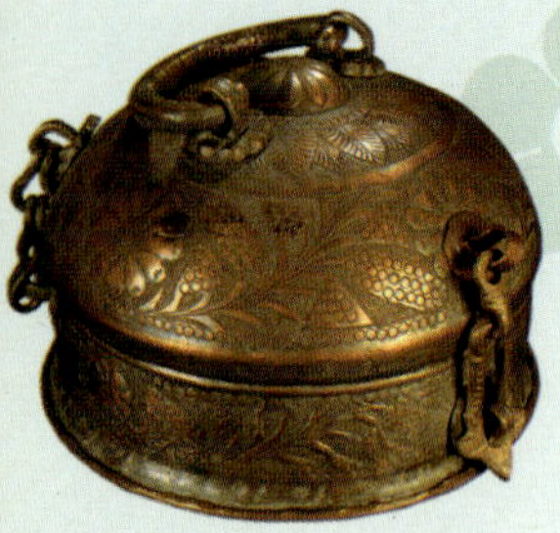

***Sarota*, betelnut cutter:** The *Kama Sutra* frequently deposes on the delights and the pleasure of sharing an evening *paan*. Placed in her open mouth, it colours the spittle a bright red, inducing all sorts of innuendoes between lovers, signalling the frame of mind, and a clear indicator, 'I am all yours'. *Sarotas*, betel nut cutters, have a considerable demand from the circles of the wealthy, who have discreet and charming alcoves hidden away, secretly set up for lovers to indulge in sexual fancies. This sharp bladed cutter is given the shape of a loving couple in a warm embrace, to enhance fantasising love play, and to add to the intense feelings aroused, when holding such a voluptuous object. *Bronze betelnut cutter, North Deccan, Maharashtra, early 19th century. Sanskriti Museum of Everyday Art.*

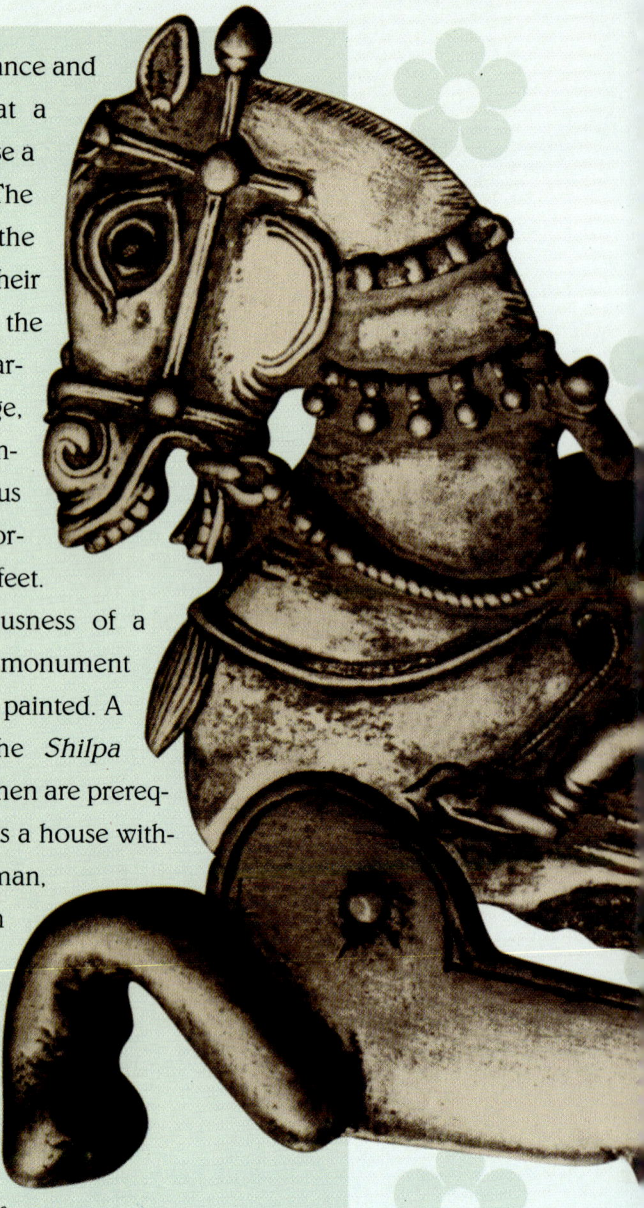

ity, which implies growth, abundance and prosperity. It was believed that a woman, by her touch, could cause a tree to blossom or bear fruit. The *Saundarya Lahiri speaks* of the radiance of Parvati's feet with their enchanting designs in henna; the poet tells us that the gods, not daring to touch them in homage, salute them verbally. Parvati's consort Shiva was inordinately jealous even of the Ashoka trees in the forest that desired the touch of her feet. In ancient India, the auspiciousness of a woman was transferred to the monument upon which she was sculpted or painted. A 10th century Orissan text, the *Shilpa Prakasa*, states that figures of women are prerequisites on the walls of temples, 'as a house without a wife, as play without a woman, so without the figure of woman the monument will be of inferior quality and bear no fruit'.

Looking at the vast repository of multiple thoughts and images surrounding the New Age woman, I am concerned not only with the extension of femininity and masculinity into cultural constructs of biological divisions but their spillover into gender negotiations. For me the feminist discourse is a limiting one femininity is about being a complete woman and living the life of a woman.

For some women, the thrill of seduction lies in the chase rather than the conquest. The excitement of wanting and pursuing someone can give a satisfaction in itself. For others, it is

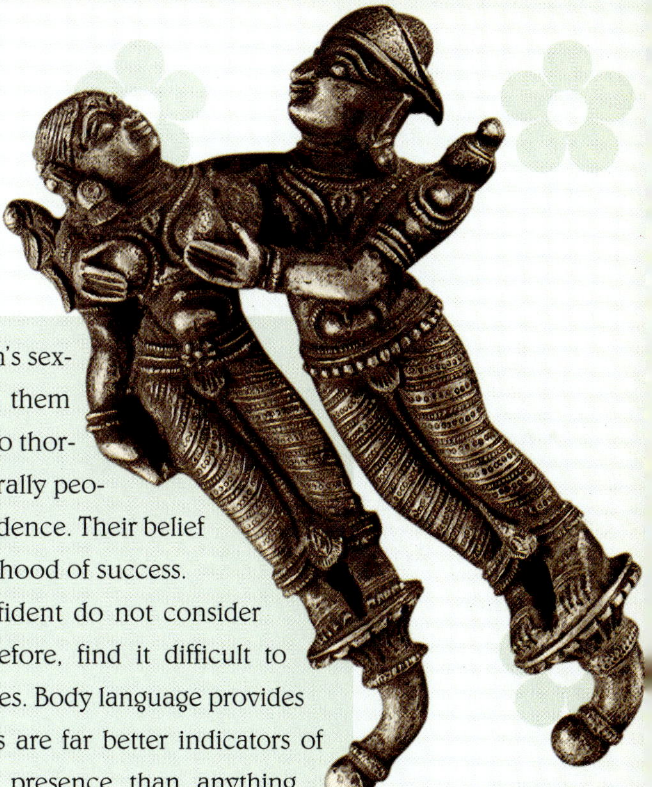

***Viddha*, pincer motions on the breasts:** *A pair of brass sarota, betel-nut cutter, Nasik or Pune, Northern Deccan, Maharashtra, early 19th century.*

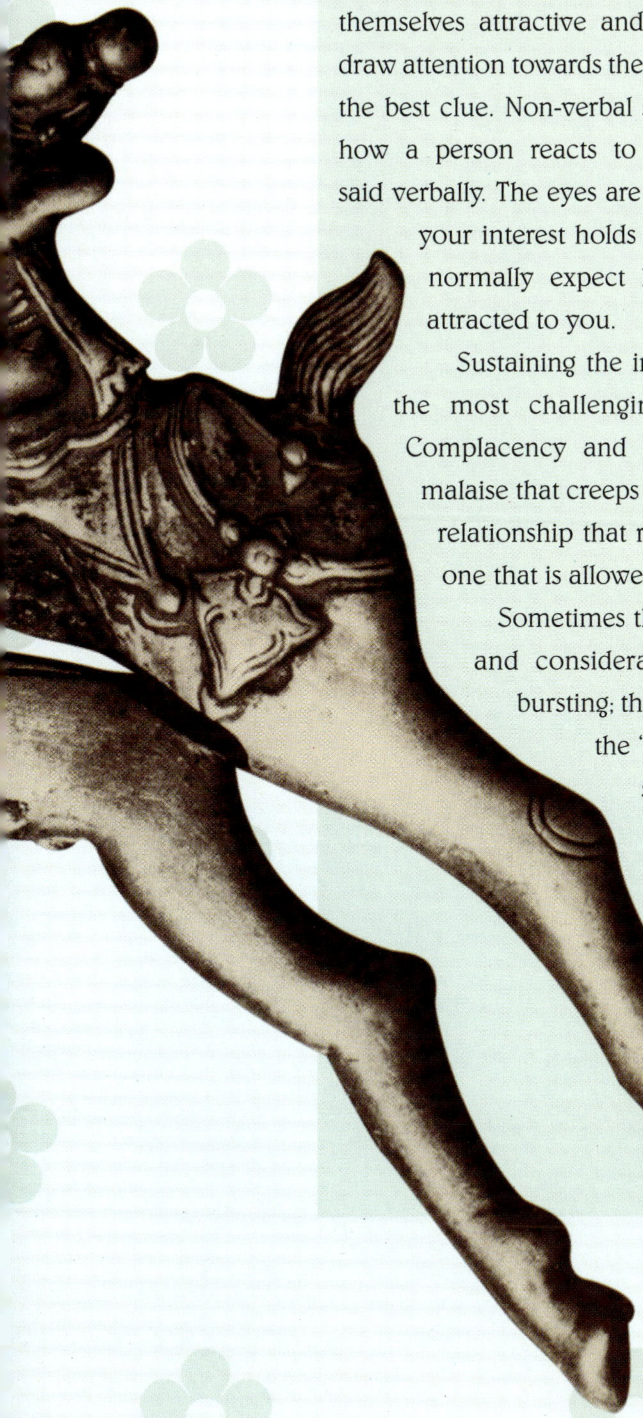

the knowledge of another person's sexual attentions being focused on them that gives them a high. Those who thoroughly enjoy the chase are generally people who have sufficient self-confidence. Their belief in themselves increases the likelihood of success.

Those who are less self-confident do not consider themselves attractive and, therefore, find it difficult to draw attention towards themselves. Body language provides the best clue. Non-verbal signals are far better indicators of how a person reacts to your presence than anything said verbally. The eyes are good indicators. If the object of your interest holds your gaze longer then you would normally expect him to, chances are that he is attracted to you.

Sustaining the interest of your partner is perhaps the most challenging aspect of any relationship. Complacency and 'taking for granted' are both a malaise that creeps into most partnerships. In fact, the relationship that requires the most nurturing, is the one that is allowed to drift carelessly.

Sometimes the answer is simple small gestures and considerations prevent the bubble from bursting; they keep the fire kindling and retain the 'special' togetherness in a relationship. We've all heard of them, suggested them to others - everything but practised them ourselves. If not sixty-four, here are at least fifty 'arts' for the woman that will go a long way towards safeguarding her relationship:

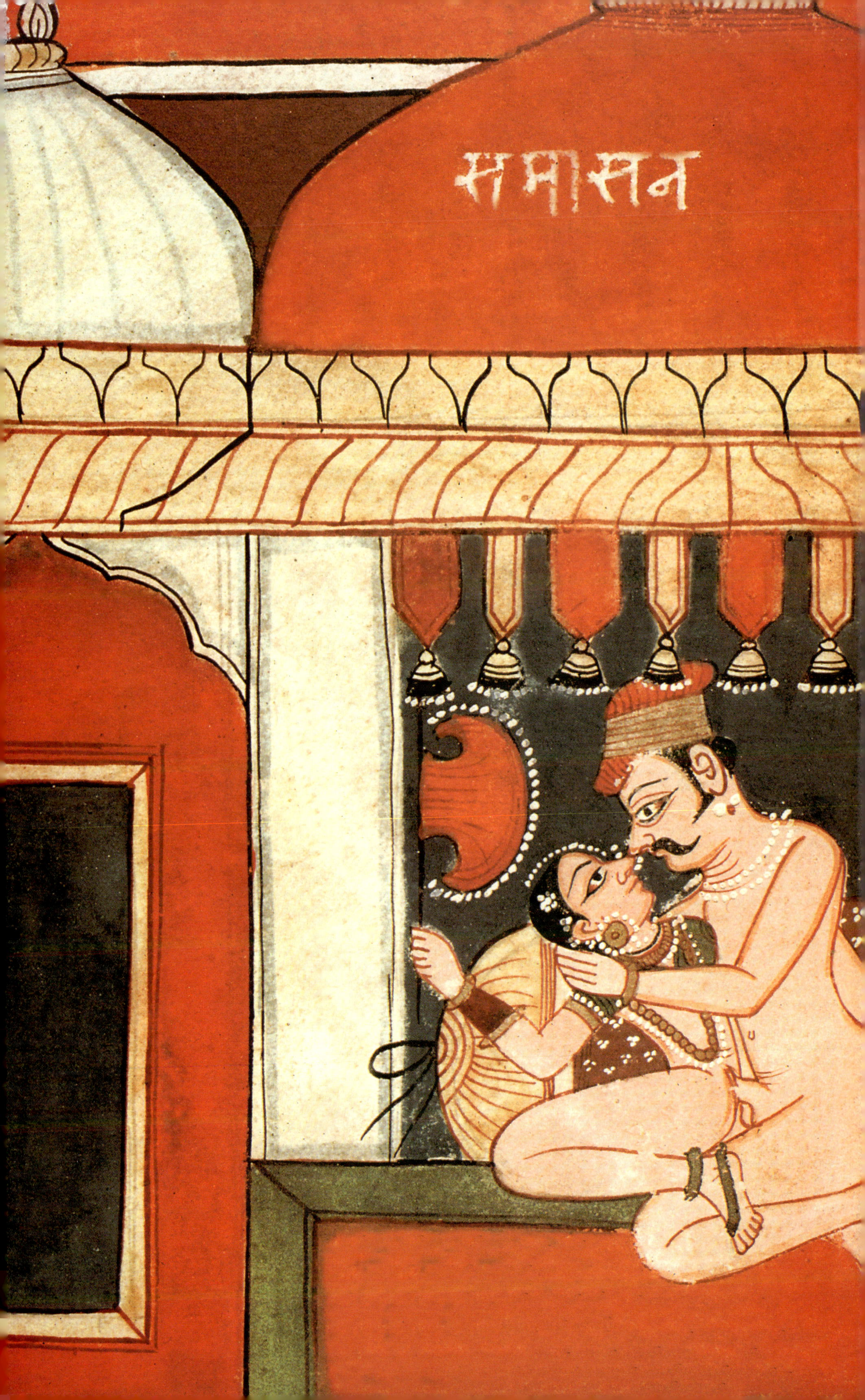
समासन

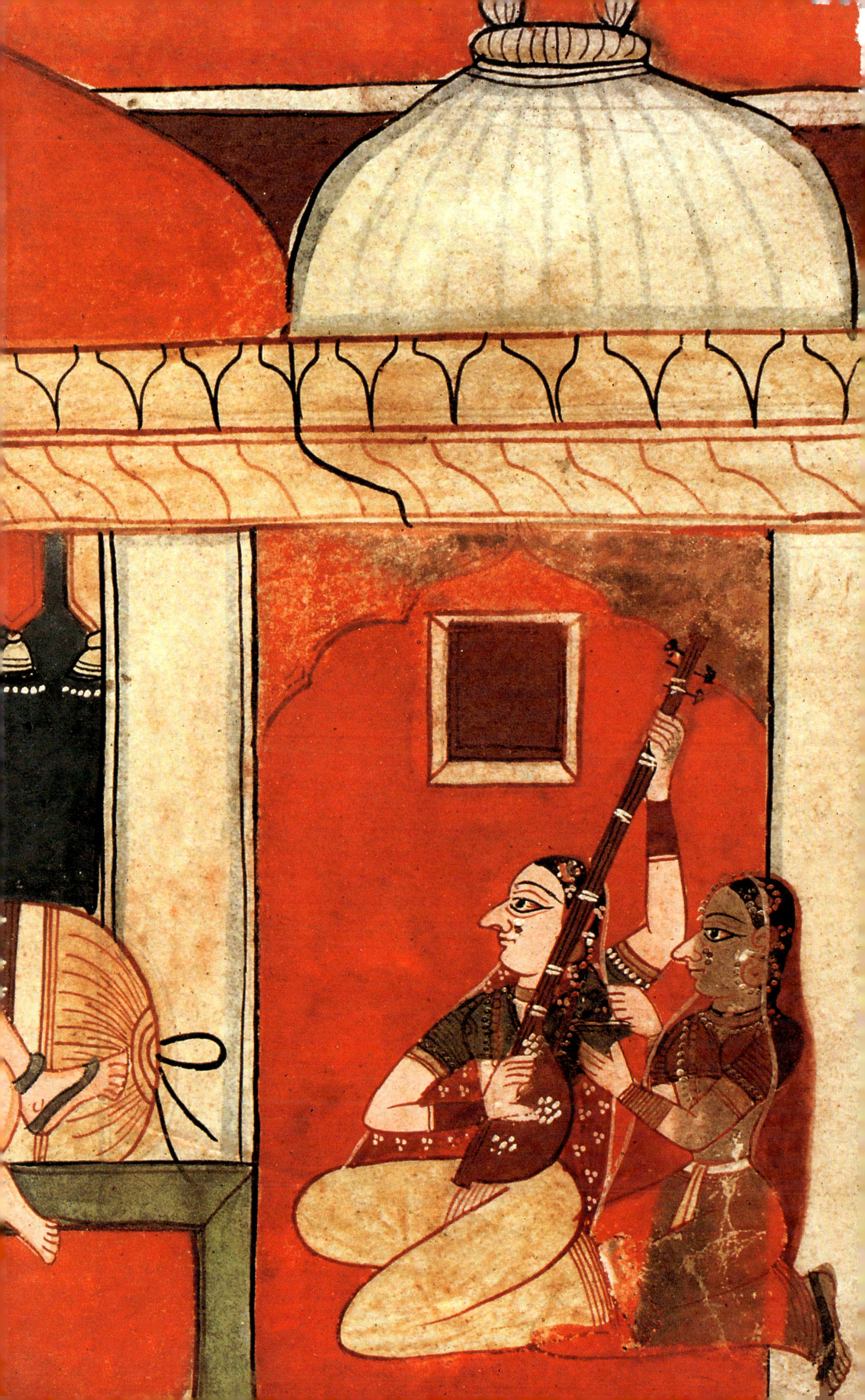

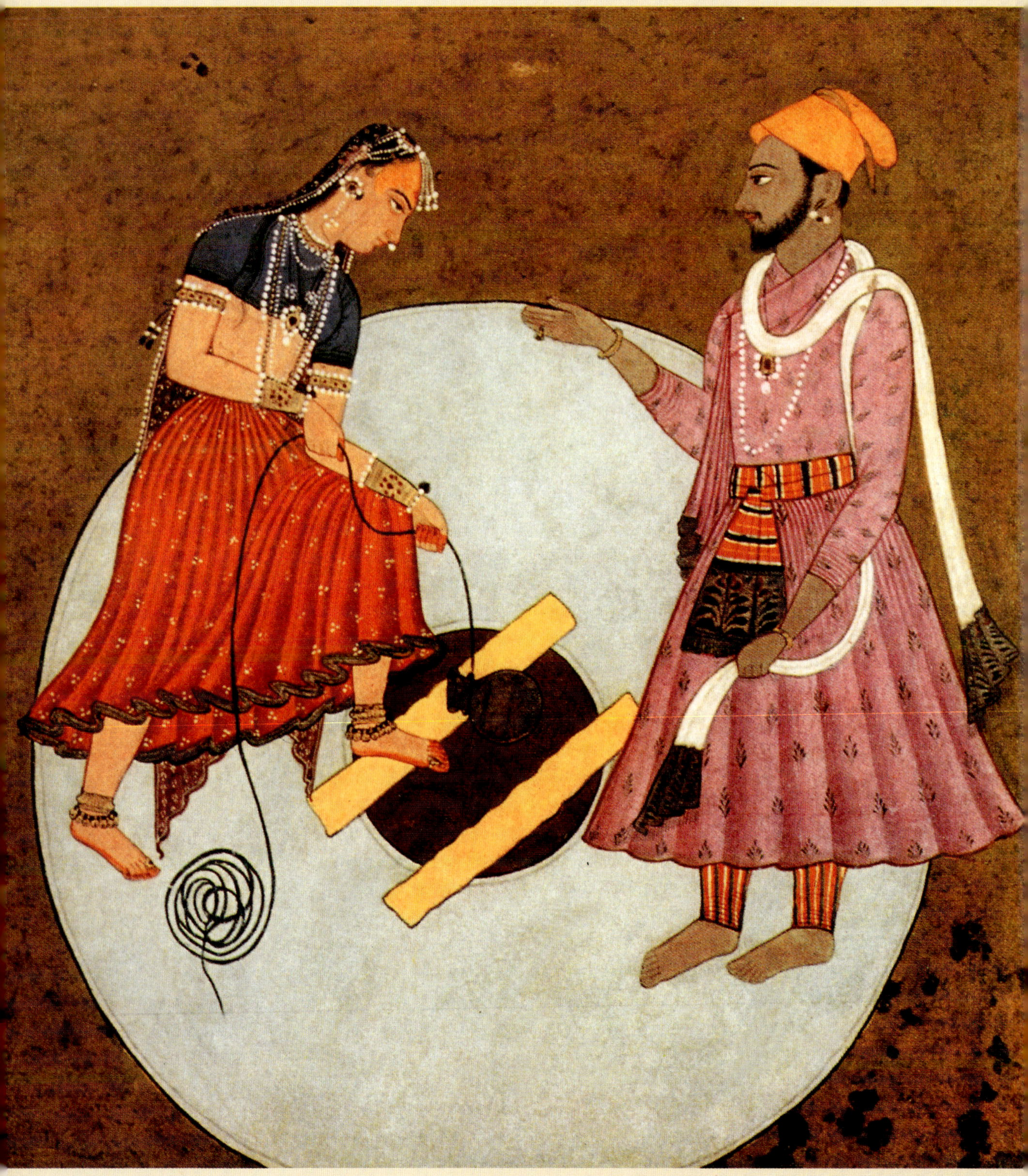

Melody of the water pot: The lovers draw water for a midnight bath. It is conjectured upon by composition of Indian musical melodies, which were written to accompany the different times of day and night, and give them a rhythmical meaning. They were called *ragas* and *raginis*. This one is the *raga kumbha*, the melody of the water pot. *Miniature painting, Mankot, Basholi, Pahari Hills, early 18th century. Bharat Kala Bhavan, Varanasi.*

Previous page: ***The widely open position:***
The heroine has thrown her legs around the hero who has the body of a bold and brave worrior. They move in a rhythmical motion in accompaniment to the throbbing plucks on the strings of the *vina*.
The widely open position presents a delightful entrance to her abode of passion. Miniature painting, Sirohi, Rajasthan, early 19th century. Private collection.

- Hug him.
- Write him a love note.
- Call him at work just to say 'Hello'.
- Give him a foot massage.
- Tell him a joke.
- Caress him with gentle strokes.
- Go for a walk with him.
- Admit your mistakes.
- Say, 'I love you'.
- Indulge in a whim.
- Listen with interest when he talks about an interest of his.
- Be trustworthy.
- Instead of complaining, tell him what you would prefer.
- Look at him directly when discussing something important.
- Send him flowers. (They're not only for girls!)
- Compliment him on something he did.
- Offer to help.
- Ask him to show you how to do some thing.
- Write him a poem about how special he is to you.
- Ask him what he'd like sexually.
- Take an afternoon drive together.
- Go away together for a weekend holiday.
- Do something he wants to do.
- Listen to him (even if he is boring you).
- Plan a candle light dinner.
- Browse through old photographs together.
- Serve him breakfast in bed.
- Take a shower together.
- Share sexual fantasies.
- Do a work project together.
- Give him an all-over body massage.
- Plan a picnic lunch.

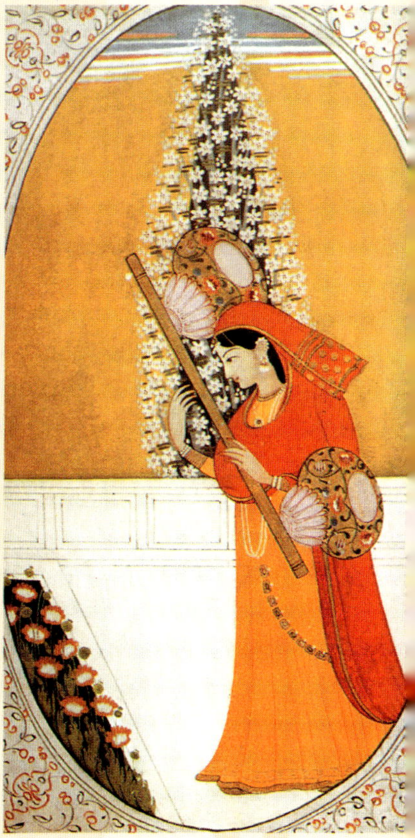

Portrait of a young heroine: She is proud and delighted with her accomplishment as a *vina* player. She is called the *Gunagarvita nayika*. *Miniature painting, Garhwal, late 18th century. Private collection. Bharat Kala Bhavan, Varanasi.*

Facing page: **The country girl:** An unusual delightful vision of a country girl moving about the markets on a festival. The movement is appealing to the eye and has a certain charm. *Wood, Chettianad, Tamil Nadu, 19th century. Private collection.*

- Repeat what he says before answering.
- Send him a card.
- Surprise him with a gift.
- Cook his favourite meal.
- Put on some romantic music.
- Compile a tape with both your favourite songs.
- Ask for his opinion.
- Ask him how he feels.
- Let him know when you are proud of him.
- Invite him to a secret rendezvous.
- Listen with an open mind to his opposing opinion.
- Watch his favourite TV programme with him.
- Watch a sunset together.
- Play a game together.
- Have him teach you something he knows.
- Go to a movie of his choice.
- Meet him for lunch.
- Let him know you care.

Whether it is the 'New Age', 'yesteryears' or 'tomorrows' - love was and will be. It needs to be revisited in thought and action. The wisdom of the ancients stays with us forever; the *Kama Sutra* manifests itself continuously amid new backdrops and new faces; gods and goddesses and figures from mythology transform into living beings, age-old potions still work their magic in their rebirth as more sophisticated trappings; feminine wiles and male expectancies merely drape themselves in more savvy attire. And at the end of the day, it is still love that is the beginning and the end.

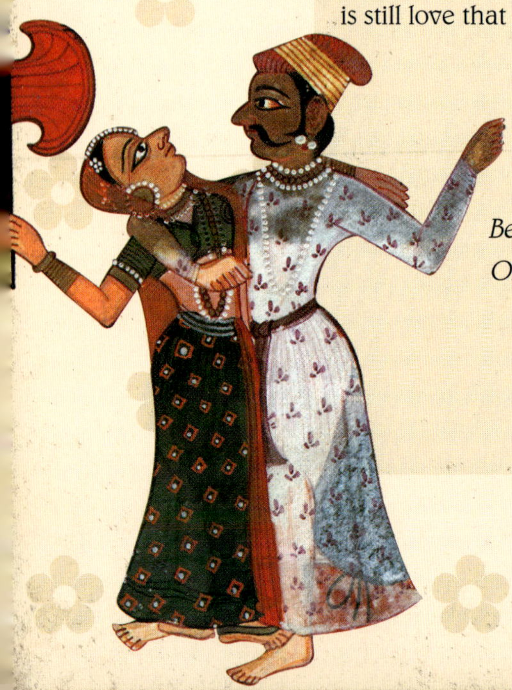

Dress in sarees, be girl,
Be wife, they said.
Be embroiderer, be cook,
Be a quarreler with servants. Fit in,
Oh, Belong, cried the categorisers.
Kamala Das, An Introduction

Following page: **Water Sports:** Any scene of a watery place conjures up the cool pleasure of immersion, added with the companionship, associated with playing together in and under the water. Skilful water sports such as striking water to make rhythmic sounds and diving in water, assuming various poses and other exercises are recommended. The *Kama Sutra* also describes love play and congress but is against the dispelling of semen in water. In this painting, the two lovers have gone under water to avoid the gaze of their friends and are then engaging in love-play. *Miniature painting, Rasikapriya Manuscript, Mewar, Rajasthan, 17th century*

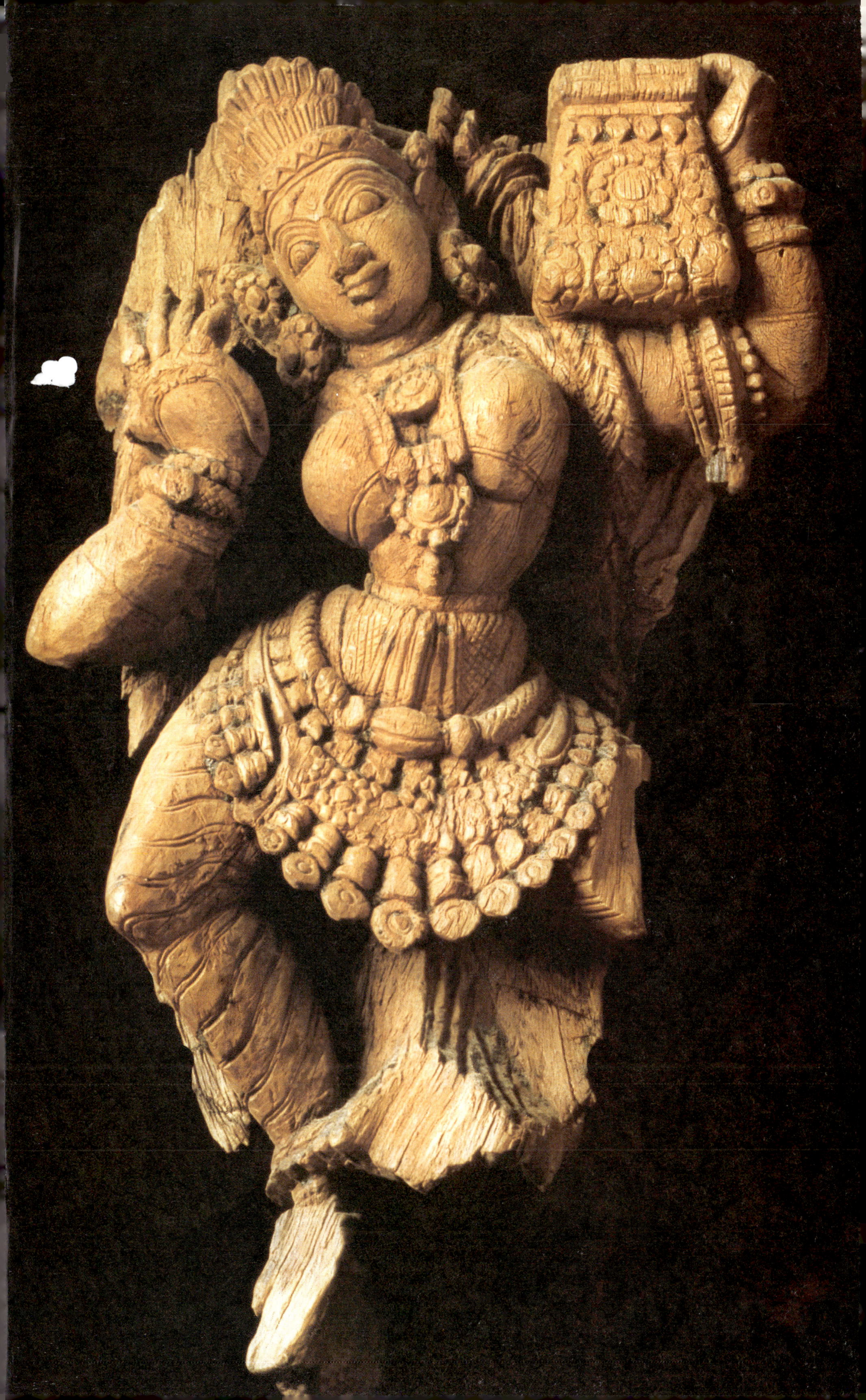

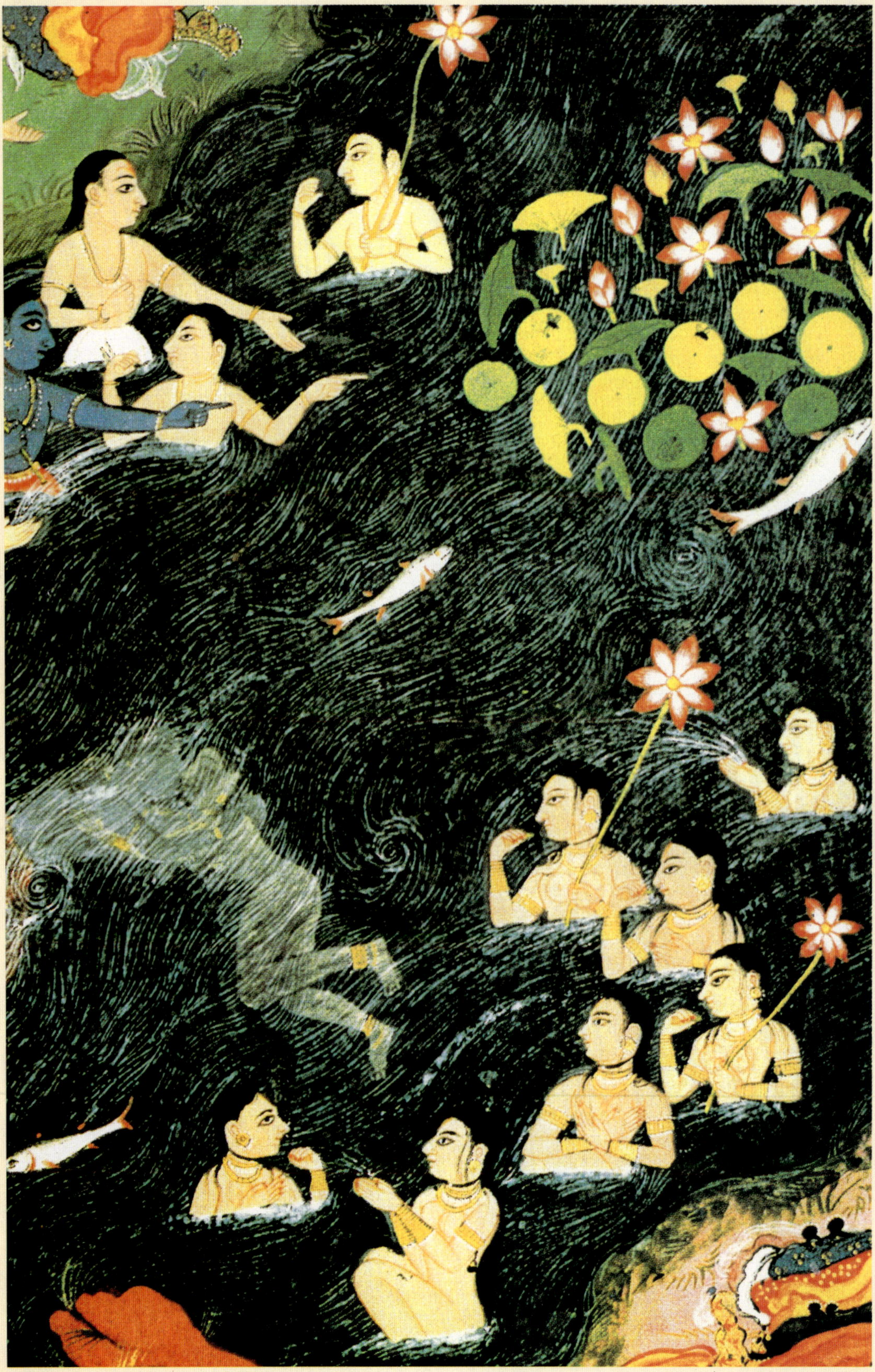

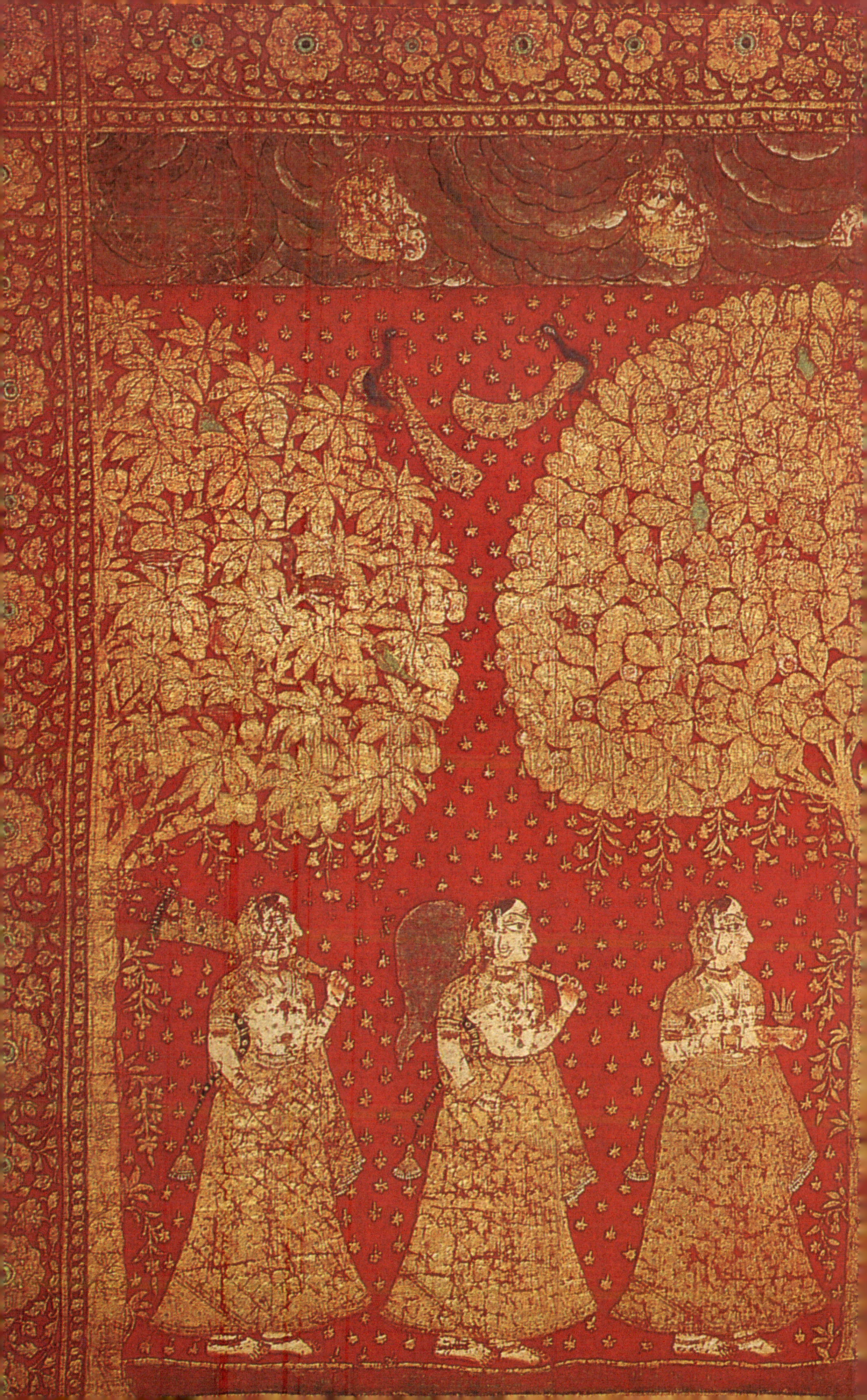